Measuring Mamma's Milk

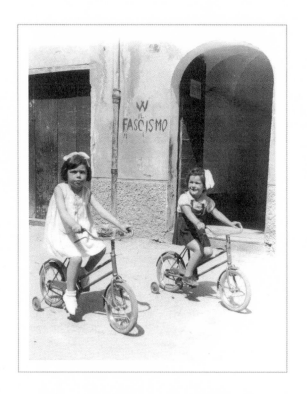

Girls on bicycles, 1938.
(From Archivio Romano Rossi.)

Measuring Mamma's Milk

FASCISM AND THE MEDICALIZATION OF MATERNITY IN ITALY

Elizabeth Dixon Whitaker

Ann Arbor

THE UNIVERSITY OF MICHIGAN PRESS

Copyright © by the University of Michigan 2000
All rights reserved
Published in the United States of America by
The University of Michigan Press
Manufactured in the United States of America
⊛ Printed on acid-free paper

2003   2002   2001   2000   4   3   2   1

*A CIP catalog record for this book is available from
the British Library.*

Library of Congress Cataloging-in-Publication Data

Whitaker, Elizabeth Dixon, 1962–
    Measuring mamma's milk : fascism and the medicalization
of maternity in Italy / Elizabeth Dixon Whitaker.
        p.   cm.
    Includes bibliographical references (p.   ) and index.
    ISBN 0-472-11078-0 (cloth : acid-free paper)
    1. Breast feeding—Italy.   2. Fascism—Italy.   I. Title.
RJ216 .W58   2000
649'.33'0945—dc21   99-050436

Contents

Acknowledgments

I am grateful to have been supported through much of the research and writing of this book by a Jacob Javits fellowship, a Fulbright fellowship, a Fondazione Giovanni Agnelli fellowship, and a graduate fellowship from Emory University. I also thank the many institutions in Italy that generously allowed me access to their resources, including the Archivio di Stato in Faenza and Forlì; the Biblioteca Comunale in Cesena, Faenza, Forlì, Mantua, and Ravenna; the Ente Casa Oriani in Ravenna; the Istituto Storico della Resistenza e della Guerra di Liberazione in Rimini; the Istituto Centrale di Statistica in Turin; and the Istituto Provinciale per la Storia del Movimento di Liberazione nel Mantovano in Mantua. I thank the preschools that allowed me to distribute questionnaires, as well as the government office in Santa Lucia that allowed me to examine the town's birth, death, and marriage registers. I thank Dominic O'Connor for helping compile data from these registers.

Several colleagues gave constructive suggestions for the project and read drafts of the manuscript. These include Walter Adamson, Fredrik Barth, Peter Brown, the late Pier Paolo D'Attore, Adriana Destro, Luther Gerlach, Bruce Knauft, Melvin Konner, Domenico Preti, and four gracious but candid anonymous reviewers. Among the health professionals, archivists, librarians, public servants, and clergy I consulted, I am especially grateful to Ennio Dirani, Anna Pia Guadagni, Giuseppe Sangiorgi, and the late Assuntina Santandrea.

I thank the hundreds of people who answered my questionnaires and conversed in interviews with patience, sincerity, and thoroughness, as well as the friends and acquaintances in Italy who have provided me and my family with unbounded affection and assistance. I will not name them, but hope that I have been successful in expressing my appreciation directly. Finally, I am indebted to my husband, Steve Whitaker, our daughters, Sarah, Emma, and Ernestine, and our extended family for their many contributions to the project. It was Emma, as a seven-year-old, who pointed out to me, "Mamma, everything you know is in the past."

Some parts of chapter 1 first appeared under the title "Ancient bodies, modern customs, and our health" in 1997 and 1999, in *Applying Anthropology* (4th ed., 36–45; 5th ed., 49–58) and *Applying Cultural Anthropology* (3d ed., 81–90; 4th ed., 67–76), edited by Aaron Podolefsky and Peter J. Brown (Mountain View, CA: Mayfield Press).

Abbreviations

CFLI	Confederazione Fascista dei Lavoratori dell'Industria
INPS	Istituto Nazionale Fascista della Previdenza Sociale; also, Istituto Nazionale della Previdenza Sociale
ISTAT	Istituto Centrale di Statistica
ONB	Opera Nazionale Balilla
OND	Opera Nazionale Dopolavoro
ONMI	Opera Nazionale per la Protezione della Maternità e dell'Infanzia; also, Opera Nazionale Maternità Infanzia

CHAPTER 1

An Unacknowledged Legacy
The Mother-Infant Relationship
in Modern Italy

Italian women who breast-feed weigh their babies before and after each feeding. Beginning in the maternity ward and continuing at home, infant meals are evenly spaced by a standardized feeding schedule, or *orario*. The amount of milk "administered" is measured in grams through the double weighing, or *doppia pesata,* of the infant at each meal. Some parents and health professionals are so exacting that they triple-weigh the child to calculate the production of each breast. If the amount consumed is too low, a precise ration of supplemental formula is given to "complete" or "make whole" the mother's milk. If the amount is too high, the mother detaches the baby earlier next time. These practices have precise historical underpinnings, but their origins have been buried with the memory of fascism.

I happened upon these methods in the early 1990s while living in Italy to conduct anthropological research on fascist demographic and health policies. My husband was conducting his own historical research on a prominent fascist leader from the region. One evening, a friend briskly broke off our conversation in her home at the chiming of the clock. It was time to breast-feed her newborn son. She undressed him and weighed him on a hospital-quality scale on the other side of the living room. She explained that she always did this and seemed puzzled when we asked why. As many others later did, she and her husband asked in return how we knew how much *our* year-old daughter took when she breast-fed, or how much her older sister had in her turn. A few weeks later, she told us that she was worried because her milk had become scarce and was completely absent in one or the other breast at certain feeding times.

I carried on with my research, but was struck by the number of references to breast-feeding in fascist-era medical and political literature. Meanwhile, I observed that our friend was not the only one to weigh her baby and unfailingly "respect" a feeding schedule. It was startling to find that parents were doing exactly what physicians had advised during the fascist period, beginning in the early 1920s. I learned that fascist leaders had hoped to reduce infant mortality rates and improve the quality of the population by eliminating alternative infant feeding methods and imposing discipline upon maternal breast-feeding. By having many children and breast-feeding them "rationally" for one year, but no longer, women were to demonstrate their commitment to the fascist nation-state. Regimented breast-feeding promised to prevent gastrointestinal disease, the main killer of infants, whereas mothers' irregularity and lack of order in breast-feeding were considered the direct cause of infant disease and death.

The practices promoted in the fascist period actually interfere with the psychobiology of lactation and significantly reduce its duration. Now that they have become commonsense behaviors, very few mothers breast-feed for more than a few months. The widespread loss of mother's milk has not gone unnoticed, for it contrasts sharply against the recent past. Yet, rather than blaming regimented infant feeding methods, people speak of the mother's insufficient desire to breast-feed or her particular physical inadequacies, reducing a social problem to individual pathology.

Women who are now great-grandmothers breast-fed for two to four years, according to the traditional wisdom that *i bambini devono mangiare poco e spesso* (babies must eat little and often). In recognition of the contraceptive effects of breast-feeding, another saying avowed that *intanto che si allatta non si rimane incinta* (as long as one breast-feeds one will not get pregnant). As more women followed the new methods, the relationship between lactation and prevention of pregnancy weakened, and its truth was rejected as just another absurd belief of the ignorant public. Breast-feeding came to be thought of as extremely exhausting, and the supply of milk fixed—and diminishing over time—in individual women and the population at large.

There is a strong sense of loss and regret regarding breast-feeding in Italy today. Cultural values continue to define a "good" mother as a robust woman who has a lot of milk, but such a woman is seen as an exceptional creature. One summer in the late 1990s, an older woman smiled inwardly when she learned that I was still exclusively breast-feeding my six-month-old daughter. She held my arm and shared her feeling that being able to breast-feed is a blessing from God. Other people offered similar praise but enjoined me to stop soon or I would be depleted by it. They unabashedly scrutinized my chest and wondered aloud that a petite mother could have yielded sufficient milk for three healthy children. One great-grandmother fixed her eyes on me and asked, "Where do you get the milk? . . . Where *is* it?"

Infant feeding is a topic of intense interest to men and women of every age and social class. Once, when I tried to put ground red pepper on my pasta, everyone at the table lunged forward to stop me. A male colleague at my side forcibly took the pepper from my hand. This generated an emphatic discussion about the passage of heat and unappealing flavors in mother's milk. My colleague and his mother-in-law also scolded me for continuing to do strenuous bicycle rides in the mountains even though I was breast-feeding, and they warned that I must not give my milk without first cooling down or taking a cold shower after cycling.

My research has revealed that the fascist intervention in breast-feeding not only imposed futuristic, rigorous methods, but also bolstered traditional values upholding breast-feeding as the essence of motherhood and the foundation of infant health. Today, this paradox finds expression in the mismatch between the near universality of maternal breast-feeding just after childbirth, and the rarity of it after the first months. The cultural concern that all women should breast-feed makes it difficult for women to renounce it without feelings of regret or inadequacy. At the same time, the disappearance of a mother's milk is accepted as an almost inevitable and even liberating event. The cause of vanishing milk is not sought in mechanistic infant feeding practices, which by now are considered indisputable necessities for ensuring infant health. A reflection of modernity and technical competence, these practices remain an unacknowledged legacy of fascism.

This book explores the way in which the underlying sociopolitical foundation for today's overlying structure of maternal and infant care practices was constructed during the fascist period to meet explicitly fascist objectives. To acknowledge the structure's origins is no longer possible because, through a complex historical sleight-of-hand, the foundation has been removed. The book explains how this cultural structure and its foundation contributed to the medicalization of maternity in Italy.

Moderating the Mother-Infant Unity

The history of breast-feeding in Italy has many dimensions. It is a complex, singular case of the cultural modeling of a universal biological process, involving subtle historical influences and an intricate shifting of health beliefs. It also resonates with wider changes affecting the modern individual's sense of personhood and self-confidence in the care of the body. This book will follow breast-feeding practices over time, as a window upon changes in health beliefs, medical care, sociocultural conditions, and political interventionism in the body and health. Some of these changes are unique to Italy; others are part of broader transformations common to the Western societies.

Over the past two centuries, Western societies have entered a new demographic regime of very low and balanced fertility and mortality rates. Differential reproduction and survival have been replaced by prenatal selection and efficacious medical intervention in many diseases and health conditions, with unknown biological consequences. For most of human evolution, prolonged on-demand breast-feeding was the only form of infant nutrition and also the main reason births were spaced several years apart. Even though ancient medical philosophers saw a connection between reduced breast-feeding and diseases such as breast cancer, modern science has only recently begun to appreciate the impacts of the worldwide decline in breast-feeding on fertility and mortality rates, and the kinds of diseases affecting mothers and infants. These impacts, and the ways in which cultural practices such as the doppia pesata and the orario interfere with lactation, are discussed in the second half of this chapter.

Compared to traditional agricultural and foraging societies, Western societies tend to meddle relatively forcibly in the mother-infant unity in breast-feeding. This is evident not only in feeding schedules, but also early supplementation and weaning, pacifiers, cribs and separate bedrooms, strollers, and playpens. It also is reflected in the tendency to focus upon the milk product rather than the process of lactation; to emphasize the benefits to infants rather than mothers; and to consider breast-feeding a simple matter of nutrition.

Cultural interference in breast-feeding seems to be much less common in societies of complex, wide families (as in many sub-Saharan African countries) than in those of predominantly simple families (as in Europe and parts of Asia). In the latter, the emphasis on women's conjugal duties allows for greater cultural intrusion in the relationship with their babies. Studies of breast-feeding in various countries verify this general scheme, but also point out subtleties and unique patterns in different cultural contexts.[1] Historical analysis can show how infant feeding patterns change with structural transformations. This book provides such an analysis for Italy, where the two main types of family and social organization coexisted until after the Second World War, contributing to significant variability in infant feeding practices.

After centuries of comparative stability, the Western family underwent profound alterations beginning in the nineteenth century, as part of the process of modernization.[2] Modernization refers to the transition from agricultural to industrial society, the subduing of former political and religious regimes by modern nation-states, and the demographic and epidemiologic transition to low birth and death rates. Modernization brought both positive and negative changes and, especially initially, extreme economic hardship.

In Italy, these changes took place much later than in neighboring countries. Although they began in the last decades of the nineteenth century, they have been telescoped into the decades following the Second World War; that is, within the lifetime of the oldest two living generations. These generations have seen a rapid increase in economic well-being, literacy, and cultural unification. They also have seen birthrates drop to the lowest in the world. The resignation and fatalism associated with the high death rates and birthrates of the early twentieth century have given way to faith in the effectiveness of human intervention. The shrinking of family size and complexity, together with the separation of men's and women's work with the decline of farming, has dropped the bulk of domestic responsibility on mothers and opened the way to scientific mothering. Traditional family, health, and religious authority has been eclipsed by the influence of medical experts as the ever more common small, simple family was opened to outside influences. These changes have contributed to the rapid rise in compliance with medical norms for breast-feeding since the fascist period.

The Western approach to breast-feeding can also be interpreted in terms of an overwhelming emphasis on autonomous individuality in industrialized society, as opposed to the more sociocentric conceptions of traditional societies. The vast research inspired by Michel Foucault indicates that the emergence of biomedicine over the past several generations incorporated the rise of an individuocentric conception of personhood. This manifested itself in the shift from empirical to clinical knowledge; the focus upon individual pathological events and processes; and the spatial and theoretical isolation of the individual patient from the familial, social, and environmental context. The focus on bounded individuals and disease agents expressed the triumph of rational science over the spiritual orientation of traditional agricultural society, where disease and disorder emerged from social and atmospheric miasmas entering a more permeable body.[3]

In fascist Italy, there arose a new understanding of the mother-infant relationship that mirrored the changes in medical organization and orientation. Until that time, ancient beliefs about human physiology still characterized women and their babies as a biological interacting pair from conception to weaning, linked by shared blood and its direct derivative, milk. Fascist-era medical ideas split this bond at childbirth and focused upon mother's milk as a product manufactured with factory-like regularity for the now-autonomous child. Interest in the impacts of lactation on mothers dwindled.

At the same time, older ideas about the noxious effects of atmospheric and behavioral imbalances were carried forward along with a rising emphasis on microbial agents of disease. This came to justify medical management of breast-feeding, for mothers were seen both as passive victims of external forces that could harm their own milk and as active agents whose disorderly infant-feeding habits could fatally endanger their children. The central importance of nutrition and digestion as the foundation of health and well-being buttressed medical authority in regulating mothers' behavior. Construing traditional on-demand feeding as uncivilized played into the cultural value of controlling nature through modernized parenting and housekeeping. Today, on-demand feeding is ostensibly promoted in Italy, but with the stipulation that babies "naturally" assume fixed daily rhythms within a few days or weeks of birth.

In addition to the general specialization and professionalization of medicine in the early decades of this century, the disciplines dealing with maternity and infancy divided in a way that corresponded with the conceptual separation of mothers and infants at birth. The hospitalization of childbirth and the introduction of more mechanistic methods in obstetrics and pediatrics reflected the affection of industrial culture for technological implements and industrial analogies for explaining bodily processes. Maternal ignorance was contrasted against medical authority, and while maternal misbehavior was depicted as menacing, medical intervention was not.

To fully explain the origins and impacts of these changes in medicine, this book links them to the expansion of medical authority and its connection to the rise of modern nation-states. Western biomedicine did wield new ideas about heredity and health to carve out a larger role for itself and exert greater influence over society, as Foucault recognized, but medicalization also depended upon a favorable social and political context. The medicalization of maternity in Italy took a particular form that was intimately connected with institutional histories and the emergence of a unique corpus of medical beliefs about lactation.

Before and during the interwar period, demographic policies were employed by governments ushering in an emerging alliance among the state, science, and medicine. It was widely hoped that the application of evolutionary and eugenic principles to the management of population could bring about not just numerical increase, but also the perfection of humanity in biological and moral terms. Medical experts were encouraged to lead public morality and oppose traditional authority by reaching into private affairs such as sexuality, procreation, and child rearing, as well as hygiene, public health, education, and work. This intrusion was more of a social than medical concern, for it began well before professional medicine had much legitimate knowledge or expertise in these areas.[4]

In the decades leading to the rise of fascism, leaders in Italy and elsewhere in the West were worried about demographic decline. Birthrates were falling from the spectacular highs that had concerned Thomas Robert Malthus a century before. The First World War and the Spanish flu caused a shocking loss of life in a short time. In an era when a large population was equated with economic and military might, Italy was particularly susceptible to feelings of demographic inferiority, in spite of its relatively high population growth rates. It was an incompletely unified nation with vast cultural and economic differences among regions, especially between the industrializing north and the traditional agricultural south and islands, and had failed to join the club of colonial powers despite prolonged military campaigns in East Africa.

Benito Mussolini enraptured Italians with his talk of rebirth and regeneration, the importance of carrying forward the glories of Roman civilization, and the expansion of the nation through population growth and colonization. Italian prolificness and virility were celebrated as supreme virtues of the Latin peoples. The overpopulation that had caused economic crisis and a massive wave of emigration beginning in the late nineteenth century in Italy would now be a factor of economic power in a mountainous country considered to be lacking in natural resources. As in France, the idealized rural economy and patriarchal family, rooted in the Catholic concept of marriage as the central institution of stable society, were exalted as the antidote to the social upheaval brought on by modernization. Europe after the First World War was compared to the late Roman Empire, and Caesar's initiatives to halt falling birthrates—along with others promoted in the late nineteenth century—were the basis of French and Italian initiatives in the interwar period.

Reproductive rights were central concerns of both dictatorships and democracies. Not only in Italy, but also in Spain, Portugal, and Brazil, dictatorships legitimized their existence with an ideology fusing pronatalism with nationalism and Catholicism. Democracies like the United States and Britain were not immune to racist fears and negative eugenic policies, and they joined Germany in contemplating or actually attempting the elimination of undesirable characteristics through forced sterilization and laws against mixed marriages. In this respect, Italian fascism had a greater affinity for French policies than German ones. Like France, Italy concentrated on rewarding parenthood through unrestricted pronatalist measures.

French and Italian demographic policies reflected not just different politicoeconomic conditions and cultural interpretations of science, but also practical considerations arising out of the need to contend with the strong political and moral presence of the Church. Even neomalthusianism in Italy reflected the influence of Catholicism. Birth control advocates argued not for zero population growth, but rather moderate procreation to reduce stress on women's bodies and thereby improve their effectiveness as mothers, and to keep population expansion in pace with economic growth. Although both France and Italy eschewed measures for manipulating heredity within the population, Italy differed from France in bringing motherhood to the center of domestic politics rather than simply forging a link between men's honor and the extent of their procreation.[5]

In fascist Italy, the politicization of parenthood, the systematic severing of women's ties to traditional medical authorities and beliefs, and the imposition of regimented breast-feeding as a national political priority had deep and long-term effects. Controlled breast-feeding and hygienic management of childhood were considered the cornerstone of fascist plans for population expansion and improvement through "state breeding." The main instrument for population management was the new Organization for the Protection of Maternity and Infancy (ONMI), which survived for three decades after the Second World War. Contradictions in fascist ideology arising from the tension between traditionalism and futurism thereby continued to affect cultural concepts about gender, nature, and the care of the body. The state medical system reached the most remote areas. Today, contact with it is close and frequent. Italy has the highest number of physicians per capita in the world.

Until the early 1980s, most historical works on the fascist period minimized or denied any meaningful effect of fascism on Italian life. This was consistent with the glorification of the Italian Resistance in politics and culture after the war. Studies of fascism tended to disregard social policy in favor of its more violent and militaristic aspects. Today's scholarship shows how fascist leaders were intensely interested in domestic matters. It documents the ways in which fascism changed the nature of state surveillance and control over individual bodies and brought both men and women into greater contact with public institutions. Fascist laws and institutions created the basis for the postwar welfare state, with a public services system that did not change fundamentally after the interwar period.[6] Yet, because fascist pronatalist programs had at most a modest quantitative impact, most studies conclude that concordance with the regime was manifested only in public rather than private behavior. That is, it is assumed that fascism's antimodern, ruralist ideology was contradicted and in the end subsumed by the practical impact of its promotion of sports, education, and industrial development.[7]

This book makes it clear that fascism did go beneath the surface and that it had a profound and enduring impact on Italian society and culture, not in spite of the contradictions but because of them. For example, the multiple-family households of sharecroppers and tenant farmers were resistant to outside intervention of any kind, including medical management of breast-feeding. Widespread poverty, illiteracy, heavy work loads, and large numbers of children did not permit most women to practice scientific mothering. Those women who did were generally the well-off urbanites most in contact with professional medicine. This was troubling to the fascists because the women who had the most children were the same ones who so obstinately refused to modernize their child-rearing behavior. This contradiction left its mark in the persistence of the coexistent cultural values of naturalistic motherhood and regimented parenting that continue to both make breast-feeding a binding obligation and interfere with women's ability to lactate.

After the Second World War, direct governmental intervention in reproduction was abandoned in most countries, as a reaction against the direction it had taken in Germany. A notable exception was France, which continued to offer economic incentives for procreation. The rationalization of child-rearing practices proceeded in Italy, but political proclamations about women's patriotic duty in the moral and physical salvation of the nation were no longer necessary. The continued expansion of the medical system, the long postwar life of ONMI, the rapid rise in economic well-being, and the simplification and shrinking of families conspired to make parents dependent upon outsiders and distrustful of the knowledge of family members or nonmedical experts. Fascist-era norms for infant feeding found hospitable territory in the civilizing traditions and food-oriented health beliefs of an ever more unified culture. The resulting conflict between biology and culture, expressed in the obstruction of the flow of mother's milk, is the outcome of Italy's unique experience of medicalization. It also reflects a crisis of confidence in the care of the body and health that affects us all.

Setting and Sources

This book focuses on the region of Emilia-Romagna, in the central-northern part of the country. The region runs west to east along the Po River, opening toward the Adriatic Sea. The flat areas around the river form one of the largest tracts of fertile agricultural land in Italy. The diverse topography of the region has created a complex agricultural history in the plains, hills, and mountains. This has involved sharecropping, tenant farming, smallholding, and large-scale industrialized agriculture. While agriculture remains strong (in part because of government support), public administration and the manufacturing, service, and oil industries have grown rapidly in the postwar period.

The political history of the region has also been complex. Once a papal state, Emilia-Romagna has long had a strong anticlerical tradition. It was a hotbed of socialist labor agitation and new political movements around the turn of the century. It was the birthplace of Mussolini and, together with nearby regions, the base of the fascist movement itself. Since the Second World War, there have been many local communist administrations in the region, but it also has rock-solid pockets of Christian Democrats. In the last decade, a new political era has begun. There was a brief experiment with populist conservative government at the national level, followed by a return to the center-left and a proliferation of opposition parties including the neofascist movement and the separatist Northern League.

Italy is divided into 20 regions, more than 90 *provincie* (provinces), and some 7,300 *comuni* (towns and their surrounding areas). I have lived and worked in the region of Emilia-Romagna on and off for more than a decade, in cities, towns, and isolated farm communities. Much of my time has been spent in a town of 3,000 in the Apennines southeast of Bologna, which I will call Santa Lucia.

Ethnographic sources for the book include participant-observation as well as formal interviews with laypersons and teachers, clerics, social service workers, a former wet nurse, and health professionals, including three midwives who have successively served the town of Santa Lucia since the 1920s. I also distributed long and detailed questionnaires about procreation and child rearing at four nursery schools (two in Santa Lucia, one each in two nearby cities), more than 120 of which were completed. More than 30 people of a wider age range answered a short questionnaire specifically about infant care.

Most of the archival research concerned the town, but I also visited archives in many cities in Emilia-Romagna and other northern regions. Using the birth, death, and marriage registers in Santa Lucia's archives, I conducted a detailed study of births, deaths, and marriages over the past thirteen decades, including an analysis of more than 1,200 infant deaths. This involved an analysis of change in the frequencies of 200 professions among 4,800 women and men. Some of the results are found in the appendix.

Many of the literary sources were written by authors from the region and gathered there. Most of the medical textbooks were or are used by practicing health professionals. Those written for the public were given to me or suggested by individuals; many can be found on the bookshelves of parents of young children. Other literary sources include novels, journals, and newspapers, as well as scholarly works by authors within and outside Italy. Among political-demographic writings I have emphasized those written by authors from Emilia-Romagna, but included others in order to weave the narrative into the national setting.

The text is organized into three periods: Unification in the 1860s to the First World War; the interwar period; and the decades following the Second World War. Medical and popular beliefs and behaviors are analyzed in each period with reference to social, economic, and political context. In addition, in the first set of chapters there is an overview of economic and demographic change, providing a background for analysis of changes in family life throughout the past century. In the second section, there is an emphasis on fascist political-demographic ideas, for they directly affected the institutions delivering medical and social assistance to mothers and infants. I include an analysis of broad cultural concepts about nature, health, and the body in the final chapters to help explain the cultural context for the medicalization of maternity in Italy.

Regarding a few of the terms used in the text, maternity refers to the phase between conception and weaning, as opposed to motherhood, or the state of being a mother, and all of the social and sentimental meanings it carries. When discussing infant meals, I use both the Italian word for schedule, *l'orario,* which corresponds better with English usage, and the plural *gli orari,* which means literally, "the hours" and refers more specifically to set feeding times. When relating medical and political ideas, I present ideas that are widely agreed upon, but would like to emphasize that in every epoch there are experts who hold contrary views and parents who do not follow cultural rules for infant feeding. Unless otherwise noted, all translations are my own.

I do not intend to give the impression of judging ideas or the behaviors they shape, especially health beliefs. I also would not want my advocacy of breast-feeding to be mistaken for judgment of anyone's choices or actions in infant feeding. I trust that my writing conveys my respect for others and the circumstances surrounding their decisions.

Breast-Feeding in Biocultural Perspective

Evolution and Health

A long-term perspective on reproductive and parenting trends will help to explain how Western beliefs and behaviors deviate from the "ancestral" human pattern. Unfortunately, the vastness of the scope of this topic precludes analysis of cultural differences within broad categories of human social formations. The benefits to mothers and infants from breast-feeding the traditional way may seem overwhelming—given that formula manufacturers have long insisted that their product is at least as good as mother's milk—but they are real and go far beyond those I am able to describe in a short discussion.

For almost all of the past four million years of hominid evolution, foraging (hunting and gathering) has been our way of life. Between thirteen and nine thousand years ago, some groups began to practice settled agriculture and animal husbandry, known as the Neolithic Revolution. Today, there are very few people who continue the foraging life-style. Those who do or did so until recently—such as the !Kung San of northwestern Botswana or the Gainj of Papua New Guinea—are considered to provide clues to the demographic and health patterns that probably prevailed through all but the latest blink of an eye in the course of human history on earth.

These past several thousand years have not been long enough for our genes to change significantly in line with our life-style, except for a few elegant adaptations. For example, some populations with a long history of dairying have a genetic variation that allows them to continue to produce lactase after infancy, allowing for lifelong consumption of milk. There is a group of blood cell defects, such as sickle-cell anemia, thalassemia, and G-6-PD deficiency, that protect heterozygotes ("carriers") against malaria in populations under long exposure to the disease.[8] Otherwise, we are carrying Stone Age genes. In fact, we are not much different from chimpanzees and gorillas, with whom we share ancestors and more than 98 percent of our genes.

While our genetic profile has not changed, our diet and exercise patterns have.[9] In contrast to what we think of as a proper diet, prehistoric and modern foragers have subsisted on a low-calorie diet made up exclusively of wild plant parts and, to a lesser extent, fish or game. Wild meat has less than one-seventh the fat in domesticated beef and a much higher proportion of polyunsaturated fat. There are no dairy products (except mother's milk); no processed grains; no concentrated calorie bombs like our junk food, except honey where it is available and can be harvested.

To collect food takes significant physical effort. Gatherers and hunters travel for six to eight hours over distances of ten kilometers or more on workdays. When averaged out with days of other activities, this amounts to more than six and a half kilometers per day, every day. Some foods such as roots require intense physical activity, while hunters must stalk, run after, and carry their prey back to camp. By the end of the day, the gatherer's bundle weighs up to 15 kilograms (almost 35 pounds) and can reach half of a woman's own body weight. Women routinely carry children up to three or four years of age, adding up to another 15 kilograms. In addition, foragers move camp several times a year. Because they work outdoors and do not have climate control indoors, they are constantly exposed to the elements.

Foraging populations suffered from degenerative bone conditions, accidents and injuries, infectious diseases, and debilitation from exposure, especially among the old. However, compared to the first agriculturalists, their health apparently was better. Agriculture brought more severe malnutrition and famine compared to the mild seasonal shortages experienced by foragers, more infectious disease since population density was greater, and more infant death apparently associated with weaning.[10] Although famines are rare now, especially in the wealthier countries, constant overnutrition produces new health problems. At the same time, the diet in many impoverished countries remains scantier and less varied than the foraging diet.

Contemporary foraging people, unlike people in affluent societies, do not experience any "natural" rise in blood pressure with age. They do not undergo hearing loss as an inevitable consequence of aging, nor does their body mass increase. The "diseases of civilization" or chronic diseases so familiar to us are very rare among them. These include heart disease, hypertension, strokes, cancer, emphysema, cirrhosis, and diabetes. While re-creating a foraging life-style would be impossible because of lack of space, we could still benefit from applying some its principles to our own behavior and strive for the best of both worlds.

All humans, past and present, share a genetic predisposition to the chronic diseases, but it is the modern life-style and environment that cause their wide expression in Western societies today.[11] Humans have the biological characteristics of foraging animals, making their bodies adept at storing fat against the likelihood of periodic food shortage. This is why obesity and overweight are so common where exercise and exposure to the elements are minimal but food supplies are abundant and steady. Similarly, we can interpret cancer as the cost of the beneficial biological adaptation of tissue repair and regeneration. In all living things, the mechanisms for regulating and suppressing cell division become less effective with age. Yet, cancer rates have risen over the past few centuries to a much greater degree than the proportion of people living into advanced age. This is not just because of exposure to cancer-causing or cancer-promoting microorganisms and chemicals. Our diet is scarce in micronutrients such as selenium and beta-carotene that protect against cancer, but overloaded in macronutrients such as fat, protein, and calories. In themselves and in relation to body composition and size, the latter promote cancer.[12]

This has implications even for infants. When human milk is substituted with fresh animal milk or formula with a higher fat and/or protein content, negative health consequences arise in the short and long term from the resulting acceleration of growth.[13] The protein content of human milk is the lowest of all mammalian milks—about one-third that of cow's milk. The kind of protein is also different, and there is less calcium and phosphorus. High protein intake is correlated with accelerated growth, early sexual maturation, and greater achieved stature in human populations, with some costs in terms of health (discussed further below).[14]

The reason why mother's milk is low in protein and fat but high in carbohydrate is that humans and other primates are born much less neurologically mature than other mammals and need more parental care. Their mothers (or fathers) carry them and sleep with them, providing transportation and warmth. In contrast, mammals such as rabbits leave their young for long intervals alone in a nest, so their milk is high in fat.

Primate mothers breast-feed their young as often as every twenty minutes, allowing them to cling to the teat in between. Some primates such as lemurs and marmosets breast-feed for only a few months, but our closest relatives do so for years. Gorillas and chimpanzees breast-feed for four or more years, orangutans for three.[15] Through breast-feeding, primate mothers protect their infants from predators and disease, both through shared and reduced exposure to disease, and antimicrobial and general and specific immunological substances passed in the milk. This is a nice illustration of convergence among behavior, physiological function, and developmental pattern. Breast-feeding has clearly been a central adaptive strategy of the class of animals known as *Mammalia*. This is reflected in the name, which comes from the Latin word *mamma* for breast.

The Human Blueprint for Lactation

Evidence of many kinds supports the view that baby-led feeding including parent-infant cosleeping has been the norm for almost all of human history. Anthropologists have sketched this ancestral or traditional pattern by observing contemporary foraging populations and studying past populations as well as other primates. Feeding is highly frequent through day and night, exclusive, and prolonged—taking place from several times an hour to every hour or two. There is no supplementation before six months and limited use of supplemental foods, such as premasticated food and very ripe fruit, thereafter. Breast-feeding lasts at least one year, but often, as was more likely in evolutionary time, two to four years. In preagricultural societies, mother's milk remains the principal food until 15 to 18 months, after which it remains a significant source of nutrition until weaning time. When these conditions prevail, infants are more likely to survive, pregnancy is prevented for two to three years or more, and births are spaced three to five years apart.

At least a year of breast-feeding remains the norm in non-Western populations today, reflecting a different understanding of the mother-infant relationship from ours (in the United States, 58 percent of mothers initiate breast-feeding, but of them only 56 percent breast-feed for three months or more; only a tiny fraction continue through the first year).[16] Far from interfering in the breast-feeding relationship, other cultures often encourage it through institutions such as milk kinship.[17] This means breast-feeding another couple's child, sometimes in the absence of any true need. In rural Italy, milk kinship persisted through the first half of this century, linking the milk child and mother, and their wider families, for life. By contrast, today's values stress individual autonomy, and this applies even to newborns and infants. Babies are expected to wait hours or days before the first feeding at the breast and for long periods between feedings from then on; to sleep through the night, alone in a separate room; and to not complain if they are not held for hours.

To illustrate how frequent feedings are in foraging populations, !Kung San women breast-feed for a couple of minutes every quarter-hour throughout the day.[18] They sleep with their children and feed them all night, but since they do not always wake up it is unknown how many times. This goes on for at least two years, and until weaning at around three and a half years feedings are less than an hour apart. The average interval between births is 48 months, and average completed fertility is 4.7 births. Similarly, among the Gainj, infants are initially fed about three times per hour, after which feedings are gradually spaced to one every hour and twenty minutes in the third year. The average interbirth interval is just over three years, while completed fertility averages 4.3 children. This would more than double if mothers stopped breast-feeding. In fact, over the 1960s and 1970s, when some of the !Kung San settled and began to adopt the practices of neighboring pastoralists—including using cow's milk as a supplement for infants—interbirth intervals shrunk. Lactation has been humankind's main method of birth control for most of our existence.

Mothers and infants are in constant contact in foraging societies. Infants ride in a sling which allows them to feed and suckle continuously. They continue to do so until weaning, which corresponds to the time when they are able to walk on their own for long distances with the foraging group. Mothers respond immediately when their children cry, but never with any kind of pacifier other than the breast. Since infants are not clothed and are cleaned immediately, wetness is not a problem. All of this adds up to very little crying. When infants do cry, they are not expected to tough it out without being held or allowed to suckle. Parents do not share the idea that infants need to be denied what they want or they will grow up spoiled and dependent.

The weaning of infants in the third or fourth year among contemporary foraging and prehistoric populations agrees with comparative data on nonhuman primates and other mammals, indicating a similar "natural" weaning age for humans. In fact, in Western populations, from antiquity until a few generations ago, women breast-fed for two to three or more years. One interesting line of evidence is based upon the correlation in mammals between age at weaning and onset of the inability to digest lactose (milk sugar). Lactase is the enzyme that converts lactose into a form that can be absorbed by the gastrointestinal tract. Unlike dairying populations, such as Europeans, most African, Asian, and Native American people have a low tolerance of lactose. They are considered "lactase deficient," even though they represent the standard rather than the variation. For them, lactase deficiency begins at around two years and intolerance is reached by three years, with a range of one to four years.[19]

In prehistoric foraging populations, birth and death rates were moderate and nearly matched each other, so population grew very slowly for most of evolutionary time. It is not clear whether population pressure forced some bands to settle and cultivate food, but it is certain that once they did their growth rates rose rapidly. Until a century or two ago, in Europe mortality and fertility rates rose, but since the latter were higher there was an explosion of population (as in many non-Western countries today). This occurred even though there were periodic crashes due to famine and epidemic disease. Then, death rates began to drop, and fertility rates soon followed their course. The shift toward chronic diseases as the major causes of death seems to be giving way now to another transition, for it is becoming increasingly clear that Western society has not, in fact, conquered infectious disease.

Changes in infant feeding practices played an important role in these historical changes. The use of animal milk and cultivated foods led to reduced periods of postpartum infertility. Substitutes for breastmilk were associated with higher infant mortality rates. This difference has been overcome only in Western societies, but significant health outcomes remain, as we shall see.

Mechanisms of Milk Production and Release

The milk of all mammals is unique to the species, but it is also unique to the individual. Its composition can vary according to the hormones and immunities the mother produces or the foods and medicines she ingests. It grows less watery and more fatty during each feeding, and fat content varies over the day and the overall course of breast-feeding. Milk production is very elastic, for some women are able to produce milk while breast-feeding several times an hour, but others, particularly after the first several months, are able to continue breast-feeding even if they only do so a few times a day or just at night.[20] Infants likewise can grow the same amount on different quantities of milk, or different amounts on the same quantity of milk. While they tend to double and triple their birthweights at similar times (5 to 6 and 12 months, respectively), growth is not usually regular from one day or week to the next, as many parents and health experts have come to expect.

Notwithstanding this flexibility, the production of milk is a highly canalized process, practically unaffected by variations in maternal condition or diet. Nonetheless, a very common "insufficient milk syndrome" has been reported from around the world. Yet, pathological conditions (from congenitally meager glandular tissue or postpartum complications) exist in only a tiny percentage of the women reporting it. Insufficient milk is a cultural phenomenon more than a biological one.[21]

On the one hand, the uniform quality of milk protects infants from protein malnutrition and many vitamin and mineral deficiencies, even in parts of the world where they are common. On the other hand, it can lead to serious caloric and mineral deficiency in the mother if she is already poorly nourished, overburdened with physical labor, and stressed further by repeated cycles of gestation and lactation.[22]

Although the breast is ready to lactate by the middle of pregnancy, circulating estrogens and progesterone keep it from doing so by blocking the effect of the hormone prolactin on breast tissue.[23] With the delivery of the placenta, progesterone levels drop abruptly, causing milk to be produced soon after. The stimulation of the nipple through nursing keeps the hypothalamus from releasing progesterone as well as the prolactin inhibiting factor. Each time the infant suckles, the anterior pituitary gland inside the hypothalamus responds after a few minutes by releasing prolactin. The posterior pituitary immediately releases oxytocin.[24]

Prolactin stimulates the lacteal or milk-producing cells in the breast to synthesize milk over the next couple of hours. These cells line the bulbous ends of the glands called alveoli or acini. Oxytocin causes the cells around the alveoli and ducts to contract and push the milk toward the nipple (the "let-down reflex"), just as it causes the uterine cells to contract during labor. The oxytocin pathway can be affected by psychological factors, for a thought, emotion, or sound or sight of an infant can cause its release. Contrariwise, fear and other stressful emotions lead to the secretion of epinephrine, which impedes circulation of oxytocin by constricting the blood vessels around the breast.

After the surge following nipple stimulation, prolactin levels drop off quickly, falling to baseline within two hours. Prolactin's half-life in the blood is 30 minutes. This means that in order to maintain continuous milk production, the mother must breast-feed at short intervals and keep prolactin levels high. This is especially true in the early months, when more frequent feedings result in greater milk production. This hormonal regulation is crucial at the beginning and continues throughout breast-feeding. Another control mechanism affects milk production more and more after the first two or three months: milk that is left in the breast has an independent dampening effect, both through a component of the milk and through the mechanical pressure of the milk itself. The more the milk is removed, the greater the rate of milk synthesis between feedings.

This negative feedback loop prevents overproduction and permits finely tuned milk synthesis. It explains why production can vary between breasts, or stop in one if it is avoided by the mother or infant. Excessive, unrelieved engorgement causes atrophy and digestion of the alveolar cells, causing the resorption of milk when the mother does not undertake breast-feeding or stops suddenly.

The importance of initiating breast-feeding right after birth is underscored by another physiological relationship as well. The proliferation of prolactin receptors on the surface of alveolar epithelial cells seems to be related to the degree of nipple stimulation and milk removal. This helps to explain why first-time mothers produce less milk in the first days than mothers who have given birth before, and why women who nurse frequently in the first few weeks produce more milk than those who nurse less often.

These considerations point to the importance of infant suckling behavior in the regulation of milk production. The readiness of infants to prefer the easy flow of the bottle and to suck less energetically at the breast is well-known, but the effect of pacifiers on reducing the duration of breast-feeding is not as widely recognized. The use of the pacifier may effect suckling, but it is also likely that infants who are given pacifiers are offered the breast less frequently.[25]

Unlike formula, breastmilk does not have a constant relationship between volume and fat or calories.[26] Both frequency of feedings and degree of milk removal are positively associated with higher average fat and calorie content. This means that infants who are allowed to breast-feed without restrictions are usually satiated and settled after feedings, whereas if they have to wait many hours they must suck longer to draw out the richer hind milk. Demand-fed infants are able to regulate their nutrition very closely over the day and night by varying feed frequencies and the extent of breast-emptying. They exercise appetite control and prevent overnutrition by leaving a residual amount of milk in the breast. Contrariwise, if they are prevented from feeding frequently or for as long as they wish, or do not remove the milk effectively because of poor attachment to the breast, the production and quality of the milk can be affected and so can their growth and health.

While the ancestral pattern of frequent, exclusive, prolonged breast-feeding provides for optimal milk production and consumption, it also prevents pregnancy. Yet, the contraceptive effect of breast-feeding has been widely denied by parents and health professionals over the past century and was not accepted by mainstream medicine as recently as the early 1980s. Many if not most people in Western societies continue to disbelieve it today. The reason is that changes in breast-feeding patterns that limited the number and duration of feedings in fact removed protection against pregnancy, as many couples found to their surprise.

In all but one family of primates (*Callitrichidae*), lactation suppresses ovulation. Interbirth intervals are as long as five years in chimpanzees and eight in orangutans. Many species of primates avoid sexual intercourse until after weaning, even though they do not avoid it during pregnancy.[27] Likewise, human populations often have postpartum sex taboos, and the prohibition against resuming sexual relations during lactation was an explicit factor in the rise of wet nursing in Europe in past centuries.[28]

The avoidance of conception, whether through biological or cultural means, protects the female during the time of maximum energy expenditure. It also protects the offspring. In humans, interbirth intervals under two years are associated with reduced chances of survival for both the first and second children in a sequence.[29]

If a woman does not breast-feed after childbirth, within two or three months the pituitary gland resumes its normal functioning, and the menstrual cycle begins anew. If a woman does breast-feed, this can be delayed for up to three or four years, depending upon the length and pattern of breast-feeding.[30] Menstruation usually begins several months before regular ovulation, and continued breast-feeding will continue to reduce the probability of conception. Nighttime breast-feeding seems to be particularly important in preventing the return of postpartum fecundity (the biological capacity to procreate, as opposed to actual reproduction, or fertility). Supplementation and weaning, by contrast, have predictable effects on its duration.

Prolactin is one of many hormones involved in preventing pregnancy. High prolactin levels inhibit ovulation. The concentration of the hormone in the blood is highest among mothers who breast-feed frequently through day and night; it can remain high into the third year. If breast-feeding is not frequent, there are periods between prolactin surges when levels are similar to those of nonpregnant, nonlactating women. Infrequent feedings and reduced time at the breast lead to a relaxation of the inhibiting effect of prolactin.

In addition, the secretion of other hormones involved in the menstrual cycle is interfered with by frequent nursing. These hormones (including gonadrotropin-releasing hormone [GnRh], luteinizing hormone [LH], and progesterone) interfere with normal follicle growth, ovulation (should an egg mature), development of the endometrium, and implantation of a fertilized ovum. Oxytocin may also contribute to keeping the endometrium from developing.

The suppression of gonadal function occurs not just in foraging women, but also among Western women who practice intensive on-demand feeding. This is important because foraging women often live in conditions of severe exercise and nutritional stress, which contributes to postpartum infecundity independently of lactation. Even moderate exercise can interfere with reproductive functioning, which accords with the theory that evolution has favored the postponement of reproduction until the woman can afford it and has sufficient nutrition and body fat.

As women space feedings at wider intervals, introduce supplementary foods, and reduce nighttime feeding, the contraceptive effect of breast-feeding weakens, and menstruation and ovulation resume.

Health Impacts of Breast-Feeding in Mothers and Infants

While any amount of breast-feeding is better than none, the greatest benefits accrue to mothers and infants when breast-feeding is conducted according to the ancestral human pattern. This pattern itself explains many of the highly publicized benefits of breast-feeding.[31]

The species-specific nutritional and immunological components of mother's milk lead to optimal growth patterns and ideal development of the body's glands and systems—gastrointestinal, vascular, immune, skeletal, nervous, and cardiorespiratory. Breast-feeding protects against a wide range of diseases. In the immediate term, these include infections of the gastrointestinal, respiratory (which includes the middle ear), and urinary tracts; neonatal sepsis, bacteremia, and meningitis; intestinal parasites such as entamoeba and giardia; botulism; and Sudden Infant Death Syndrome (SIDS).

In the long term, breast-feeding has been found to reduce the risk of inflammatory bowel disease and other gastrointestinal disorders, vasculitis, juvenile diabetes, lymphoma, breast cancer, multiple sclerosis, chronic respiratory disease, coronary artery disease, psychomotor and neurological disorders, allergies and autoimmune diseases, malpositioning of the teeth, and, possibly, paralytic poliomyelitis, liver disease, reduced bone mass in females, and exposure to radioactivity. These health benefits are not limited to poor countries, where differences in infant health and survival are extreme. They also apply to wealthy nations, where bottle-fed infants are hospitalized up to five times more often than breast-fed or mixed-fed infants.[32]

The flesh of breast-fed infants feels firmer and more solid than bottle-fed infants, reflecting differences in endocrine and metabolic processes. Bottle-fed babies and breast-fed babies who receive supplements before six to nine months often develop iron-deficiency anemia because there is less iron in formula and cow's milk, and it is less readily absorbed. Unlike mother's milk, formula does not contain lactoferrin, which binds iron. As a result, putting more iron into formula only makes matters worse, as the iron will remain free to bacteria.[33]

Colostrum, the yellowish fluid that is secreted in the first few days, helps to purge the dark sticky meconium from the newborn's digestive tract. Meconium contains bilirubin, the waste product from the destruction of red blood cells, which is responsible for the jaundice that many babies present in the first few days. Colostrum and the milk that replaces it beginning on the second or third day contain nutrients such as zinc which protect against infection, as well as many bioactive compounds including enzymes, hormones, peptides, and amino acids that optimize the development and functioning of the pancreas and gastrointestinal tract.

Colostrum and milk also deliver immunoglobin molecules and general and specific antibodies, lymphokines, epidermal and nerve growth factors, and anti-inflammatory substances. Some of these exert a local germicidal effect and protect the gut against injury and disease, while others pass into the bloodstream to defend against diseases and strengthen the immune system. The bacterial cultures and pH levels in the gut of breast-fed babies are very different from those of babies who receive other foods, and they protect against many pathogens.

The nutritional-immunological protection conferred by breast-feeding is important because the immunity acquired through the placenta lasts only a few months and is limited and imperfect. During the five to six years it takes to reach full competence, the immune system seems to need stimulation and training. The immunological protection provided by breast-feeding can last for years after weaning.

Poor nutrition can shorten the period of "inherited immunity" (passed from the mother during gestation) to a few weeks rather than months, while extreme nutritional deficiency in the first year can permanently compromise cell-mediated immunity. But even without nutritional deprivation, artificial feeding seems to interfere with proper immunoregulation later on. Bottle-fed infants are less resistant to disease, and their immune systems may develop inadequately. Ineffective immune response may permit tumor initiation or growth, or it may fail to defend against viral infections associated with cancers such as lymphoma. Children who are breast-fed for more than six months have a lower risk of cancer in general before age 15 than those breast-fed less or not at all, due largely to increased incidence of lymphoma (by six to eight times) in the latter.[34]

Some studies have found an advantage in the performance of breast-fed children on intelligence tests, but one found that the association vanished when it accounted for pacifier use: this study suggested that the home environment in which the pacifier is used, the pacifier itself, or both, could be the cause of lower scores.[35] The physical and cognitive interactions favored by breast-feeding could explain those studies finding an intelligence advantage. Also, the placenta and then breast provide certain essential nutrients for developing brain and nervous tissue that are especially needed by preterm infants, but that might also benefit infants born at term.

Breast-feeding seems to prevent or at least postpone the development of allergies, for allergic reactions during breast-feeding are very rare. This is important because cultural conventions have often limited what breast-feeding mothers could eat for fear of causing an allergic reaction or simply displeasure in the child. It is true that some substances ingested by the mother can pass in the milk and cause an allergic reaction in a susceptible child. By far, the most common of these is cow's milk, but even this is rare.

Unfortunately, the response is often to switch to formula rather than eliminate cow's milk from the mother's diet. There is no need for mothers to do
this or restrict their diet in other ways unless the child shows clear signs of
a reaction.

Compared to the impacts on children, the benefits of breast-feeding
to women receive much less attention, even though they are significant.
When it conforms to the ancestral pattern, breast-feeding prevents pregnancy. It also reduces the risk of breast and other reproductive system cancers, as discussed in the next section.

Two benefits that have been publicized are quicker weight loss after
childbirth and the earlier return of the uterus to its normal size and position. The hormones prolactin and oxytocin, mentioned above in the discussion on fertility, are secreted at higher levels in breast-feeding women.
Oxytocin causes the myoepithelial cells in the uterus and blood vessels to
contract, favoring the expulsion of the placenta and its residues, and
reducing bleeding and the risk of hemorrhage. Prolactin favors the metabolism of fat in peripheral tissues and its uptake in the breasts, where it is
used in milk synthesis: women who breast-feed more frequently than others show a greater reduction in upper arm fat.[36]

The two hormones also promote nurturing behavior, reduce anxiety,
and moderate mood swings, which help make the child feel accepted and
nurtured in turn. Sedative substances in the milk that calm the infant and
help it to sleep, especially in the first months, may contribute to a peaceful
relationship between mother and child.[37]

Other ongoing effects of lactation include higher body temperature;
higher blood flow to the chest, gut, liver, and skin; reduced urinary excre-
tion of calcium; and changes in the levels of hormones associated with
digestion and metabolism. Metabolic efficiency improves, helping to moderate the demands of lactation on the mother. Bone mineral density also
improves over the long term, reducing the risk of osteoporosis and hip and
other bone fractures later in life. This means that, as in children, in mothers the benefits of breast-feeding extend far beyond the time of weaning.

Breast-Feeding, Breast Cancer, and SIDS

Breast Cancer

Until the mid–nineteenth century, medical philosophers in Italy wrote that
well-off women who lived in cities were much more susceptible to breast
cancer than women who lived in the countryside. They attributed this difference to the decline of breast-feeding in the urban and upper classes,
which, they noted, caused numerous other maladies and grave health

effects. Even today, not only is breast cancer much more common in affluent societies, but within them it is more frequent among the wealthy.

The decline in breast-feeding has been part of a broad change in reproductive and child-rearing patterns since the Industrial Revolution. Urban women were the first to undergo the secular trend of earlier maturation and greater achieved stature (height). They experienced earlier puberty, delayed marriage and first birth, fewer pregnancies, and reduced or forsaken breast-feeding. Over time, these patterns diffused through the entire population.

Many of the things we consider "natural" are actually aberrations or deviations from evolution's path.[38] To illustrate, a typical woman of a foraging or preindustrial society reaches puberty and her first menstrual period (menarche) at the age of 16 to 18. She becomes pregnant within three or four years. As we have seen, she breast-feeds for three or four years and has a subsequent child four or five years after the first. This sequence repeats itself between four and six times before she reaches menopause in her early to middle forties. As a result, she has about 150 ovulations in her lifetime, taking account of nonovulatory cycles at the near and far end of her reproductive years. Periodic nutritional and exercise stress reduces the number of ovulations even more.

In contrast, Western women enjoy a stable food supply, including foods concentrated in fat, protein, and calories, and experience very little stress from exercise or exposure. Over the past centuries, this has caused them, and men, to grow taller and to mature sexually at an earlier age. Menarche begins at the age of 12 or 13, while menopause is delayed to 50 or 55 years. Significantly, the first birth is postponed for 13 or 14 years, to the age of 25 or 26, or later. The total number of births is low, averaging under three in most Western societies. Mothers breast-feed for a few months, if at all. Because they space feedings at long intervals and supplement with other foods, breast-feeding does not prevent pregnancy for long. These differences mean that if she does not take oral contraceptives, the Western woman will ovulate around 450 times over her lifetime. Ovulation will rarely be suppressed due to physiological constraints associated with nutritional or exercise stress. This amounts to at least three and perhaps up to nine times as many ovulations over the lifespan.[39]

As recently as the early twentieth century rural women's reproductive development in Italy was similar to the ancient pattern.[40] The average age at menarche for rural and working-class women ranged as high as 16 to 18 in the northern regions as recently as the 1930s. Since the 1960s, the average for all women has fallen to 12 or 13, with a range of about 9 to 14, which had been the norm for elite women for several centuries. In contrast, the increase in age at menopause has taken place mostly over the past few decades. Through the 1950s, the range remained between 40 or 45 and 50 years, but today the average is around 55. Meanwhile, the duration of postpartum amenorrhea has fallen drastically, from as long as a few years to 40 to 60 days if the mother does not breast-feed, and 60 to 90 if she does.[41]

The differences in reproductive patterns between women in foraging as opposed to affluent societies match some of the currently known risk factors for women's reproductive cancers (breast, endometrium, ovary), including age at menarche and menopause, parity (number of births), and breast-feeding. Differences in diet and exercise, as well as body composition, also agree with identified nonreproductive risk factors such as fat intake and percent body fat. Together with other factors, they give Western women, especially below the age of 60, at least 20 times the risk of reproductive cancer. The risk for breast cancer may be more than 100 times higher.[42] In nonhuman primates, these cancers are extremely rare.

For all three cancers, earlier age at menarche and later age at menopause increase risk, while greater parity reduces risk. In addition to these factors, breast-feeding is protective against ovarian cancer because it inhibits ovulation. This reduces the monthly mechanical injury to the ovarian epithelium and the release of hormones by the follicle, the main elements in ovarian cancer. For breast cancer, lactation and earlier first birth are also protective factors.

The breast's susceptibility to carcinogenesis is directly related to the rate of epithelial cell proliferation. In breast tissue, cell proliferation is promoted by exposure to estrogen, apparently in concert with progesterone, and cell division rates are highest during the first five years after menarche. The expansion of the period between menarche and first birth widens the window of time in which undifferentiated structures destined to become secretory glands are vulnerable to carcinogenic agents and therefore the initiation of tumors. With pregnancy and lactation, these structures differentiate and develop, devoting themselves less ardently to cell proliferation. Their cell cycle is longer, and they are more resistant to chemical carcinogens. Subsequent pregnancies may also be protective because they increase the proportion of fully differentiated secretory lobules, until in advanced age, pregnancy increases risk by favoring the expansion of initiated tumors.

While age at first pregnancy seems to be of primary importance and may even modulate the protective effect of breast-feeding and later pregnancies, breast-feeding in itself provides protection in step with the number of children breast-fed and the cumulative duration of breast-feeding. The reason some studies have found no effect or a weak one is that they were based upon Western women, who do not generally conform to the ancient pattern. Short periods of breast-feeding may in fact provide very little protection.

Besides systemic protection, breast-feeding protects the breast directly. Among women in Hong Kong fishing villages, where it is customary to breast-feed only from the right breast, cancer in postmenopausal women is much more common in the left.[43] There are lower levels of a potential carcinogen, cholesterol-epoxide, as well as cholesterol, in the breast fluid of lactating women, a reduction that persists for two years after childbirth or breast-feeding. Estrogen levels are also lower, protecting the breast tissue directly as opposed to systemically through variations in blood estrogen levels. Breast-feeding also affects the turnover rate of substances in the breast fluid, so that prolonged breast-feeding reduces exposure of the breast epithelial tissue to potential exogenous carcinogens.

Other aspects of the ancestral life-style are protective against breast and other cancers, including high levels of exercise, high consumption of dietary fiber, and low fat consumption and body fat. High dietary levels of fat and protein (especially from animal sources) and total calories are associated with higher levels of breast cancer across populations and within subpopulations of single countries. Dietary protein promotes tumor development while restriction of protein intake inhibits tumor growth. The enzymes in fat tissue convert precursor adrenal hormones into active estrogens, while dietary fat raises serum estrogen levels. This promotes the development of tumors and may play a role in originating them. In contrast to Western women, foragers have low serum estrogen levels.

Western women's skinfold thickness (a measure of the proportion of body fat) is almost twice that of preagricultural women. Compared to college athletes, women who are not athletic in college (and less active in adolescence and somewhat less active after college) have two to five times the rates of breast, uterine, and ovarian cancer. Women in affluent societies consume 40 percent or more of their calories in the form of fat, against 20 to 25 percent among preagricultural women, but only 20 as opposed to 100 grams of fiber per day. Dietary fiber is protective because it reduces free estrogen levels in the blood. It helps to prevent bowel dysfunction, which has been associated with breast cancer, and the severe constipation that can lead to the migration of mutagenic substances from the gastrointestinal tract to the breast fluid.

The protective effect of breast-feeding goes beyond the current generation to the next one, for early nutritional influences have an important effect on later susceptibility to cancer. Breast-feeding contributes to the development and regulation of the immune system, which plays a central role in suppressing the initiation and growth of tumors. It prevents overconsumption of fat, protein, and calories. This influences body size and composition, the baseline against which nutrition works throughout life. Breast-feeding prevents the accelerated growth of muscles and fat stores associated with breast cancer risk factors: faster growth rates, earlier menarche, and increased stature and size. Women who have been breast-fed themselves are less likely to develop breast cancer.

Breast-feeding benefits both the mother and child with respect to breast cancer. In the mother, breast-feeding the traditional way influences systemic hormone levels and the microenvironment of the breast tissue, reducing exposure to exogenous and endogenous carcinogens. In the child, breastmilk provides an appropriate balance of nutrients and prevents overnutrition and rapid growth and development. This two-way protection is an elegant expression of the mother-infant dyad as a biological interacting pair. The concept is also fundamental to the following discussion of sleep.

Sudden Infant Death Syndrome (SIDS)

From a global perspective, Western society's expectation that infants should sleep for long hours away from their parents stands out as anomalous, even if it fits well within its cultural context. One unfortunate consequence is the rise in the frequency of infant death from SIDS, which may be related to the diffusion of lone infant sleep over the past several generations.[44]

While there seem to be many intrinsic and secondary factors that affect infants in different ways to bring about SIDS events, one common factor is that they usually happen during sleep. Breast-feeding in itself reduces risk, but it is frequent, intensive, prolonged breast-feeding (implying mother-infant cosleeping) that may provide the best environment for avoiding the disease.

The meaning of reproduction and child rearing changed with the emergence of industrial society and the predominance of small, simple families. In this kind of society, the crib symbolizes the child's place, usually in a separate room. By contrast, in rural preindustrial Europe and in over 90 surveyed contemporary non-Western societies, infants invariably slept in the same room or bed as their parents. SIDS does not appear to have existed in these societies, nor is it found among nonhuman primates or other mammals. In many Western societies, SIDS is the major cause of infant death, though rates are very low among subpopulations in which there is cosleeping and noctural breast-feeding. Peak mortality is between the ages of two and four months, with 90 percent of all deaths before the age of six months.

When babies sleep with their mothers, they lay on their backs or sides with their heads turned toward the breast. They feed through the night, often without waking their mothers (who may also not be aware of the number of times they open their eyes to look at the baby). Even newborns and very young infants are able to attach to the breast on their own, provided it is within reach. In nonindustrialized societies, it is rare for infants younger than one year to sleep long hours with only a few awakenings for feedings. They do not increase the length of their longest sleep episode within the first few months, nor do they stop feeding at night, as parents in Western societies expect.

These same patterns are observed in sleep laboratories, where mothers report waking up and feeding their children many times fewer than the number recorded on the monitors. They and their infants move through the various stages of sleep in synchrony, shifting between them more frequently and spending less time in the deep sleep that makes arousal more difficult. If in the laboratory the cosleeping mother spends the night in a separate room from her child, on average she breast-feeds less than half as often. She also tends to put the child on its stomach when leaving it to sleep alone. Notably, breast-feeding mothers who routinely sleep in a separate room from their infants actually sleep for a shorter overall time period than mothers who cosleep.

One factor common to a majority of cases is that the infant had been placed on its stomach to sleep: the opposite of the position used by babies who sleep with their mothers. This may be due to suffocation because the child is unable to move out of pockets of its own carbon dioxide in puffy mattresses, pillows, bean bag cushions, or heavy blankets. Over the past decade, campaigns against the face-down position have been initiated in many European countries, the United Kingdom, and, more recently, the United States.[45] These have been followed by huge reductions in SIDS rates.

The crib itself may be the villain, since it implies isolated, prolonged, deep sleep. Like adults, infants are able to fall into deep sleep, but they are less equipped to arouse themselves out of it. All people have temporary lapses in breathing during the night, but their brains generally respond to them appropriately. Infants are different, for they are born at a much earlier stage of neurological development than other primates, even our closest relatives.

During sleep, infants may need frequent arousals in order to allow them to emerge from episodes of sleep apnea or cardiorespiratory crisis. External stimuli and parental monitoring in cosleeping and breast-feeding give them practice at doing so and keep them from spending long periods of time in deep stages of sleep. SIDS deaths peak at the same age at which the amount of deep sleep relative to rapid-eye-movement sleep increases dramatically, at two to three months. Moreover, at this time infants begin to exercise more voluntary control of breathing, as parents notice in their more expressive cries. This is a step toward the speech breathing they will use later, but may complicate breathing in the short term.

The rhythm of sound and silence in the mother's breathing gives the infant auditory stimulation, while contact with her body provides tactile stimulation. The carbon dioxide which her breathing releases into the air they share induces the infant to breathe. Frequent waking for breast-feeding is a behavior common to primates and prevents hypoglycemia, which has been implicated in some SIDS deaths. Mother's milk also provides immuno-logical protection against several infectious organisms (and preparations of them given as immunizations) considered responsible for some deaths. This protection is especially needed after two months, when inherited maternal antibodies become scarce but the infant's own immune system is not yet developed. Breast-feeding and constant physical contact prevent the over-heating and the exhausting crying spells which seem to be occasional factors in the disease. In addition, the infant is sensitive to other aspects of its microenvironment, including temperature, humidity, and odors.

While many experts and parents advise against or avoid cosleeping because they fear suffocating the infant, in fact this risk is very low, espe-cially where people sleep on hard bedding or the floor. Modern bedding is dangerous because of the conformation of bed frames and the use of soft mattresses and heavy coverings. Yet, these factors are at least as relevant to cribs as parents' beds. On the other hand, some parents should not sleep with their infants, such as those who go to bed affected by drugs or alco-hol. Cigarette smoke in the sleeping room could cancel the benefit of cosleeping.[46]

Isolated infant sleep may be consistent with parents' desires, the pri-macy of the conjugal bond, and other Western values, but it is a new behavioral norm in human history and does not represent a natural need. It is neither in the infant's best interest nor in conformity with behavioral patterns and biological conditions established long before our time. By contrast, parent-infant cosleeping matches evolutionary considerations such as the need for temperature regulation, frequent nutrition, and pro-tection from predators and disease. There may be some wisdom in the popular term *crib death* or *cot death,* for it points to the crib and the West-ern concept of infant independence as major factors in the disease.

The discussion of breast cancer and SIDS has shown that mothers and infants are physiologically bound together from conception to wean-ing, not just conception to birth. The Western ideal of the autonomous individual, which is even applied to the neonate, is not shared by other societies today or by those of the past. Evolution has favored frequent, exclusive, prolonged breast-feeding. This entails constant physical con-tact, parent-infant cosleeping, and nighttime breast-feeding. Through massive social transformation, the Western societies have moved far away from this pattern. In Italy, this change has taken a particular form that reflects both cultural patterns and structural changes associated with industrialization and political consolidation.

CHAPTER 2

Blood and Milk

Medical and Popular Beliefs
before the First World War

The fascist period was pivotal in the abandonment of prolonged, on-demand breast-feeding, in favor of a regularized, regimented method of infant feeding. During that time, old ideas about the body and health were upset, and the way people thought about their relationship to state and medical experts was transformed. Yet, the new outlook was shaped by pre-existing beliefs and socioeconomic conditions. In the same way, fascist-era beliefs and behaviors have had an enduring impact beyond the interwar period and continue to influence Italian culture today.

We will begin with turn-of-the-century health concepts rooted in the empirical knowledge of the ancients. These ideas touch upon not only the nature of knowledge in the past, but also the eternal truth of the physiological interdependence of mothers and infants from conception to weaning. According to traditional health beliefs, breast-feeding was as much a part of gestation as pregnancy. Mothers and infants were directly linked in their material and moral essence through the blood and its purified product, the milk. To deviate the milk away from breast-feeding had harmful consequences for both.

This conception fit within an understanding of the body that emphasized atmospheric and humoral influences on health. It assumed that all humans were homologous in form and function, making the moderate and regular use of all bodily functions essential to the health and life of everyone. Secretions including blood and milk were not suppressed or released excessively. Diseases derived in an essential way from their causes, making it vital to avoid disequilibrating forces by practicing moderate behavior.

Until the nineteenth century, the only condition precluding breast-feeding was an imbalance of the constitution, for it was assumed that all women were naturally able to breast-feed. Then, over the course of the century, the list of contraindications grew, as did medical advice about breast-feeding, weaning age, supplementation, and "artificial feeding." Medical beliefs began to detach themselves from popular knowledge. Well-off urban women most in contact with professional medicine learned of the necessity of scheduling feedings, initiating supplementation earlier, and weighing infants more often to monitor their growth. The rest of the population was slower to be absorbed into the national culture, economy, and health-care system. In the interwar period, the blood-milk bond between mothers and infants would be broken. A single method of breast-feeding would be proposed that no longer honored individual variation in constitution or daily needs, the health consequences of climatic and seasonal variations, or economic or social class differences.

Through the early twentieth century, there was still significant variability and little outside intervention in women's behavior in reproduction and child rearing. The medical system remained largely a dispersed network of local physicians and midwives together with independent professionals. This contrasted with the centralized state medical system soon to arise. Most people relied on traditional and family authorities when they needed health advice and care, and sought medical help only as a last resort. These characteristics of health beliefs and practices were consistent with a sociocultural system that stressed geographical diversity and family autonomy as opposed to national cultural uniformity, and networks of human relationships as opposed to a cultural ideal of autonomous personhood. As we will see, both health beliefs and sociocultural systems changed over the following decades, leading eventually to realignment of medical and popular belief and behavior.

Ancient Understandings of Maternity and Lactation

Blood and Milk

Breast-feeding has been a central survival characteristic of humans and other primates. Cultural beliefs have upheld its importance, especially in past times when alternatives presented real dangers to health and life. In Italy, the core concept about the mother-infant relationship was a unity between blood and milk. It derived from ancient Greek and Roman ideas that persisted through the nineteenth century and into the twentieth. These beliefs emphasized the permeability of the body to atmospheric influences, and the importance of regularity and moderation in all bodily functions. This meant that maternity was extremely beneficial to women.

The endurance of ancient beliefs through the beginning of this century is documented in contemporary books about medicine, hygiene, and child rearing. These books were generally written by classically trained physicians and social reformers of the upper classes, given that very few people in Italy were educated beyond the fifth grade at this time. While not every author agreed in every respect with the main ideas presented below, there was a relatively high degree of conformity among them, and between their beliefs and ancient knowledge. Medical ideas converged with those of the public, as seen in historical works on nineteenth-century popular health beliefs and the recollections of older Italians.[1]

As Mercurii explained in 1601 in the first obstetrics text written in Italian, mother's milk (*il latte materno*) was a direct product of the same blood that had nourished the fetus. To give the milk was to complete the work of gestation, whereas to abstain from breast-feeding was to have a *birth* that was "against nature, imperfect, halved." Such a birth was against nature because no other animals delivered offspring without intending to raise them; imperfect because no other woman could nourish the infant as well as its mother; halved because

> the woman had willingly nourished [the child] in her abdomen with her own blood, not knowing if it were male, or female, or monster; and now that she sees it, and recognizes it as her child, indeed with its cries, and with its sighs she feels it asking her for help, nearly cutting it in half . . . she sends it into exile, content-ing herself to have given it its being, and enduring, that others give it a good existence, as if the breasts were given to her by God, and by nature only for the ornamentation of the chest. (1601:105)

Citing Aristotle, Hippocrates, Avicenna, and Galen, Mercurii de-scribed how the blood that nourished the fetus was the mother's menstrual blood diverted to and mixed directly with the fetus's blood in the placenta. After birth, this blood was drawn into the breasts, where it was cooked, whitened, and changed to become milk. While there were good and bad elements in the menstrual blood, only the best part became the material of the milk. Compared to regular blood, the blood destined to become milk was purer, sweeter, less fatty, and only moderately cooked.

This cooking, called coction (*cottione*), involved a number of steps and had all kinds of health effects. For example, during illness, the blood heated up and expelled disease. In milk production, the cooked fraction of blood was sent to the breast by the veins for a final cottione. This step did not add heat, but purification, making the milk cooler than blood. Blood that was pungent or hot, too thick or viscous, or unequal in all its parts was distilled and perfected in the process. This is how dangerous men-strual blood became virtuous milk. Through the early twentieth century, milk production was known as "the separation of the milk."

Through the nineteenth and early twentieth centuries, medical thought held that the creature once born was more perfect than the unborn and fed with a more perfect food. The overall experience of gesta-tion, birth, and breast-feeding influenced lifelong health, while mother's milk was the very foundation of health and life. The milk even endowed the child with moral qualities and values, while its physical characteristics mechanically influenced the development of the organs. Mother's milk was such an ideal, even magical food that popular and medical remedies for sickness in children and adults frequently involved taking it as a medicine. Two feedings from a wholesome woman would restore health and happiness in cases of lost strength, organs oppressed by humoral intemperance, recent weight loss, or a disheartened nature. Moreover, it was widely noted that animals rarely died in the time of breast-feeding, and the same held for women even though they often died in pregnancy and childbirth. Nature also spared women many diseases until after breast-feeding was terminated.

Breast-feeding was given many exalted names: it was a natural duty, a sacred obligation, one of the first laws of nature, and a fundamental aspect of the arrangement of the animal economy. To abstain from breast-feeding for frivolous motives or unashamed indifference, as bourgeois women had long done, was not to deserve the name of mother. This betrayal of nature and religion would be avenged sooner or later. Instead of protecting their beauty, abstention destroyed women's looks and health, slowed the expulsion of the uterine residues, or lochia, after childbirth, turned the skin a pallid moldy or yellow color, withered the breast, slackened the limbs, and depressed the morale. It deprived women of other benefits too, such as the favorable evolution of the constitution to greater strength and better development of the organs, and the reduction or complete disappearance of any predisposition to nervous afflictions.

The imprudent, violent retropulsion of the milk also brought more serious, even fatal, consequences, including puerperal fever. It increased susceptibility to the ill effects of the so-called *febbre lattea* (milk fever, discussed later in this chapter) that killed so many city women. It not infrequently led to the growth of tumors that could degenerate into breast cancer, especially among women with a gracile (frail) and sickly constitution. Since the breast was in intimate relationship with the uterus and ovaries, its morbid alterations often diffused there. In addition, the sending back of the milk could accomplish what other causes could not, bringing about the development of latent diseases to which puerperal women were predisposed by heredity or environment, such as tuberculosis or scurvy. That more women died in the city than the countryside was considered the consequence of city women's refusal to breast-feed. The same reason explained why, within the city, more wives than husbands died.

Lactation, Menstruation, and Fertility

Since breastmilk derived from the same blood as menstrual blood, the two were temporally incompatible. This explains the age-old practice of waiting to feed the infant until the mother's lochia had stopped, and the concern with the lochia being of moderate quality and quantity. It also explains why the return of menstruation during lactation was considered pathological, and pregnancy even more so. Lactation was said to exert a strong effect on the entire reproductive system and to normally prevent these events for the duration of breast-feeding and some time afterward. When women did not breast-feed, they saw the return of menstruation after six to eight weeks, an event known as the *capoparto* (*capo* for head, *parto* for childbirth). This term marks the end of the puerperium after 40 days (the *quarantena,* from the word for 40), a number with strong ritual and religious connotations. The Old Testament says that the state of impurity brought on by childbirth lasts 40 days after the birth of a boy, 80 after a girl.

Activities such as exercise and sex were to be avoided because they provoked menstruation, which dried the milk and led to a new pregnancy. Menstruation during lactation would reduce the quantity of milk and change its quality, making it more serous and turning it a bluish color. The breasts would refill poorly, while the child's features would change and its skin become hot, and it would suffer from colic often accompanied by diarrhea. Similar, but more mild effects would be seen during the missed menstrual period even if the mother had not resumed her cycle.

Pregnancy had even more pernicious effects, if not in ceasing the production of milk then in reducing and altering it dangerously. Wet-nursing contracts specified that nurses (*balie*) must report a new pregnancy to the parents and authorities. A woman in the public health service explained to me with reference to her aunt—who was born in 1848—that wet nurses would often become pregnant, "which makes the milk stop." Rather than telling the parents and losing their jobs, the balie would put the nursling at risk by feeding it other foods. Nineteenth-century regulations of the foundling home in Faenza specify that the wet nurse must maintain a "temperate and honest life" to keep her milk "pure and nutritious" and inform the director of the wet-nursing service should she take ill, become pregnant, or lose her milk.[2]

The belief that pregnancy harmed lactation backed up the idea that breast-feeding women should practice sexual continence. This belief, upheld by the Church, had fueled the wet-nursing business for centuries and contributed to some couples' preference for keeping the wet nurse in the home in order to better oversee her actions. Experts argued that sexual relations in themselves could harm the milk, while those who disagreed said that they were not damaging so long as they were not conducted with "extraordinary frequency, and excessive rapture."[3] Yet, because to not have sex would represent a physiological deficit and therefore be harmful to the woman, some physicians permitted "discreet and moderate use of conjugal pleasures: excess, as everyone knows, is reproachable in all circumstances of life."[4] The softening of the belief in the danger of sex during lactation was essential to the return to maternal breast-feeding among the bourgeoisie and aristocracy.

Over the nineteenth century, physicians grew more likely to argue that the return of menstruation did not affect the milk secretion, or if it did it was not serious enough to change the nurse; that pregnancy did not always disturb breast-feeding; that women were able to successfully breast-feed twins or a series of children each to the moment of the labor pains announcing the next birth; and that the infant could be breast-fed by a pregnant mother so long as it showed no alteration of health. Today, while there are some experts who oppose the old ideas about the discordance between lactation and reproductive functioning, many health professionals and parents continue to believe them and to act accordingly.

Humoral and Atmospheric Influences on Health

The ideas we have discussed so far hint that general health beliefs stressed moderation and balance in all aspects of life. Though an ancient one, this is still a central cultural value today. It is a primary tenet of classical medical philosophies, which merged over the centuries and even accommodated the ascendant germ theory of disease in the latter half of the nineteenth century.

Through the middle of the nineteenth century, it was usual to think of diseases and causes as a single phenomenon. For example, the public-hygiene expert Francesco Ballotta classified occupational diseases in the following way: an excess or defect of exercise, an absence or lack thereof, or a penurious position of the head, trunk, or limbs; the condition of the air, whether hot or cold, or humid-hot, or humid-cold; and the qualities of mineral or vegetal substances that entered the lungs in the form of vapors or powders (1857:312). Similarly, social miasmas such as jealousy and rivalry could cause illness through means such as evil eye. The way to protect against them was to minimize exposure. These concepts matched a sociocentric notion of personhood typical of social systems in which people are linked through complex networks of responsibility and obligation.

As the social system changed over the second half of the nineteenth century through industrialization, agricultural intensification, and the progressive isolation of ever smaller and simpler families, concepts of personhood became more individuocentric. Diseases were separated from their causes and embodied in microorganisms. Once it was socially acceptable, the practice of autopsy gave rise to a new focus upon the connection between the living body's disease response and tissue changes observable after death. Family members and traditional medical authorities were passed over in favor of mainstream physicians, who understood illnesses less in terms of reciprocal disease-causes, whether of atmospheric or social origin, than specific responses to particular pathogens. However, the older understandings of illness have never been successfully overturned by the laboratory and germ-focused medicine of the late nineteenth and twentieth centuries. Instead, agents of disease would ride upon the wings of ancient atmospheric and behavioral influences to enter the body and cause illness.

The ancients believed in the permeability of the body to atmospheric forces, as Hippocrates explained in his famous essay on "airs, waters, places." The position and altitude of the house, the direction of prevailing winds, the orientation of the sun, the variations in temperature and humidity, the climate, nearby bodies of water, and the water used by the household all impacted upon health and well-being. Depletion, whether from sweating, childbirth, or sex, exposed the person to illness, especially if confounded by exposure to environmental insults. Loss of equilibrium through excesses in diet, drink, sleep, sex, exercise, or the passions (which ideally would be lacking entirely) had the same effect, as did *colpi di aria* (gusts of air), *colpi di vento* (gusts of wind), *correnti* (drafts), sudden temperature changes or atmospheric events, sunbursts, and excessive humidity, heat, or cold.

Another paradigm still in force today is the classical concept of the constitution. The theory of the four humors, which holds that the balance among blood, bile, phlegm, and lymph is the foundation of the constitution, commingled with the more ancient view to yield four main categories of atmospheric influence: heat, cold, humidity, and dryness. This implied a greater scope for human control of health and illness through limitation of excess, but expanded the field of possibilities for compromising the equilibrium state.

There were direct implications of these beliefs for the treatment of mothers and infants in the nineteenth century. Physicians argued that in order to treat any mother or child during gestation or lactation, it was necessary to obtain unequivocal knowledge of their constitution. Certain female constitutions were associated with specific qualities and quantities of milk, while excessive milk production would exhaust and deplete a weak woman whose constitution was the cause of the excess secretion in the first place. Women should not leave milk in the breast too long, as the stagnation and retropulsion of the milk would be harmful and it would lose its good qualities. Mothers were warned that if they did not swaddle the infant's head, it would grow precociously while its dangling would cause the accumulation of abundant humors. On the other hand, they must not swaddle the body too tightly, for to do so would obstruct the free circulation of humors.[5]

The requirement of practicing moderate behaviors was imposed with increasing rigidity in the late nineteenth century, at least in part because of the widespread perception that women—especially urban women—were getting out of control. Their new, self-interested ideas were producing an abominable decline in fertility, and they were not living up to the ideal image of girls and wives, which held that they should be simple, servile, hard-working, modest, and not at all demanding. In contrast to the sober, active life of the countryside, life in the city was unhealthy, depraved, and idle, causing women to commit innumerable errors of regimen. They read improper books that excited the passions, engaged themselves excessively in the social life, and stayed up too late or slept too much. Unlike country women, who reproduced and breast-fed in conformity with natural instinct and the balance of female secretions, they compromised their maternal instinct and threatened pregnancy and the postpartum period with illness and death for themselves and their children. They also complicated menopause with reproductive system disorders and nervous and spasmodic ailments.

Homology and Utility in Form and Function

Another central component of the traditional belief system was that all people—male or female, young or old—were anatomically and physiologically homologous. For example, male and female genitalia were drawn in exactly the same way.[6] This meant that the laws of health maintenance and treatment of illness applied equally to everyone. All people needed to exercise moderation and circumspection in their behavior and maintain balance in their secretions, in conformity with ideas about atmospheric and humoral influences on health.

For example, infants' convulsions could arise from the suppression of diarrhea or sweat, as well as "excesses of anger" or the abuse of food or drink by the wet nurse or mother. Convulsions also resulted from the "incautious retropulsion" of an eruption on the skin such as smallpox, ringworm, or the *crosta lattea* (literally, milk crust, this skin ailment was said to cover the head and face often at the time of dentition; cradle cap was and still is blamed upon defects in the mother's milk, just as dandruff after infancy is attributed to liver problems due to an improper diet). Women's maladies could result from the suppression or overproduction of secretions such as menstrual blood, milk, or the lochia following childbirth.

The concepts of homology and balance in secretions converged in the idea that the regular and moderate use of sexual and reproductive functions was a universal necessity for good health. Every part and function of the body must be utilized, or else noxious substances would accumulate in the blood. If a weakened or atrophied organ did not take its ration of materials, they remained in and obstructed the circulation, compromising well-being and bringing feelings of weakness, heaviness, and irritability.

This was why widows and nuns were especially prone to noncongenital anatomical disorders of the uterus. It was also the basis of neomalthusianist criticism of traditional brakes on population control such as institutionalized celibacy and the indissolubility of marriage. Several of the more popular contraceptive methods were also denounced, even though they were considered moral and Christian, because they interfered with normal sexual function: these included withdrawal, the rhythm method, and prolonged breast-feeding. The latter caused undernutrition in infants and depletion in mothers since most mothers were not strong and healthy enough for it. These pitiful "beasts of burden" found in prolonged breast-feeding "the precocious twilight of their youthful floridity and health."[7]

Women's sexual and reproductive functions were all mediated by the blood, making menstruation the most important function for their lives and well-being. Although governed by universal principles, the blood underwent specific transformations in women, for they were cooler than men and did not convert all of their food into meat and body substance through the third coction.[8] The excess blood was transmitted to the uterus little by little until it was expelled each month through menstruation (in other animals, the material of menstruation was converted into hair, nails, and horns). Puberty began when girls cooled down in adolescence, while menopause resulted from a natural reduction in the amount of blood in older age, and a weakening of natural heat resulting in a lack of force to push the blood from the uterus. Given these sex differences in blood and heat, Hippocratic theory held that certain foods, exercises, and drinks could be used in pregnancy to determine the sex of the child: cold-humid for girls, hot-dry for boys.

Menstrual blood, like other humors, was secreted in proportion to constitutional and other factors. Beyond the effects of the inborn constitution, it could be suppressed, interrupted, or diminished through transgression of the rules of moderate behavior. In healthy women, the menstrual cycle lasted two to three days, but in sick women it could go on for months or years. The quantity was greater in virgins and sanguinous women, lesser in old and phlegmatic women. Women who did not have menstrual "purges" lived short lives and suffered all kinds of infirmities. These encompassed difficulty in urination and pain in the kidneys; white or yellow discharge with unbearable itching in the genitals; inflammation of the reproductive organs; hemorrhoids; uterine cancer; fever; and death. Other afflictions included nervous disorders such as madness, melancholy, convulsions, and hysterism.

Given these serious consequences, it was important to avoid interfering voluntarily with menstruation. This could happen if one became hot through sunbathing, running, dancing, drinking heat-producing liquors, or using a foot warmer. It was also risky to allow the skin to be exposed to sudden cold, to live in humid rooms, and to take cool drinks when sweaty. Excessive physical activity or overly long periods of wakefulness, and their opposites, together with sad passions, violent grief, surprise, anger, or fright, had to be scrupulously avoided. Not coincidentally, the menstrual period was and still is called *il tempo delle regole* (the time of the rules), or simply *le regole.*

The suppression of menstruation would lead to menstrual scarcity, hysteria, and genital disorders such as *leucorrea* or *fiori bianchi* (white "flowers" or secretions). These ailments had many other contributing causes besides imbalances in sleep, exercise, and emotions, or predisposing conditions such as blood defects, constitutional factors (weak or lymphatic for menstrual scarcity, labile constitution for leucorrea), or unhealthy housing or climate. They included insufficiency or insalubriousness of diet; unhealthy waters; an overly soft or hard life; excessive or inappropriate clothing, including wearing metal corsets or dressing out of season; excesses in bleedings, bodily functions, or bathing; lust or frustrated or unhappy love; novels that excited the imagination; and exposure to acute odors or the sight of something disgusting or revolting. The primary treatment for all of these disorders, as well as the opposite condition of excessive menstruation, was a "moral" cure, or the establishment of correct female behaviors.

The necessity of exercising prudence, moderation, and circumspection applied equally to menopause, when good behavior would prevent common disturbances such as inflammations and frequent loss of blood. The menopausal woman should severely and soberly regulate her diet, physical activity, social life, relationships, dress, sleep, habits, and the physical and moral agents acting upon her. She must not think of trying to enjoy the time ahead of her by abandoning herself to social or physical pleasures and new licentious practices—reading obscene books and consuming foods and beverages that excite the appetite of concupiscence—nor should she overindulge in folk cures such as baths, enemas, purgatives, and bleedings. As in her younger days, the aging woman must always preserve balance and regulate behavior in order to maintain health and avoid disease and discomfort.

Medical and Popular Ideas about Maternity and Breast-Feeding

Moderation and Maternal Behavior in Pregnancy

It is little wonder that nineteenth-century medicine considered the transformative events of maternity extremely disequilibrating. Even if the woman were of robust constitution, pregnancy modified the reproductive system and overall organism. This, combined with the fierce labors of childbirth, caused intemperance and a state of elevated sensitivity, nervous irritability, and impressionability. After childbirth, the exuberance of humors beyond what was needed for organic reparation created an imbalance between solids and fluids and therefore *disordini* (disorderlinesses) in the health of the *puerpera* (postpartum mother).[9] Pregnant women always fed this imbalance through their behavioral excesses, but provident nature realigned the discordant secretions by eliminating them in the lochia and milk.

It was said that pregnant women's behavior could be responsible for sterility, birthmarks and birth defects, and loss of pregnancy, among other negative health effects. According to folk belief and linguistic conventions, conception was linked to the spinning and weaving of cloth—the child grown from its mother as the spider makes a web from its own substance. Consequently, a woman who worked hastily, distractedly, awkwardly, or with frigid repetitiveness could cause a difficult or delayed pregnancy and even sterility. A restrictive set of rules for pregnancy and childbirth respected a symbolic association between strings and the umbilical cord, and prohibited women from wearing necklaces or jumping over strings or ropes. During childbirth, all such things were banished from the house, and the skeins were removed from the distaffs.

Folk belief and mainstream medicine were in complete agreement about maternal responsibility for birth defects and miscarriage. Because the unborn child was considered more a simple receiver of messages than a person in its own right, mothers had to avoid anything that would give them strong emotions. This included crowds, funerals, reading romantic literature or any other source of moral sensations, and the sight of deformed people (from whom the child would develop the same deformity). If the mother committed a sin such as adultery, she would have a difficult birth. If she ate a wild rabbit (*leppre*), her child would be born with harelip (*labbro leporino*). To influence hair color, she could drink white or black (red) wine, according to her desire.

Most importantly, she must not touch herself in the case of an unsatisfied *voglia* (desire or craving). If she did, the image of the thing she so ardently desired would form itself in the blood, be pulled to the part she touched, and indelibly imprint itself on the part of the infant's body corresponding to the place where she touched herself, as the ancients had explained. According to the logic of disease-causes, the word for birthmark is the same as the word for its cause. The mark could simply be a spot with the appearance of a fruit or other object, which usually disappeared over time; but it could also be grotesque and life-threatening. A prominent Neapolitan physician described the case of a woman who heard about a child born without arms or legs in the first few days after she had conceived a child. She was traumatized by the story and later took to touching her breasts and thighs. Her female infant was born without humeri, and on her thighs there was a breast complete with a nipple. The baby died after a few hours.[10]

Mothers could also cause *aborto* (loss of the embryo or fetus), premature birth, and stillbirth. In popular belief, women could purposely end an unwanted pregnancy by eating a lot of parsley or other herbs considered abortifacients, making repeated leaps on hard ground, or breaking other rules for a safe pregnancy. The other side of this was the medical view that most cases of aborto, whether intended or not, were entirely the fault of the mother: a crime voluntarily committed. "Abortion is always a grave accident for which the sagacious and Christian woman would not be able to give herself peace, [considering] how many times when inspecting her way of life could she say to herself that she had been its cause."[11]

Physicians allowed that some children were lost due to causes which could not be helped, such as imperfections of the reproductive organs, chronic weakness, disease, gracile temperament, or other maladies or misfortunes. But the majority of cases were the result of behaviors that interacted in a dangerous way with atmospheric and constitutional influences. For example, abortion could be caused by clothing worn tight around the chest or abdomen; exposure of certain parts of the body, especially in variable weather; exposure to inclement weather; and baths that were too cold or footbaths that were too hot. Other causes included the suppression of sweat; use of strong purgatives; excessive pleasure in sex, or sexual relations in the first and last months of pregnancy; protracted periods of wakefulness; tumultuous passions; and bleedings. Yet others were any forceful physical activity, violent movement, or jolting, whether from running, jumping, horseback riding, traveling in poorly suspended carriages, or dancing. However, since laziness was also a great evil, moderate exercise in spring and fall was recommended—as long as it was not done to the point of tiredness.

Loss of pregnancy and other disturbances in pregnancy were considered much more common in the city due to its greater disorderliness of life, its contradiction of the rules of hygiene, and its unhealthy morality. Drinking and eating between meals ruined the constitution; hot drinks and heat-provoking liquors caused inflammation, while cold drinks could cause aborto. Foods such as fennel that affected the urine also affected the menses and consequently were damaging to pregnancy. Stimulating and highly seasoned foods were absolutely forbidden, while wine, coffee, and tea had to be used with great circumspection in order to avoid accelerating the circulation and harming the fetus.

Care of the Mother and Infant after Childbirth

After childbirth, maternal behavior continued to be a dangerous influence on the health and life of the mother and child. Inflammatory peritonitis and other serious infections could be caused by taking cold, abusing food, experiencing vivid moral impressions, or being covered excessively to the point of great sweating. Puerperal fever was caused by weak organic tonicity and self-abandonment to idleness or sloth, voluptuousness, or voracity in diet during pregnancy. In the days after childbirth, it could be caused by the woman's lack of attention to herself and her cleanliness, getting up too soon, putting her bare feet on the ground, not giving needed fresh air to the room, taking stimulating foods and drinks, suspending the secretion of lochia, or refusing to breast-feed.

To avoid these and other disorders, the new mother was to sleep in a room with pure, temperate air. Hot air excited excessive sweats and inflammation of the organs; cold air impeded the transpiration of the skin; and humid air favored the corruption of the humors. The mother must not take cold, especially at the abdomen or breast, and these parts must be wrapped in warm fine cloth each morning to avoid stretch marks, support the organs, and avoid the pooling of blood in parts susceptible to inflammation.

Because of the new mother's extreme weakness and sensitivity, she was given neither good nor bad news, since upsetting her could cause grave illness. Funeral bells and the sounding of mortars for festivals would be silenced for a new mother, and if her infant were deformed it would not be shown to her. For several days, she was given scarce, easily digested food such as chicken broth and a small amount of wine and water, as well as a bland purgative the morning after the birth. Her genital secretions were favored with infusions and lotions, and the cloths were changed frequently to keep her clean and to signal hemorrhage. This also prevented the lochia or her body from emanating "disagreeable flows" that would sicken the circumambient air. In summer and under mysterious atmospheric conditions, this air had been enough to cause epidemic puerperal typhoid.

After the milk arrived, the food ration was increased, but the puerpera was not to get up for 10 to 12, or even 20 days. She could sit in an armchair for at most two to three hours a day. If she impetuously abandoned the bed, she would remain exhausted of strength, with swollen limbs and a face of persistent pallid-yellow color, and become extremely prone to convulsions. After a month, she could return to her usual activities.

Women who had the leisure and domestic help would stay in bed for three or four weeks. The popular ideal was to remain in semidarkness for

as long as possible. However, most women had to get back to work immediately, and several older women have told me that they or their mothers
were up the day after childbirth to do whatever chores they could around
the farm, house, or family business. Some people speak of women's prac-
ticality and physical stamina with pride, but many disdain their getting up
so soon after childbirth as an animalistic practice that caused prolapsed
uterus.

In popular tradition, puerperal women were extremely vulnerable to
malevolent forces such as wind, cold, or sorcery. Just like menstruating
women, they were also dangerous to others and were not permitted to prepare the family's food or eat at the family table (which would make the
bread turn black and the wine acidic). As in menstruation, during childbirth their heads were covered to avoid losing any hair at the moment of
maximum impurity. The laundry from the birth was washed immediately
in running water, or the water was thrown in a sandy place where the
blood would promptly disappear, for this would protect the mother from
sorcery aimed at taking away her milk.

For the first 8 days, the puerperal woman did not change clothes or
brush her hair to avoid headache, and she did not swaddle the child herself. For 40 days, she would not bathe, wash her hair, go outside the house,
have sex, or cook food. She had to be very careful to avoid drafts, taking
cold, or exerting herself, for it was thought to be very difficult to recover if
one got sick during this time. Once "outside childbirth," the mother could
return to family life, society, and church (the latter through a purification
ritual discussed below).

During the quarantena, the mother was allowed to eat well, and relatives and friends would bring gifts of the more highly valued foods such as
capons or chickens. There were many ritual means of protecting the milk
supply, some of which were seconded in medical texts. Given the jealousies
and rivalries in multiple-family households (see chap. 3), women feared
that if they drank from the same glass as a sister-in-law, she would take
away their milk. The family avoided lending out anything, as it could be
used for sorcery.

Even in mainstream religion, there were rituals to protect breast-feeding women, especially on February 5, the Feast of Saint Agata. This saint
was the chaste woman whose breasts were severed after she refused the
advances of a Roman official in Sicily.[12] In Forlì, the powder (known as
the Virgin's milk) which came from drying the roses that had been placed
on the Virgin's altar in May was distributed throughout the city that day.
Artistic depictions of Sant'Agata's breasts on a tray in her hand had long
been interpreted as symbols of bread, and in one valley in Romagna nursing women ate "bread of Sant'Agata" that had been blessed by some
nearby monks. These monks also distributed small glass beads with white

and red veins that had been blessed in the Church, which nursing women wore on a string. Interestingly, Mercurii suggested wearing the rock *agata* (agate) at the collar to favor milk production when it was deficient or lacking (1601:251).

In caring for the newborn, the mother had to be extremely careful about maintaining humoral balance and avoiding exposure to atmospheric dangers. After birth the child was washed with butter, egg yolk, and olive oil, then covered and swaddled. The newborn had to be protected against any sensations from the air, and especially from being struck by cold. A warmed cap prevented premature growth of the head, while faithful swaddling of the legs made them grow straight; crooked legs were considered the fault of a sloppy mother. When one woman's physician recommended leg braces for her child in the 1930s, her mother criticized the way she had been swaddling him.

Infants were completely swaddled for at least six months, more if they had been born in summer and had to wait for the following warm season. Rousseau had campaigned against the practice in the eighteenth century, and Italian reformers continued to take his lead, but the practice endured until after the Second World War in Romagna. Similarly, there was a common practice of rushing infants into walking while not permitting them to crawl. This was supported by some physicians but criticized by others. The reluctance to allow infants to crawl has persisted to the present day.

Nineteenth-century medical experts and social reformers increasingly advocated putting the infant in a crib to sleep. They argued that this protected the child from suffocation and harmful fumes from the mother's secretions. The crib should be next to the mother's bed, though, as it blocked air currents and bright light, and the child should be put often in the mother's bed to benefit from her heat, especially in the early days and weeks. The child should be turned from side to side so that light hits the eyes equally. However, rocking the baby to sleep was not humane, for it would have no hope of escaping damage to the brain. Physical and psychological stimulation were harmful; scaring the infant with noises and shouts could easily cause convulsions. Neither should the baby be left to cry for hours, as this could damage the trachea and cause hernia. Experts criticized other traditional popular practices besides sleeping with infants and rocking, such as giving infants opium tea (to calm them or induce sleep), pacifiers made of sugar or sugar soaked in wine and wrapped in a cloth, or wine at mealtime.

While experts and parents agreed that infants must be protected from the cold, nineteenth- and early-twentieth-century physicians and reformers began to scold parents for "excesses" which had been in complete harmony with medical recommendations until then. Now, infants should be washed every day or every other day; not covered too much, either by day or night; and allowed free movement and exposure to fresh air and sunlight. They should become habituated to the elements—even fog and wind. Instead of keeping their infants indoors for three or even six months, and rendering them so very gracile that the slightest atmospheric variation made them fall ill, mothers should go out for walks with their infants after the first month. With this kind of care, even infants born gracile could be rendered robust.

Qualities of Mother's Milk and Characteristics of Milk Production

Since the milk directly transferred material and moral substances to the child, it was more important to focus upon the qualities, constitution, and behavior of the mother or nurse than the technique of feeding—the opposite of today. The former had a much greater impact than feeding technique on the milk secretion and the health of the mother and child. This way of thinking also favored attention to the health problems deriving from milk caught in the breasts, which was a problem for upper-class women who hired wet nurses, or from imbalance and intemperance manifested in overproduction and underproduction of milk.

For a few days after childbirth, women were given a mostly liquid diet in order to prevent an imbalance between solids and fluids due to the loss of liquid. The febbre lattea that accompanied the arrival of the milk after two or three days brought symptoms of fever such as shivers, weakness, headache, thirst, and accelerated pulse. It diminished the secretion of the lochia and made the breasts hard and knotty. Some experts believed that colostrum was formed only after the fever ended, while others said that it was secreted immediately. The fluid became true milk within ten to fifteen days of childbirth.

The disequilibrium of the milk fever required special precautions. If the woman did not breast-feed, the diet had to be more severe and minimal to cause the excess to pass, while more liquids and diuretics favored the secretion of urine rather than milk. The breasts were kept warmer, rubbed often with tepid almond oil, and covered with a wet plaster containing laudanum (a tincture of opium) if the pain was excessive. If the woman did breast-feed, her breasts were supported and the cloths changed often to keep them dry. They were kept uniformly warm with cotton wool and preserved from all contact with the air, especially if cold and humid. A tranquil and well-regulated life hinged upon a proper diet allowing for no deviations. The diet was light and delicate but substantial, including small amounts of meat beginning on the fourth day. However, if the breasts were swollen it would have to be reduced.

A serious condition called phlegmatic inflammation of the breasts illustrates how important it was to behave correctly during breast-feeding. This disorder arose most often in the first few months of breast-feeding but especially when it was "difficult and poorly directed."[13] The inflammation rarely resolved itself, but instead led to ceased milk production, abscesses, and destruction of glands and tissue. It could be caused by the action of cold, pressure, or the declivity of the breast by its weight pushing downward and outward, but also moral factors, general disposition, or breast-feeding itself.

Unlike other bodily secretions, the milk did not continue indefinitely once established. It depended upon the stimulation of suction, being produced in proportion to the "excitation" it aroused in the breasts: a stimulus so powerful that it had been known to cause milk secretion in virgins, decrepit old ladies, and even men. The milk produced in the morning was considered superior in quality to that of the evening. That which remained in the breasts became more serous, while that which was extracted last in a feeding was richer in creamy material. While earlier medical experts had not put a limit on milk production, late-nineteenth-century writers said that the stimulus could maintain milk production for 18 to 20 months, but that milk diminished in quantity and quality around the twelfth month. There could be exceptions, such as women who nursed several infants in a row with the same milk, or the same infant for six or seven years. On the other hand, some women lost their abundant milk secretion after only two or three months.

Although reproductive history and age mattered—first-time mothers and women under 18 or over 40 years produced less milk—the most important factor was the strength and development of the constitution. "Lymphatic" women produced a lot of milk, but it was serous and less nutritious. An intemperance affecting the liver would be mirrored in the quality of the blood and milk. The worst was hot and dry, making the blood "choleric [hot], and almost angry"; the poisonous milk made the infant sicker the more it nursed.[14] The imbalance could be caused by anger, rage, much exercise, little sleep, abundant wine, salty foods, or onion, garlic, and many other herbs and vegetables. For this and other kinds of intemperance, the cure was an opposite way of life and the administration of medicines that purged the guilty humor. The traditional way of testing was to leave drops of milk on a white cloth to dry in the shade. The dried milk retained the color of the "sinning humor": yellow for choleric intemperance; black for melancholia; moldy spots, bad odor, and bitter or other than sweet taste for phlegmatic.

The quality of the milk could be compromised by excessive exercise, insufficient sleep, rabid anger, fright, displeasures or other vivid passions, and poor or insufficient nourishment. The milk would then become noxious to the child, causing loss of sleep, continuous agitation, colic, and diarrhea. The taste, color, and smell would be affected by medicines, excessive amounts of wine, and foods such as absinthe, onion, garlic, saffron, many herbs and greens, and salty dishes. If emotions were very strong, the milk secretion would be suspended for a day or two, while extraordinary physical efforts would cause the heating of the milk and lead to ringworm and skin ailments in the child. Effects such as these could be judged by the infant's behavior as well as the taste and color of the milk.

Overproduction and Underproduction of Milk

We have seen that retention or retropulsion of bodily fluids was thought to cause grave harm. Milk, as one of these, was to be secreted neither too much nor too little. The ancients had discussed how an abundance of milk deriving from humoral imbalance caused great infirmity in the child, oppressing it with convulsions. The excess milk could not be digested, and so it filled the head with vapors that followed the nerves down the spine. The disorder, rooted in excessive blood, was typical of sanguine women of hot and humid nature—generally young women who lived an idle life and enjoyed the best foods and wines. The remedy was to "slow down nature" and repress the "exuberance" of the blood and milk.[15] This was done with hot drinks and a severe diet; exercise; purgatives, diuretics, and sweat-inducing substances that favored other secretions; and massage and topical remedies applied to the breasts. The breasts were supported with cloths looped around the neck, while the arms were kept immobile since they drew the blood and milk toward the chest. They might even be bled if necessary.

Medical experts wrote that in some women breast-feeding brought better health and a favorable evolution of the constitution, while in others it caused health problems. Most women lost weight during breast-feeding, which could hasten the development of incipient diseases such as pulmonary tuberculosis. These women were moreover susceptible to phlegmatic abscesses of the breasts and a greater organic vulnerability, as if prolonging the puerperal state. Then there were women whose weakness, unfavorable hygienic conditions, overly abundant milk secretion, or excessive zeal in caring for their children, especially at night, determined "a grave cachexy, which could even produce death, if they did not stop breast-feeding."[16]

Overproduction was clearly a serious condition, but some physicians in the nineteenth century argued that it was not a disease after all. In any case, it was rare, and much less prevalent than underproduction. Some women lacked milk entirely because of an intemperance of choleric or dry humors due to pains and fevers of a bad birth, their own temperament or disorderly way of life, or some external cause. To correct this, a cold and humid life would be instituted, together with increased sleep (since staying awake dried the body), forsaken sex and exercise (they provoked menstruation and dried the milk), and purgatives and other medicines taken internally or applied to the breasts. Rarely, lack of milk was also caused by an intemperance of cold and humid humors. The coldness would lead to insufficient blood generation or thick blood obstructing the veins, and was treated through remedies to heat up the blood.

Milk insufficiency was caused by weakness in the attractive virtue of the breasts, narrowness of their veins, a bad pregnancy, or bad blood heated by fevers, exertions, or birthing pains. Excessive pain in childbirth consumed heat, leaving little to conduct the blood to the chest and transform it into milk. Eating sorghum bread all year, as some farm women did, was also a factor in poor milk production because it made the blood scarce or thick. Lymphatic women and those who were weak and noticeably losing weight were prone to milk insufficiency and would have to stop breast-feeding if the condition persisted. Other causes included fevers and ailments before or after childbirth, insufficient or poor nutrition, abuse of venereal pleasures, forced periods of wakefulness, vivid emotions such as anger, love, or jealousy, the desire to breast-feed more than one child at once, and very prolonged breast-feeding. If treated under the surveillance of the physician, the condition would go away with the cause, although some causes of milk insufficiency were not curable. These included incomplete development or atrophy of the gland and a defect of vital energy.

To increase milk production, women were advised to avoid exertions and exercises that caused too much sweating, renounce frequent amorous encounters, and eliminate violent passions. Their diet should contain food of good substance such as chicken, capons, and veal. Foods that increased milk production included rice flour, sheep's milk, sweet peeled and sugared almonds, and broths and milk drinks made with melon seeds and sugar taken after dinner to induce sleep. Moderate amounts of white, subtle, and not sweet wine were permissible, but too much black wine was harmful to nursing women because it interfered with sleep. Even though they were hot and dried the body, salted meats and fish could help because they increased the appetite. Finally, the midwife could put a cupping glass under the breasts to pull the blood there, and massage them with hot white wine boiled with herbs, followed by oil of white lilies (associated with virginity) prepared with moss and laudanum.

Contraindications to Breast-Feeding

Over the nineteenth century, the list of contraindications to breast-feeding grew, as did the authority of physicians in matters of maternal and infant care. Until this time, the principal contraindication had been extreme humoral intemperance. Rather than emphasizing women's or children's potential inability to breast-feed, the discussion of contraindications had focused upon treating the retention and stagnation of the milk since they would lead to serious health problems in the mother.

This treatment continued to be relevant not only in the case of humoral intemperance, but also because noble and well-off women often chose not to breast-feed. If left in the breast to congeal and harden, the milk would drive the mother mad, in addition to causing aposteme, cancer, and death. To avoid this and the intemperance behind it, it was necessary to minimize sleep; increase exercise; eat hard bread and thick, roasted meat, but little liquid; and possibly bleed the woman from the feet and legs to keep the blood from going toward the breasts. The woman should live above the ground floor in airy bright rooms facing the sunset. The hardness of the breast was dissolved with hot remedies to melt the congealed milk. Vigorous medicinal massage followed by oiling and covering with a wax poultice disassociated the blood from the breast and sent it back to the uterus.

While constitutional factors persisted as reasons for not breast-feeding, other contraindications such as illness, ailments, and mechanical obstructions appeared more and more in the medical literature. These included maternal weakness, recent weight loss, and thinness; breasts that produced insufficient or inadequate milk; and milk that, after previous births, remained suspended in the conduits and glands and created puddles. Others included cracked and damaged nipples that caused pain and rendered the infant's suckling useless; a grave illness in the puerperium, such as an organic heart defect or any contagious disease; and bad maternal humors that could infect the infant's liquids and body through the milk. On the other hand, women who had syphilis were obliged to breast-feed their infants, in whom the disease may not manifest itself for three or four months. Treatment benefited both mother and infant, and wet nurses were protected.

As the contraindications multiplied, physicians spoke in stronger terms about their role in deciding whether a woman may or may not breast-feed. Balocchi's obstetrics text argued for dissuading women from breast-feeding if they had an infirm constitution, even in the absence of any appreciable disease, were under 16 or 17, or over 40, or were exhausted by a bad or complicated pregnancy. Women who had a hereditary predisposition to tuberculosis, scrofula, skin diseases, or mental illness were to be strongly discouraged. Those who actually had one of these diseases, or were subject to violence, hysteria, or epilepsy, were to be absolutely excluded from breast-feeding (1847:622).

When breast-feeding was inadvisable, a wet nurse would be hired, or, particularly among the common people, a friend or relative would be asked to help out. In the case of humoral intemperance, the nurse had to have the correct constitution to balance it. For example, an infant born to parents with rickets, cachexy, or tuberculosis would be given to a very robust balia with a sanguinous temperament, dark skin, black eyes, and masculine features. The idea that infants could be matched up with more ideal nurses led to their being switched around for many different conditions. For example, a new mother with small nipples pulled back further due to engorgement would nurse a three-month-old baby, whose greater force would empty the breast and reconduct the nipple to the proper dimensions. The mother of the three-month-old child would, in turn, nurse the newborn. As we will see, this kind of remedy involving wet nurses, relatives, and friends soon gave way to artificial feeding methods—a shift from human to mechanical solutions that was entirely consistent with wider changes in infant care practices.

Techniques of Infant Feeding

Breast-Feeding, Supplementation, and Weaning

Cultural rules postponing the newborn's access to colostrum or milk seem to be a universal of Western society, and Italy is no exception. This is because traditional European medical beliefs held that the overexertion of childbirth had a noxious effect on the secretions of both the uterus and breast (accounting for the particular color and consistency of colostrum). Sorano d'Efeso, writing in Roman times, said that breast-feeding should begin on the third day, with the child taking boiled apple until then—a practice older Italians today remember as common, together with the use of sugar syrup. Other purgatives recommended in the medical literature included tepid wine with cinnamon and sugar; radicchio; and a mixture of cow serum and purified apple. Ancient wisdom held that purgatives were necessary to prevent the meconium, which came from the humors mixed with pancreatic juice and bile, from remaining stuck in the gastrointestinal tract. Ancient wisdom also held that it was necessary to wait until the mother's lochia stopped, or four days in the case of wet nursing, before initiating breast-feeding.

In the nineteenth century, experts tended to advocate earlier attachment of the infant to the breast, beginning around 10 or 12 hours after birth, but still emphasized that the baby must not suckle until it eliminated the meconium. They argued that before then, the infant absolutely must not be fed by its mother, but to wait too long would be to lose the purgative advantages of colostrum, make the breast distend to the point of obstructing suckling, and not permit the infant's suckling to moderate the

febbre lattea. This was a tacit admission that medical advice had been contributing to the severity of milk fever and to problems in milk production,
particularly among the women in contact with physicians.

The writings of nineteenth-century medical experts make it clear that
women were breast-feeding on demand and without any restriction of the
time spent at the breast. Now, they were urged to resist ignorant traditions
like responding to crying by offering the breast. Giving milk too often burdened the stomach and gave rise to many disturbances, while excessive
amounts of milk that could not be digested were the cause of abdominal
colic, diarrhea, worms, inflammation of the intestines, and convulsions.
Consequently, physicians advised feedings for short periods separated by
discrete intervals in the first days or weeks, or they permitted frequent
feeding without regimen for a time. By six to eight weeks, the "dose"
would be increased, as would the interval between feedings—generally
three or four hours by day, and six by night.

Another popular habit seen as odious was to sleep with the child and
keep it attached to the breast all night. Both mothers and wet nurses were
criticized for this and told that their misguided love or laziness in trying to
placate the infant exposed it to suffocation—especially if the baby slept
between the parents. Breast-feeding on demand was said to make the
infant fat, with soft and flabby flesh, but this apparent beauty would disappear at the slightest disturbance. The child would also be prone to a
greenish diarrhea that rapidly altered its health.

Women were scolded not only for breast-feeding too often, but also
for doing so too long and introducing supplemental foods too late. Before
the nineteenth century, very little had been said about how often or how
long women should breast-feed, except that it should go on until the child
had a full set of teeth and could be nourished in another way. But weaning
was now to take place between 15 and 18 months, with outer limits of 12
to 20 months. As the century progressed, expert advice tended toward the
lower limit of 12 months.

Physicians who advocated exclusive breast-feeding for many months
were criticized for privileging mother's milk too much. It was argued that
infants would prosper better if given softened supplemental foods as early
as the fourth or sixth month, and that mothers too would benefit from
being spared bites and other discomforts. If the child were permitted to
breast-feed exclusively for 10 or 12 months, it would remain obstinately
attached to the breast and refuse other foods. Yet, it should continue to
take some breastmilk to ensure the eruption of the teeth and prevent illnesses associated with earlier weaning.

The experts' recommendations for weaning foods mirrored those
recorded by local historians and remembered by older people. They
remain the base for today's practices as well, though they have been

modified by modern food processing and packaging. These foods included premasticated meats, fruits, or breads. The first paps were made with toasted breadcrumbs or rice, barley, oat, or other flour cooked with milk, salt, and sometimes olive oil to make something similar to béchamel sauce. Sugar, butter, and parmesan cheese could also be added, and the base would soon be changed to meat or vegetable broth. The next foods were soft and well-cooked meat, mature fruit, and lightly cooked or warm freshly laid egg, though some people say that eggs and egg pasta were avoided until school age. Pasta, legumes, leafy vegetables, and prosciutto were popular foods for older infants, as were coffee or barley-coffee mixed with milk, wine mixed with water, and abundant garlic (to combat worms).

Though they enthusiastically welcomed the switch to other foods, experts warned that to precociously wean the child on pap was to provoke indigestion, colic, diarrhea, and other intestinal disorders. Foods should be introduced gradually, not only to prevent food poisoning or disease, but also to avoid disturbing the mother's spirit since anger or fear could alter her milk and render the child convulsive or epileptic. Complete weaning could be done when the child had four upper and four lower incisors; it should take place in spring or fall to avoid the high mortality of summer and winter. Even after the child had joined the family routine, it was prohibited all foods that were stimulating, very spicy, or difficult to digest.

Infant growth has always been a subject of great concern to parents and health professionals, but it was not measured instrumentally with much precision or frequency before the twentieth century. After the initial weighing at birth, infants were weighed every few months, if at all. When they were weighed at home, they were put in a sack and placed on an agricultural or household scale. One city woman showed me one of these scales, which had been used to weigh her father in the 1880s. She used it again in the 1940s to double-weigh her baby, as part of what she describes as the *avanguardia* in infant feeding. However, the scale did not work at low body weights, and she had to use the one at the clinic until her baby weighed ten kilograms. The home scales were soon abandoned and replaced by more exact ones for rent or purchase at pharmacies. With the old home scales went an approach to breast-feeding that was comparatively naturalistic, unregimented, and free from medical intervention or surveillance.

Wet Nursing

Until the nineteenth century, the main alternative to maternal breast-feeding was wet nursing. Since it too involved a human source of milk, the qualities and behaviors of the nurse assumed utmost importance com-

pared to the technique of feeding. Bad qualities in the balia's milk were
considered the cause of every childhood disease, for children "suck the
germ of every infirmity with the milk."[17] The child's health, constitution,
and life itself depended upon the good character and constitution of the
nurse. Given the extreme importance of choosing the right wet nurse,
experts warned that this responsibility must rest with the physician, not
the mother.

The balia's age, constitution, manners, cleanliness, breasts, and milk
must be optimal, for any defects were passed on to the child. For example,
bad breast-feeding by a "choleric, salacious, disorganized wet nurse"
caused ringworm, while milk from an angry nurse caused "atrocious col-
ics" and even immediate death.[18] Convulsions, hysterics, and epileptic
seizures were passed almost instantaneously to the child, for which reason
the nurse must not be too impressionable or nervous. Her husband must
not mistreat her, be a member of a suspect group, or be prone to vice, drink,
philandering, anger, or laziness. She should not be a first-time mother, as
this would make her more distracted, less prudent, and more interested in
socializing. Best of all was a mother who had recently lost her own child,
for there would be no competing claims on her milk or attentions.

The nurse should not be pregnant, too young or old (under 20 or over
35 or 40), or too fat or thin, but fleshy, robust, and rich in good humors,
with a large chest and lively but not red coloring. Her physical and moral
health would be evident in the condition of her skin, eyes, and mouth, and
the absence of any bad odors emanating from the mouth, nose, skin, or
lungs. She must be sexually continent, have dry genitals free of any discharge, and not be menstruating, but have regular menstrual periods in the
nonpregnant, nonnursing state. The nurse was expected to inform the parents in the case of resumed menstruation, any disturbance to the health,
and, above all, pregnancy, for which breast-feeding would immediately be
suspended and the balia changed.

The breasts should have bluish veins and be elastic, moderately sized,
well-formed, and free of scars indicating disease. Overly large breasts usually betrayed a true poverty of milk, for the heavy fat parts impeded the
separation of the milk and its free passage through the narrow conduits
leading to the nipples. The nipple must be rose-colored, firm, and the right
size: if too long, too wide, very limp, or flabby it could interfere with suction and be fatal. Pear-shaped breasts gave the most and best milk. The
milk production itself should be between six weeks and four months along
to suit the tender digestive organs of the newborn. "Younger" milk still
contained traces of colostrum, and the nurse was not yet able to give the
child sufficient attention. However, because most wet nurses had to wean
their own child before taking on another, the upper limit was extended to

eight months, beyond which the milk was too rich and made the infant's stomach swell.

Since rural women were considered healthy and robust, their life-style more in conformity with nature, it was common to send babies to country wet nurses. However, some nineteenth-century observers began to point out the dangers of this practice and advocate bringing the nurse into the home. They argued that the country nurse's robustness was outweighed by her tiredness, dangerous deep sleep, coarseness, poor nutritional status, and distraction. The infant was exposed to cold, heat, sudden changes in weather, horned animals, and noises from guns and animals, especially if the nurse left it on the threshing floor or in the doorway while she was far away working in the fields. Indeed, there is no shortage of stories of unscrupulous and irresponsible wet nurses in the literature and the memory of older people today.[19]

The rules for the wet nurse's behavior were essentially the same as those for breast-feeding mothers. The house should be dry, healthy, and ventilated, the nurse and her clothes clean. The balia must avoid exposing herself to colpi di aria and other atmospheric perturbations, strong anxieties of the spirit, theater productions and dance parties, or any morbose condition residing in herself. A daily walk in the open air was necessary for all nurses, but especially those that came to the city from the country. The nurse should know how to cook and nourish herself well but with sobriety, sleep moderately and avoid tiredness, and be fit to care for the infant lovingly and diligently. She should not overeat or indulge in wines, liquors, or aromas, as these excesses harmed the milk and caused the child colic, inflammations, and convulsions.

The diet was to be regular, habitual, and of easily digested food. Meat, especially rich red meat, was to be avoided, but the balie apparently had trouble complying with this prohibition. The nurse must not become hot in any way, for her heat made the milk noxious to the infant, especially during dentition—a delicate time during which the nurse had to drink more to dilute and sweeten her milk. Constipation and diarrhea altered the milk and were passed on to the child. Certain foods caused colic or diarrhea, in which case the nurse would have to completely stop eating them.

The nurse not only had to regulate her own behavior, but was watched over carefully if she lived in the infant's house. The rules and regulations for wet nursing were a subject of great concern to medical experts, who usually devoted many more pages to it than to maternal breast-feeding, even while lamenting the practice and admonishing mothers to breast-feed their own babies. Some physicians discussed rules for breast-feeding only in sections on wet nursing, in which they referred to mothers and wet nurses together as *nutrici.* This attention to wet nursing reflects its social significance, particularly among the elite, literate classes in closest contact with the authors.

Artificial Feeding

From its earliest days, the subject of artificial feeding has evoked both enthusiasm and regret or disdain. For many centuries, there had been glass and metal instruments for pumping milk in cases of overabundance or other special conditions, as well as bottles for serving human and animal milk. But these were used very rarely since wet nursing was much more common. Artificial feeding was necessary when a mother or nurse died or lost her milk and another could not be found. There was a strong belief that the same animal should always provide the milk, and in Santa Lucia a farmer kept a single cow for local infants into the 1970s. Animals such as donkeys, goats, and cows were the main sources of nonhuman milk. The donkey was believed to have the constitution most similar to ours, but older people recall that the goat was used most often if the child was fed directly by the animal. Sometimes, a cow would be used for an older infant. An early-twentieth-century text illustrated the story of a sow that heard a baby's cries and came to succor it (fig. 1).

In the early decades of this century, parents and health experts preferred artificial feeding through a sponge, from an adult's mouth, or directly from an animal, for bottle feeding was associated with the spread of disease. The new implements were too expensive for the poor and not needed by the rich, for it was better to feed the infant directly from mouth to mouth. To help administer the milk in small quantities, the loving man or woman could use a piece of sponge or a bundle of hemp parts to form a nipple between the two mouths.

An animal's health and disposition were investigated in much the same way as those of a potential wet nurse. The goat was considered ideal because it required little care, ate indifferently of coarse and fine plants and consequently could live anywhere, and was not strongly affected by atmospheric conditions. Just the same, it had to be treated well, for if people abused and threatened it, the milk acquired pernicious qualities. The goat should be young and free of disease, have recently given birth (but not be a first-time mother), and preferably be experienced in feeding another child. White goats were preferred because they produced an almost odorless milk. The goat must drink adequately and enjoy cleanliness and walks outdoors. As in women, the breast must be completely emptied so that excess humor did not collect or retreat. Initially, the animal would be pastured on fresh vegetable foods, passing thereafter to bran, oats, and clover. Later, for milk more abundant in solids it would eat dried hay.

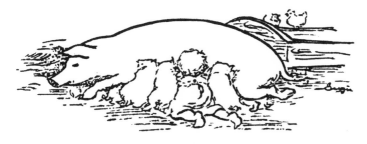

FIG. 1.   Illustration by the Countess Augusta Rasponi. (1914:40)

As time went on, bottle-feeding became more acceptable, indeed advisable. Experts expressed the opinion that direct animal feeding was barbaric or animalistic. However, they recognized that although bottle-feeding was successful in the countryside it was dangerous in the city, where general hygienic conditions were poor and the dairies were especially filthy. Experts warned that in certain cases such as extreme weakness or a delicate constitution, bottle-feeding would be fatal.

The rules for artificial feeding foreshadowed the technicism and regimentation that would later be applied to breast-feeding in the interwar period. Beyond the techniques of milk extraction and sterilization, there were complex rules for the dilution of the milk, the removal of fat, and the addition of sugar, salt, or other substances (though some experts recommended giving the milk in its intact form). Feedings were to be spaced according to a schedule and "dosed" with a bottle or an "English" spoon, which was more precise than an Italian spoon. Infants were weighed frequently to be sure they grew in a controlled way. Pamphlets and medical texts on artificial feeding were illustrated with not only bottles and other implements, but also babies being weighed on home scales.

While some experts wanted to reserve artificial feeding for infants with syphilis or a defect of the palate or lips, others thought it could be used more widely. The Romagnan countess Augusta Rasponi considered bottle-feeding of goat's milk superior to wet nursing and even maternal breast-feeding. She argued that many children thrived on animal milk after being fed by a series of wet nurses, and their mortality and morbidity rates were better. So long as the public learned about hygiene, sterilization, and the mechanisms of contagion, bottle-feeding would be safe.[20]

No doubt, artificial feeding was attractive to reformers and medical experts because it promised greater control over the way infants were fed. Rasponi justified it on the basis of the variability of mother's milk and its susceptibility to alteration: mother's milk could be too scarce or too rich, cause colic and degradation of infant health, and make the infant excessively and fatally fat.[21] Since any mother might suddenly lose her milk due to emotions or fright, it was only prudent to get her to begin using the bottle early on, for after three or four months it would be too late to habituate the infant. Arguing that mortality was higher for infants breast-fed by their own mothers or by balie than mixed or bottle-fed, she suggests that "perhaps the absence of nerves in the bottle makes it superior to woman?" (1914:43).

This query contrasts cultural control against natural vulnerability and hints of an emerging tendency to disparage women's bodies and traditional ways in favor of instrumental approaches and modern scientific rationality. Mothers were held directly responsible for disease and death through the harmful effects of immoderation and also seen as helpless victims of circumstance including the constitutions, hygienic conditions, and atmospheric influences. This paradox filtered into the fascist approach to infant feeding and has contributed to the power of symbolism surrounding breast-feeding to the present day. The great importance of mother's milk and the potentially lethal consequences of breast-feeding improperly were highlighted in order to ensure that women complied with medical management.

Medical Care

The Relationship between Medical and Popular Belief and Practice

Before the second half of the nineteenth century, medical knowledge, especially that related to maternity and infancy, derived primarily from empirical observation and converged with popular belief and practice. For example, expert advice to avoid weaning in summertime reflected the public's observation of higher risk of gastrointestinal disease in the hot months. The popular practice of prolonged baby-led breast-feeding for the dual purpose of protecting infant health and preventing subsequent pregnancy found confirmation in medical theory about the discordance between lactation and menstruation. The belief that skin ailments in infancy were caused by defects in the mother's or wet nurse's milk was rooted in old ideas about the noxious effects of humoral, atmospheric, and behavioral imbalances on the milk secretion. Other examples of medical and popular agreement include the *voglie* (cravings) in pregnancy, the choice and order of supplemental and weaning foods, and the protection of pregnancy and the milk supply through avoidance of imprudence and immoderation as well as malevolent environmental and social forces.

On the other hand, there were areas in which most women did not comply with medical or traditional ideals, such as complete inactivity for weeks after childbirth. Likewise, they were unable to heed the rules for rest during pregnancy. Women worked at the hardest agricultural tasks until the moment of childbirth, often miscarrying or giving birth in the fields. One seventy-five-year-old woman recalls that her mother was plowing with the cows and oxen when she had a miscarriage. She and the others immediately buried the "creature" under the clods of earth they had just churned up. This woman explains that compared to today, "*non c'era questo riguardo per la donna allora*" (there wasn't this consideration for women back then). Around the same time, another woman's grandmother gave birth in church on All Soul's Day. She notes that today a woman would not go out so close to her due date.

A midwife we will call Giuliana remembers being called to a large farmhouse in the mountains in the early 1920s. She was greeted by a pregnant woman, who was setting an enormous table for the day laborers. When she asked her to come aside for an examination, the woman responded that she did not have time yet, for she had to feed all of the workers and take drinks out to those in the fields. By the time she finished and went inside, the birth was already nearly complete.

For most women, childbirth was the only time they saw a health professional, for prenatal care really did not exist before the present century. This was recognized as a major impediment to the spread of new medical ideas in the late nineteenth and early twentieth centuries. In fact, rural women usually went through childbirth alone or with the assistance of female in-laws and a local lay midwife. The latter was known as a *donnina* (little woman), but was admired for her experience even if she had "nothing" in the way of education. If there were time, money, and inclination, the trained midwife might be called, and with luck she might arrive in time. Husbands were present during childbirth, and some would help by holding their wives in their laps. It was believed that their presence hastened labor and delivery, but a few older women have told me they thought husbands brought bad fortune. In that case, the woman would wear her husband's clothes, belt, or hat for protection.

A popular preference for upright birth position was rooted in an ancient tradition, which had held that even for caesarean section the woman should be strapped to a board held upright.[22] One woman recalls a poor neighbor who had no bed or other appropriate furniture and was completely alone for childbirth. She put a pot of water over the fire for use afterward and squatted before it to let the heat draw the baby out. When a great-grandmother gave birth to her eight children over the 1920s and 1930s, she did so over the bedpan. In general, women who gave birth alone or with relatives or a lay midwife used the bedpan or a low "birthing chair." Those who called a trained midwife used the bed. The supine position grew in favor as the influence of professional midwives and physicians increased around and after the turn of the century.

By around 1930, there were some hospital births in Santa Lucia, though urban women had begun to use hospitals and clinics decades earlier. There, the upright position was banished, as were untrained attendants including husbands, and in the process the experience of maternity was transformed. One of the first mothers in Santa Lucia to give birth in the hospital was also one of the first to use formula. This is an early example of the connection between the hospitalization of childbirth and the medicalization of infant care and feeding.

Beginning in the late nineteenth century, medical writings had begun to diverge from popular knowledge and practice, as professional medicine sought to distance itself from its unspecialized, empirical base. New concepts arose that had little basis in common practice. For example, while the supplemental and weaning foods recommended by physicians matched those in current use, the timing of supplementation and weaning was different. Experts wanted to shorten the period of breast-feeding and would soon disregard the knowledge that it was best to avoid weaning in summertime. Though most families slept together in the same room, physicians recommended isolated sleep for infants and children. Women should not offer the breast on demand around the clock, but at discrete intervals. Those using animal milk should choose only certain animals and serve the milk according to a specified method.

The stage was set for the rise in medical intervention in infant feeding in the fascist period.

The Organization of Nineteenth-Century Medicine

A major transition in medical care began in the nineteenth century with the emergence of the germ theory of disease and the growing emphasis on clinical medicine. The old orientation toward social and environmental contexts for illness began to shift toward individual patients and their disease histories, while long-term care of sick patients shifted to short-term treatment of signs and symptoms. Medical practice was increasingly focused in urban clinics, hospitals, universities, and laboratories.

In the nineteenth century, there were very few medical specializations, and the term did not have the narrow meaning it came to have in the early twentieth century. Even the specialized physicians were generalists compared to their successors and ranged freely beyond their chosen fields. In the mid–nineteenth century, there were four main specializations: physician, surgeon, oculist, and phlebotomist (who bled patients).[23]

The new medicine sought to increase the level of specialization, deny or eliminate traditional interpretations of disease, and convince people to stop seeing charlatans and traditional healers of both sexes—a complaint repeated often in turn-of-the-century literature. The meaning of the hospital would also have to change. For a long time, hospitals like the one in Santa Lucia had been considered hospices where people went to die or to be isolated because of contagious disease. Public authorities and professional medicine were now taking over these hospitals from the religious or local guild or trade associations that had created them. People were encouraged to see the hospital as a place where they could hope to recover from disease.

Yet, the dreams of medical reformers were not realized for many decades, especially in the rural areas. The main (and in many places only) providers of medical care remained the local *medici condotti* (district physicians) and *levatrici* or *ostetriche* (midwives). They were assigned by the municipalities to a particular geographical area, and their poor compensation (often in the form of eggs or whatever else the patient could afford) was usually offset by their high social position and, if they were amiable and capable, the goodwill of the community. "Liberal professionals" (*liberi professionisti*) such as surgeons were not bound by geography; they provided private, often more specialized and expensive medical care.

The district health workers served many people dispersed over a large territory. In Santa Lucia, until the Second World War there were two ostetriche and one medico condotto plus one or two liberi professionisti serving the town and country population of 5,000 to 6,000 people. A physician- or midwife-to-population ratio of 1:2,500 was not uncommon in rural areas in the region.[24] The scarcity of assistance was made worse by the lack of roads and bridges, making it difficult if not impossible to reach many patients. Moreover, during the latter half of the nineteenth century many communities were reducing the number of medical positions, reflecting a lack of public and administrative support for the medici condotti.

At the turn of the century, one-fifth of the communities in Romagna completely lacked a midwife, or the midwife was not authorized by the public authorities. There were four times as many district physicians as liberal professionals in the region, and as many phlebotomists as the latter. There were more veterinarians than either liberal professionals or phlebotomists. Pharmacies were ill-equipped and insufficient in number. Hospitals were located mainly in city or town centers, in unhygienic ancient buildings. Although cemeteries had been moved out of the churches to the outskirts of towns, population growth had filled in the areas in between so that they were no longer at a safe distance. The author of a study on the geography and history of the region concluded that the success of vaccination and the draining of marshes to eliminate malaria were counterbalanced by the inadequacies of the medical system, particularly in the countryside (Rosetti 1894:362–63).

Medical Specialization and the Attack against Midwives

In the first decades of the twentieth century, the main discipline dealing with the care of mothers and infants from conception to weaning remained the general science of *puericultura* (also spelled *puericoltura*). Obstetrics had been considered a medical-surgical discipline since the 1820s, but had remained in the hands of women and was therefore less attractive than specializations such as internal medicine or cardiology. At the scholarly level, the emphasis was similar to that of ancient times, when medical experts had included some practical notions in their writings, but were more interested in eugenics than technical considerations.

Pediatrics and the new science of *nipiologia* (care of the nursling) were not glamorous specializations, either, and were slow to attract physicians and patients. Contemporaries noted that scientific progress was not benefiting everyone, leaving out in particular mothers and children. There were still grave problems of infection in the urban obstetrics clinics and hospitals, and a lack of proper conditions and adequately supplied personnel in the countryside.

Beginning in the eighteenth century, women had begun to give birth with the assistance of folk midwives (*comari*), rather than alone or attended by neighbors or relatives. Then, over the nineteenth century midwifery became a schooled profession. Some people considered midwives (now called *levatrici*) on a level with priests and landowners as the leading members of society. Others, especially physicians, wrote that they were the worst of ill-mannered, uneducated malefactors.

Physicians claimed that everyone knew that the public held midwives in low esteem but continued to call them out of habit or prejudice. The "*comari ignoranti*" (ignorant midwives) and the backward women they served were the direct cause of infant death. The midwives' mistakes were the cause of avoidable operations physicians were called upon to perform. Balocchi wrote that "the destruction of the sweetest hopes, of the happiness of a mother and a family, the indispositions, the painful and often disgusting infirmities, death, pains even more terrible than death itself, are the ordinary consequences of the ignorance, inability, and negligence of the midwives" (1847:xxii). He added that they were mostly immoral, bad women disposed to helping women induce abortion or sending their legitimate infants to an institution.

While some experts looked forward to the day midwives would no longer exist—when women would realize that they were destined for something other than being health professionals—others sought not to eliminate but to improve the profession. They suggested giving midwives a true education in obstetrics, but one that matched their more "limited minds," meaning a lesser one than physicians received. This would attract women of the upper classes, whose youth, health, education, and morality would elevate the profession. Yet, midwives would be confined to the simple surveillance of the natural progression of childbirth, leaving everything else to the true *perito dell'arte* (expert in the art), the physician.

Although in theory midwives were excluded from performing caesarean section or using forceps, as well as other more violent instrumental means of extracting the fetus, in practice they often had to do tasks reserved for physicians. One midwife remembers performing many kinds of surgery she was not authorized to do, because the district physician had been trained as a lung specialist and was squeamish about and uninterested in obstetrics. Moreover, midwives continued to learn the different kinds of *rivolgimento* (manual turning or "version" of the fetus), which was considered a difficult procedure and the fundamental base of obstetrics.

Midwives have remained the principal caregivers during pregnancy and childbirth to the present day. Rather than being eliminated or marginalized, they, together with the socialist district physicians, were absorbed into the state medical system in the interwar period. This is reflected in the new title of *ostetrica,* which midwives began to use in the 1930s to reflect their higher degree of training. In this way, they became agents of the national medical culture and propagated its ideas and practices, including infant feeding methods.

We will return to these topics after examining how infants were actually breast-fed in the nineteenth century, and why there was so much variation and so little medical intervention in infant feeding practices compared to today.

CHAPTER 3

More Arms, More Land
Turn-of-the Century Feeding Practices, Culture, and Demographics

The infant feeding practices of a century ago had two main characteristics that set them apart from today's: they were affected rather little by expert intervention, and they varied widely with socioeconomic status, family size and structure, urban or rural environment, and regional and local culture. To understand these differences, we will examine some of the vast transformations that have taken place over the past several generations. These include an expansion of governmental authority and activity, a transition from subsistence or local agricultural production to an urban industrial or postindustrial economy and a rapid rise in material well-being (especially since the Second World War). In some regions such as Emilia-Romagna, the ancient sharecropping system persisted into the twentieth century alongside new economic developments. Overall, Italy remained a predominantly agricultural country until the 1930s, and a rural one through the 1950s.

Economic changes brought a distinction between unpaid domestic labor and paid wage work, creating a more pronounced gender division of labor. Close and constant physical proximity but emotional detachment gave way to greater physical separation but more emotional closeness between spouses and between parents and children. This was the result of work and schooling away from home, together with the simplification and shrinking of households.

In the late nineteenth century, a sense of little control over vital events and a relatively weak cultural ideal of maternal devotion were reflected in the abandonment and suppression of newborns, child labor, and harsh relations between children and adults. There did not seem to be any escape from the cruelty of nature or the will of God. Three trends arose in opposition to this culture of resignation and fatalism: neomalthusianist and feminist ideas that procreation can and should be approached conscientiously; bourgeois social and medical beliefs about the importance of informed and attentive maternal behavior in pregnancy and child rearing; and expansion of the role of medicine together with rising faith in its effectiveness.

Although relatively limited, post-Unification governmental intervention in Italy included data-gathering, support of industry, and nation building through infrastructural development. Increasingly, the state encroached upon the Church's activities, such as education, medical and hospital treatment, care of mothers and infants, and general moral authority. In part because of the urban focus of professional medicine, and in part because of the awareness that industrialization was being fueled by cheap female labor, there was legislation to protect women (and children) in the workplace. Meanwhile, the institutions for infants began to change from foundling homes to day-care centers for the children of working parents or overburdened mothers.

Beginning in the last decades of the nineteenth century, mortality rates fell dramatically. Fertility and infant mortality rates followed a generation later. This time lag caused a rapid expansion of the population, which continued for many decades more. Because fertility rates were falling, leaders in the interwar period would fear the biological decline of the nation. One major goal of their "demographic battle" would be to rationalize breast-feeding, for infant sickness and death were blamed upon mothers' ignorant resistance to modern medicine.

By now, differences in infant mortality rates noted at the turn of the century as having to do with factors such as season or social class have evened out. Infant health and survival are considered to be relatively unaffected by feeding method. The connection has faded as differences in infant feeding practices have diminished, while the surveillance of medical experts has become close and uniform.

Infant Feeding Practices

Maternal Breast-Feeding

One of the clearest differences in infant feeding practices was rooted in geography. In the urban areas, where households tended to be small and simple (a couple and its children), the voice of physicians and fathers in infant feeding decisions tended to be rather strong—especially regarding the choice of mercenary feeding and the selection of a wet nurse. However, this was accompanied by reduced paternal involvement in actual infant and child care.[1]

Urban couples were more likely to use alternatives to maternal breast-feeding, separate sleeping arrangements for their children (with reduced nighttime feeding), and new birth control methods that reflected both a different kind of conjugal intimacy and a desire to limit family size. When they did choose breast-feeding, they followed a schedule for meals and the early introduction of supplemental foods. They also tended to disbelieve the postpartum sex taboo, which had long existed alongside the notion that infant feeding meant breast-feeding only. Both of these beliefs eroded over the nineteenth century, first in the urban and nonfarm population, then in agricultural households as well.

Rural households were often made up of multiple or extended families less likely to be influenced by medical opinion (which was directed at urban, literate parents anyway). Breast-feeding was considered extremely important and lasted much longer. Mothers slept with their babies, feeding them whenever they cried. If a substitute nurse was needed, the child and its family developed a lifelong relationship with her and her family. The intervention of fathers and outside experts in infant feeding decisions was minimal. Yet, fathers had a much greater presence in the life of infants and children due to the organization of work and family life, and the lesser participation of children in formal schooling.

Through the first decades of the twentieth century, maternal breast-feeding lasted for two or more years. Contemporaries noted that this had been the case since antiquity, according to poems and literature.[2] Today's parents of young children say that their mothers and grandmothers breast-fed for years. One woman's father, who was born in 1918, suckled at his mother's breast until he was six years old, sharing the milk with his younger siblings. Several people in their forties and older remember hearing their siblings say, "*mamma mettiti a sedere che voglio del latte!*" (mamma sit down because I want some milk!), an expression also recorded by local historians.[3]

A great-grandmother explains that "*qui in campagna c'era la miseria ma il latte non mancava*" (here in the countryside there was poverty but milk was not lacking). A man in his nineties is perplexed by the apparent lack of mother's milk today, for in his youth this problem hardly existed. Instead, women breast-fed with almost no supplementation for 17 or 18 months. One woman's 94-year-old mother was an exception: she had milk for "only" six months, a period now considered a long time to breast-feed. There were many popular remedies for stopping milk production at weaning time, suggesting that running out of milk was not a primary reason for weaning, as it is today.

Breast-feeding was conducted without any method, except to follow the traditional wisdom that infants should be fed *poco e spesso* (little and often), meaning every two hours or so. Farm women would take their children with them wherever they went, or an older sibling would bring them out to be fed whenever they cried. An observer noted in 1909 that it was a "much used system in the countryside" to breast-feed for two or three years to prevent pregnancy, saying, "Everyone knows that when a woman breast-feeds she is very unlikely to become pregnant."[4]

Then, after the turn of the century, the feeding schedules and earlier supplementation popular in the cities began to spread through the countryside. The midwife Giuliana was taught in the early 1920s that women had to wait at least three and preferably four hours between feedings in order to *rifare il latte* (remake the milk). Otherwise, it would just be water. It should not surprise us that many women became pregnant while breastfeeding: *"tante rimanevano incinta senza vederle"* (many became pregnant without seeing them [their menstrual periods]). As a 90-year-old city woman explains: they did not feed their babies "little and often." A country woman in her eighties recalls that *"quasi tutti gli anni c'era un figlio"* (there was a baby almost every year).

Early supplementation and weaning had become so diffuse by the early twentieth century that some experts cried out against the practices. They blamed gastrointestinal diseases on the "too abundant and disorganized paps," the "too precocious paps given in exuberance!"[5] A woman born in 1900 says that women who did not have milk early this century gave their infants to the balia for three months rather than a year or more, then used a spoon to feed them paps and milk from a cow or goat.

We can gain some idea of the variety and frequency of infant feeding methods from an analysis of infant mortality from early this century. The Countess Rasponi (1914:42–47) divided over 4,200 infants into nine categories. Five of them involved maternal breast-feeding: maternal breast-feeding only (2,269), mixed feeding (115), breast-feeding followed by in-house wet nursing (134), breast-feeding followed by external wet nursing (207), breast-feeding followed by bottle-feeding (178). The other four involved wet nursing and/or bottle-feeding: in-house wet nursing only (820), external wet nursing only (254), wet nursing followed by bottle-feeding (25), and bottle-feeding only (237).

These numbers alone show that more than two-thirds of the mothers breast-fed, at least for a time. We cannot learn much about social class differences because the Countess did not separate the two classes of infants for each method. It is revealing that more than twice as many of the children studied were "well-off" (2,922) as "not well-off" (1,317). Further, the "not well-off" infants were likely to be of the laboring classes in the towns and cities, rather than children of country women "far from observation." The latter would continue prolonged breast-feeding for another generation or two.

Rasponi does tell us that no infants in the poor class were mixed-fed or wet nursed in the home; that external wet nurses were used more often in the poor class; and that the wealthy were more likely to use the bottle. This means that more than one-third of the wealthy infants were mixed-fed or wet nursed in the home, sometimes after maternal breast-feeding. It suggests that less than one-half of the wealthy class breast-fed, but well over half of the poor class did.

These proportions agree with other data indicating that breast-feeding was still very common, and mixed and artificial feeding were relatively rare. The pediatrician Angiola Borrino (1937:56–60) reported studies showing that, out of 4,631 infants born in 1903 in Milan, 77 percent were breast-fed, 5 percent were artificially fed, and 17 percent were mixed-fed. In Rome, 75 to 80 percent of 3,344 children of women of the poor population were breast-fed by their mothers, 10 to 15 percent were mixed-fed, and 5 to 10 percent were artificially fed. Even in institutions in Turin, artificial feeding was practiced in 22 to 27 percent of cases, whereas exclusive or mixed maternal breast-feeding was practiced in 73 to 78 percent of cases in 1905 through 1910.[6] In her pediatric clinic in that city, 93 percent of the 1,110 infants born between 1913 and 1915 were breast-fed by their mothers. It was necessary to use artificial feeding immediately or after a few days in 7 percent of the cases, while mixed feeding was utilized in 10 percent of the cases because of demonstrated milk insufficiency.

In neighboring countries, the frequency of maternal breast-feeding was much lower, according to Borrino's sources. In Berlin, in 1885 only 55 of every 100 newborns were breast-fed; in 1892, only 44; and in 1900, not more than 32. In Monaco in 1900, only 36 of every 100 women breast-fed, and 62 never tried. In Germany, alarming infant mortality rates had led to the opening of institutes to reduce the damage of artificial feeding, but these only promoted the method. Then, the Great War had imposed a general return to breast-feeding. In Italy, where there were stronger family traditions, a lesser participation of women in industrial labor, and the opposition of university pediatrics departments, the same experiment was not made. Even in the industrial cities of Milan and Turin, artificial feeding had remained within the limits of 4 to 5 percent of legitimate births in 1904 and 1910 through 1918, respectively (though illegitimate infants were likely to be fed artificially in institutions).

Alternative Infant Feeding Methods

There were two main types of wet nursing. The institutional *baliatico* had been a response to the large-scale abandonment of infants in past centuries and involved wet nursing within or outside the *brefotrofio* (foundling home). The second kind of wet nursing was that practiced by the elite social classes in Roman times and revived by the aristocracy in the eighteenth and nineteenth centuries. From the very beginning, it was associated with high infant mortality rates and difficult relations between the balia and the family. As Marcus Aurelius complained, "it is more vexing to satisfy balie than to marry off daughters!" A woman who lost her infant at the hands of a balia cried, "there must be a separate hell for the balie!"[7]

Yet, there were *balie di latte* (wet nurses) and *balie asciutte* or *balie senza latte* (dry nurses) into the 1930s and 1940s, and as late as the early 1950s in Santa Lucia. Wet nurses had a definite, established role in the family and society, expressed in a particular uniform that varied from region to region, and in their place in literature and the popular memory.[8] Often, the *figli* and *mamme di latte* (milk children and mothers) as well as the *fratelli* and *sorelle di latte* (milk brothers and sisters) developed close, lifelong relationships, whether the nursing lasted years or just a few months.[9] One man born just after the turn of the century was taken in as a foundling by a farm family in which the mother had "lots of milk" after her own child turned one. Even though he was later reunited with his natural mother and half-siblings and lived in the same town as his natural father, he remained closer to his milk brother and has returned to the latter's home in his old age.

The aristocracy also led the way in ending the practice of wet nursing, beginning in the late nineteenth century. Reformers now complained that it was bourgeois families who hired wet nurses for frivolous motives, and working-class families who did so out of necessity. For centuries, physicians had blamed the practice on modern culture and the demoralization of urban women, noting that these egoistic women preferred to shop and socialize rather than endure a noisy house.[10]

However, there is evidence that the motives were different from these. Mothers who worked in industry would lose their jobs if they tried to breast-feed. New laws required rooms and breaks for breast-feeding, and even nurseries in large firms, but compliance was rare in the extreme. Women were criticized for turning to mercenary breast-feeding or the help of a relative, when they could have been using the (admittedly imaginary) nursing rooms.[11] The city wet nurses, wives of day laborers or industrial workers, did not know how to raise children and lived in unsanitary houses lacking air and sunlight.[12]

It seems that bourgeois women chose wet nursing or artificial feeding because of the advice of their physicians, not because they were vain and self-indulgent. Rasponi (1914:42) reported that 25 percent of wealthy mothers breast-fed happily, but 35 percent could not continue after a short while or were only able to feed some of their children. Forty percent did not even try, but few for good reason. The majority of women reluctantly declined breast-feeding, "*per espressa volontà del medico*" (by the express will of the physician). The main reason was gracility or a gracile constitution. This vague condition that could simply mean thinness or apparent weakness was considered an unbeatable defect in the mother, requiring the physician to dissuade her from breast-feeding and suggest the choice of a wet nurse.[13]

That women were frequently discouraged from breast-feeding was evident in the admonitions of reformers such as Rousseau and Belaxarde that wet nursing was much worse than breast-feeding by a gracile mother. Pretexts such as gracility may have excused women in society's view, but they never excused them in nature's view, and the woman would suffer from the deviation of the milk.[14] Even today, older people say that lack of milk is caused by gracility, other constitutional factors, or misfortunes such as being an orphan.

However, physicians put "gracile" women in an impossible position by scaring them and their husbands away from bottle-feeding. Rasponi described a gracile woman whose gracile infant died. The second child, another "victory of the physician," died at 10 months, suffocated by the balia in her sleep. When the third child was born, the mother recoiled at the word *balia* and refused to give up her child. It survived. "If only we at least always let the mother try, except in exceptional cases!" (1914:15). Rasponi asked why it was that the infants of the wealthy almost never could "drink *their* milk in holy peace?" Because, "depending on the epoch the physicians permitted it more or less. '*Latte di donne più robuste!*' [Milk of more robust women!]" (1914:12).

While there was enthusiasm for artificial feeding among some reformers and physicians, most experts reported poor growth and high death rates. Infant mortality rates around 1920 were still much higher with artificial feeding than a good balia; while maternal breast-feeding brought the lowest mortality rates.[15] Even in the 1930s, when formula was becoming more available and was considered superior to animal milk, medical texts contained photographs and illustrations showing that formula-fed infants were half the size of those breast-fed by their mothers.[16] This is the opposite of what happens today, when infant formulas are better tolerated and cause an acceleration of growth.

A Different World

Political Unification and Economic Transformation

In only a hundred years or so, life and living conditions have changed almost beyond recognition in Italy. Where I live in Santa Lucia, there is a 50-meter drop out the back window to a very steep road leading down to the river. One of my neighbors told me a story of his great-uncle, whose job it was to bring 100-kilogram stones from the river up that road, to make buildings like ours. The men would tie the stones on their shoulders with their coat sleeves and march up the hill in line. One day, the man behind him didn't answer when he spoke. He could not turn to look, but when he headed back for another load he found that his friend had lost his footing and been crushed to death under the weight of the stone.

This was a physical burden, but there were others just as real, if of less substance. Sharecroppers (*mezzadri*) enjoyed certain protections (housing, dowries, medical care, credit, and risk protection—together with protection against economic gain!), but remained under the thumb of the landowners (*padroni*). They could keep kitchen gardens and a few animals, but in return had to give a large number of eggs and their best produce to the landowners at certain times of the year. They also owed the padroni free labor in the house and gardens, as well as laundry and kitchen services.

Sharecroppers could not vary the number of family members during the contract period (one year in Emilia-Romagna), and no one could marry (or in some cases even court) without the padrone's permission (this lasted until around 1920, with landowners continuing to have a say for another generation). At the same time, farmers owed gifts of eggs and other foods, as well as the *decima* (10 percent of income), to the local priest. Until Unification, sharecroppers had been required by law to baptize their children and could be dismissed by the padrone for refusing.

Things began to change in the second half of the nineteenth century, with economic, demographic, and epidemiologic transitions that had already been under way for generations in northern Europe and the United Kingdom. The changes away from herding and subsistence farming initially brought economic crisis and social disruption. With the rise of a relatively strong Italian nation-state came the appropriation of Church and common lands, the breaking up of the *latifondi* (large agricultural concerns employing day laborers) in the south, and the abolition of feudal rights and privileges in the sharecropping system typical of the central and northern regions.

The poor found themselves worse off than before. Privatization meant that even firewood became scarce in areas rich with forests. Families would spend up to 90 percent of their money on firewood and corn, which was often the only food they ate. Corn had been brought to the Old World without its New World processing technique and without the custom of eating it with complementary foods. As a result, the nutritional deficiency disease pellagra became endemic in corn-producing regions such as Emilia-Romagna, Veneto, and Lombardy, known as the pellagra triangle.[17] This disease is pertinent to our discussion for two reasons: it gives an idea of how poor living conditions used to be; and it underscores a persistent cultural concern with food and eating that is rooted not only in "high" cuisine but also in deprivation.

In the decades after Unification in 1861, high taxes on small landowners, combined with the milling tax on grain, worsened debt and led to many dispossessions. Much of this land, together with former Church and common land, was consolidated into large capitalistic agricultural enterprises, especially in the Po Valley. These farms were worked by a growing class of landless day laborers, called *braccianti* after the word for arms (*le braccia*), their only assets. A new term arose, *dipendente,* which today describes many jobs but at the time reflected a new total dependence upon the employer and cash to provide for all necessities.

Contemporaries in the pellagra triangle observed that day laborers often had nothing to eat for the entire day, while farmers ate nothing but corn porridge (*polenta*) or bread made of corn and a little wheat. They would prepare the bread once a week and take it to the public ovens for baking, but by the end of the week it would be moldy. The families of a young professional man's grandparents in Lombardy used to suspend an anchovy from the ceiling above the table and season their corn bread by rubbing it against the fish. In fact, corn was a common form of currency, and workers were paid in it. Many families could afford to eat meat only on Sundays or feast days, or when it could be caught. As more and more land was converted to cash crops, this left only frogs in some areas. By contrast, a century earlier there had been many times more farm animals than people in the region.

The changes of the late nineteenth century eliminated the protective characteristics of the sharecropping system but maintained the most repressive ones. Sharecroppers and smallholders were forced to devote more land and resources to cash crops and sell everything but the least valued product, corn. They suffered from pellagra, as had laborers in the plains beginning a generation or two earlier.

There were many different kinds of households and large variations in the number of children among social or occupational classes. For sharecroppers, it was best to have a large family, and many households were multiple-family groups of parents, sons, and their respective wives and numerous children. There was a saying: *più braccia, più terra* (more arms, more land). Younger brothers could stay on the farm only if it would support more laborers. Women, whether in farming or elite families, could not marry if it meant leaving their fathers or brothers alone, a tradition that has remained in many families.

Day-laborer, merchant, and artisan families were often simple or extended (usually by a widowed parent of one of the spouses), with few children. Landowners included simple, multiple, and extended families, usually with a small or moderate number of children. They had the economic resources to raise more children than artisans or day laborers, especially if they desired a male heir, but they often restricted their number in order to be able to afford to send them to school and university.

The categories were not fixed, however. Some families owned land and also worked as sharecroppers. Others sent a few family members out as agricultural or industrial day laborers, or hired day laborers during the busiest times. Piecework in the home with silk, weaving, and clothing also linked agricultural families to the world of industry. Similarly, there was no consistent relationship between family simplification and urbanization and industrialization. Industries often located their plants outside urban areas, and migration between city and countryside went in both directions. The change in family organization was more a matter of shifting proportions than a definitive break with the past.

The extremes in economic well-being were very far apart and continued to be so until the postwar period. While a tiny percentage of the population had the means to live off its own wealth, large numbers of workers and farmers had literally nothing to eat, and when they did eat it was a single food for months or years on end. Sharecroppers lived in notoriously bad housing, but it was much better than that of tenant farmers or day laborers, who slept 10 or 12 to a room in dark airless buildings literally on the edge (on or around the walls) of town. By contrast, some landowners owned more than 100 farms and lived in huge palaces in the towns and cities. One woman in Santa Lucia explained that her father's family had 70 farms. Her mother's had a house with more than 30 bedrooms and a restaurant provisioned by their farmlands. For six months of bombing during the Second World War, 80 people lived in their basement and risked going out only to get meat and salt. The poor people went out of their much more crowded hovels to gather chestnuts and lard.

Modernization and Miseria

Modernization in Italy meant a combination of changes. There was economic change through agricultural intensification, industrialization, and internationalization, together with political consolidation and administrative expansion. Cultural unification came about through increased literacy, education, and diffusion of cultural products through literature and radio. In the nineteenth century, modernization's mixed effects were already clear. Improvements in transportation, agricultural and industrial production, and labor organization had not been enough to eliminate *la miseria.*[18] *Miseria* is a word that means poverty, ignorance, ill health, and disempowerment all at once. It comes up often when people in Emilia-Romagna talk about the past.

Post-Unification governments followed a classical liberal political philosophy that permitted some intervention in the economy but limited social and health services to a minimum. The state administration remained weak, the economy fragile, and regional differences marked. The nation-builders sought to overcome these obstacles with improvements in health care, employment, and sanitation, which turned out to be very modest, and patriotic but financially doomed attempts at colonization in East Africa. A significant effort was made to know about and characterize quantitatively the new society. The state commissioned or performed unprecedented statistical studies on the land, population, and economy.

In the 1880s and 1890s, grain imports from the United States, Russia, and India led to deep agricultural crises. The government responded with tariffs and other protections, contributing to economic stagnation. Over the last three decades of the nineteenth century, the contribution of agriculture to national income declined, and that of industry remained stagnant. Growth came from the governmental and service sectors. This infrastructural development paved the way for rapid industrial growth in the years straddling the turn of the century, especially in the northern regions.

By the first quarter of the twentieth century, most regions in the northern half of Italy devoted a larger proportion of their working population to industry or services than farming, the opposite of the southern regions. In the 1930s, the nation as a whole crossed the 50 percent benchmark, but remained predominantly rural until after the Second World War. Today, one-third of the population lives in cities of over 80,000 inhabitants and only 6 percent in communities smaller than 2,000.[19]

In Santa Lucia, from Unification through the Second World War, the proportion of the adult population employed in agriculture remained about three-quarters among men and two-thirds among women. However, there were shifts in the relative number of sharecroppers as opposed to tenant farmers, day laborers, and smallholders. The proportion of landowners and servants dwindled, as did the number and types of artisans: an old shoemaker points out that there used to be more than fifty cobblers in Santa Lucia alone. New businesses such as bars and restaurants increased in number, reflecting a rise in cash and leisure time. After the war, the proportions in agriculture rapidly dropped to below one-fourth, but when all age groups are considered they remain more than one-third of men and somewhat less than one-third of women. Overall, there has been a shift to an expanded and more specialized range of professions in industry, services, and government at the same time as differences in living conditions have narrowed.

Industrialization did not immediately bring economic well-being: quite the opposite. It was fueled by cheap female labor in all areas including metalworking, printing, and construction, but especially textiles, rice processing, silk spinning, and cotton processing.[20] This was regrettable to some observers because it took women and children away from the home, and to others because it was unwholesome: female workers were badly paid, ate almost nothing, were exposed to dangerous substances and physical activities, and lived and worked in deplorable hygienic conditions. While in agriculture female day laborers earned two-thirds to three-quarters of the male wage, in industry the proportion was smaller and reached a low of about one-half in the interwar period. It is likely that women who worked in the informal economy earned even less.

There were signs of economic improvement and better health by the beginning of the twentieth century. In 1910, an institute for preschoolers in Forlì eliminated shoes from the supplies it distributed to children each year, due to improvement in the economic conditions of area workers.[21] Infant mortality rates began to decline. Average consumption of wheat flour, fresh fruit, olive oil, meat, and dairy products increased while that of corn flour, rice, and chestnuts decreased.[22] Pellagra was rapidly disappearing among laborers and industrial workers, though it would still afflict sharecroppers into the 1930s. The First World War relieved pressure on the labor market, provided conscripts an adequate diet, and gave their families cash.

Improvements in literacy contributed to the development of a national culture. Before Unification, each of Italy's twenty regions had been a separate country with its own language. More than 90 percent of the population did not speak Italian, and 75 percent could not read. Particularly since the 1880s, formal education and literacy have increased steadily. Literacy rose first and most rapidly in the school-age population, except for the children of sharecroppers, who continued to be involved in productive labor and did not receive much formal schooling. The most industrialized regions showed the earliest and most rapid improvements. Among them, the more agricultural ones such as Emilia-Romagna were slower to reduce illiteracy rates. By the 1930s, the illiteracy rate was only 5 percent in Lombardy and 15 percent in Emilia-Romagna, compared to around 50 percent in southern regions such as Calabria. These differences have since evened out a good deal, and the present national average is around 2 percent.[23]

These economic, social, and cultural changes imply a radical transformation in worldview. The rural sharecropping system had stressed obligation, resignation, permanence, and agricultural or climatic time-scales. The industrial system stressed mobility, autonomy, and industrial concepts of work and time. The two worldviews coexisted for many decades, thanks to the economic stagnation and cultural isolation of the rural areas. Their population enjoyed comparatively little access to cultural products such as radio and literature due to unfamiliarity with the national language, lack of leisure time, and geographical barriers to communications and transportation.

Family Relationships and the Treatment of Infants
and Children

The large, complex households of the old agricultural system in Emilia-Romagna were like worlds unto themselves compared to the simple, mobile families favored by industry and industrialized agriculture. In the former, husbands and wives contributed to a single economic enterprise and shared economic rights and responsibilities. All members of the household worked for a pooled annual income of food, firewood, housing, clothing, and cash. Farm and domestic work was hard physical labor for women and men. In the evenings, they continued their work by the fireside or in the barn if they could not afford a fire, making clothing or farm implements. The hearth was a central symbol of family unity, the focus of prayers and rituals for overcoming problems or maximizing success in breast-feeding.

Farm families slept in a single room or were separated at most by lofts. Spouses were constantly together physically, but they shared relatively little conjugal intimacy. Combined with the idea that one must submit to God's will, a taboo against talking about sex or bodily functions—even between spouses—led to what older women remember as a state of extreme ignorance about sex, reproduction, and the body (sustained at least in part by ideas about the impurity of reproductive events, which excluded men from contact with women and their knowledge). Likewise, there was relative emotional distance between parents and children, in spite of their close, continuous physical proximity. Landowning, commercial, artisan, and professional couples also worked together in the management of properties or a business, usually having less economic cooperation but more conjugal intimacy than among farmers.

Rural children were resigned, shameful, and shy outside the family circle and remained this way as long as they were kept from attending the schools the state was opening in the countryside. Children addressed their parents, and adults their in-laws, with the highest level of linguistic formality. They might have kissed their mother or father for the first time when the body was being laid out for burial.

As in other places in Mediterranean Europe, the multiple-family household fostered a hostile, competitive atmosphere between daughters-in-law and mother-in-law.[24] The mother-in-law, being the senior woman on the farm, governed the house and the daily schedules and behavior of the daughters-in-law. The latter did not eat at the family table, but sat on the stairs or in a corner with the children, eating leftovers. Young women were expected to contribute labor inside and outside the house as a natural extension of their role as wives, but, in a typical expression of the breadwinner syndrome, it was the men who got to eat first and most.

The mother-in-law and her husband would encourage or coerce their daughters-in-law to have many children, but reproach them if they had too many girls. The productive and reproductive capacities of girls were lost upon marriage, but boys brought these resources to the family enterprise. The mother truly demonstrated her worth during breast-feeding, for a good mother was one who had a lot of milk and breast-fed a long time. One without milk was a failure as a mother and wife, for her condition would either require money for a wet nurse or cause the child to develop poorly or die.

This kind of family was relatively closed to outside influence, as medical and other reformers noted with great disdain and frustration. Mothers-in-law enforced traditional behavioral prohibitions during pregnancy, childbirth, and breast-feeding, though this was the only time younger women were allowed or encouraged to eat well, for the sake of their babies. The *voglie* (cravings) and *quarantena* (40-day period after childbirth) compensated women to some degree for the increased restrictions on their behavior by giving them an opportunity to demand special attention and cherished foods. On the other hand, their food rations dropped just when their caloric needs rose, for at 40 days they resumed hard work and their usual diet, even if they were breast-feeding.

Senior women also controlled young mothers' access to health professionals. Women were sometimes left to suffer and give birth alone, both to demonstrate their worth and because the birth could cause jealousy and rivalry among the sisters-in-law, especially if it were a boy. These are the words of a woman who gave birth early this century, recorded by Ulivieri (1988:199):

> I had worked until I felt the pains, I was very afraid. Oh for goodness sake, I felt that it would have gone badly. I was laying on the hay, with the cows' sheet under me . . . I was suffering a lot . . . I implored: "go and get the midwife" . . . And my mother-in-law repeated to me: "I have always done this all by myself and I have had fifteen of them." Then they hung a rod from a cord: "Grasp at the rod," shouted my mother-in-law. With the force with which I clenched the rod I broke four teeth and my gold wedding ring. Eh, it was like that. They left me to cry out for three days and three nights. And then the baby was born dead, asphyxiated.

Young mothers were expected to maintain a harsh, hurried relationship of few words and little affection with their children and were chastised for wasting time in foolish pursuits if they did otherwise. Small infants were neglected for hours at a time if they had no older siblings to care for them. They would be left on a blanket or in a basket filled with hay. When their parents returned from the fields, they would be covered in excrement and surrounded by flies (see Camprini 1978:59). One woman remembers her neighbors leaving their infant in the furrow left by the plow, sometimes forgetting where they had left it and having to wait to hear its cry.

Children were put to work at an early age. As one woman said, *"appena camminato il bambino diventò uno schiavo"* (as soon as it could walk the child became a slave). They began with chores such as sweeping the manure out of the barn, barefooted, at four or five, then took on harder work at six or seven. At this age they could be sent out to work as servants on another farm or in the city, often far from home. They tended sheep or cared for small children and earned little more than the polenta they were given to eat: a pair of shoes a year, if anything at all. Calculations presented to the government in the 1870s gave an average value of 75 lire for infants and 1,600 for children up to ten. Twenty-year-old men, by contrast, were worth 5,000.[25]

This treatment indicates something other than the "natural" love and assiduous care that would come to be expected of parents, and especially mothers, with the bourgeois ideals of the late nineteenth and early twentieth centuries. It was only then that upper-class mothers stopped sending their newborns off to wet nurses for a year or more. Even when they did hire wet nurses, they brought them into their homes along with several other servants including nannies, seamstresses, cooks, and housekeepers. It was not until after the Second World War that all of the responsibilities of caring for children and household fell upon the mother.

In many cases, wet nurses and foster parents treated their charges well, but there were also cases of abuse. Dissatisfaction with wet nurses caused some parents to send their infants to six or seven different nurses in a row. Nurses who were very poor would try to trick parents by giving the child to someone else, feeding more than one child at once, or weaning precociously. One family of ten children in Santa Lucia was supported entirely by the income they received from taking in a foundling, the father of a woman now in her seventies. Working-class mothers were forced to send their children to day-care centers or even less well-off wet nurses. It was not uncommon for working-class couples to abandon their legitimate infants to the brefotrofio and reclaim them a few years later.

Through the 1920s, as many as one-fourth to one-third of all children in Italy were considered illegitimate (compared to 7 to 8 percent today). This must have been due in large part to the fact that from Unification until the Lateran Pacts of 1929, the state did not recognize Church marriages unless they had been followed by a separate civil ceremony.[26] In strongly religious areas, couples often did not undergo the civil ceremony: their children were considered illegitimate unless the father legally recognized them. In anticlerical areas such as Emilia-Romagna, many couples did away with ceremonies altogether and lived in common-law marriages. Even today, Emilia-Romagna's proportion of civil marriages is among the highest of all the regions.

In Santa Lucia, one-fifth of the children born during the half-century before 1920 were illegitimate. Two-thirds of these were born to common-law couples. Another 5 to 7 percent of all newborns were abandoned to the *ruota*. This was a "wheel" or revolving church door, from which the infant would be taken to hospitals or foundling homes in Florence or in cities in the Po Valley. There were seven of them in the eighteenth century, and one as recently as the Second World War. On a hillside in a nearby district, women left their newborns on a parish well known for its beauty and rang the church bells to call for the priest before running away. They did so into the 1930s and 1940s.

There were many methods of avoiding a birth in the first place, by inducing abortion chemically or mechanically. Beginning early this century, midwives and physicians used the safer method of curettage. Sometimes, a child would be killed shortly after birth. Because women concealed their pregnancies, authority figures including priests and even midwives often did not know about infanticide. One retired midwife was shocked to hear the stories her housekeeper told. A friend of this woman gave birth one Sunday and killed the newborn in time to go to mass (where she fainted). A relative killed three newborn infants while her husband was away in the Second World War. According to tradition, they, like aborted fetuses, were not fully human. She buried them in the space under the gutter, that margin between the house and the wild. Presumably for the same reason, stillborn infants were not given names until the late 1890s in Santa Lucia, but listed simply as "*nato-morto*" in the birth registers.

Infanticides were often interpreted as misfortune or chance, such as involuntary suffocation in sleep, drowning in the bathtub, or an accidental fall in the fire. Mothers who intended to abandon or kill their child would not clean it and often would not tie off the cord. They would not baptize the child, unless they were very afraid of divine retribution, and would not put it to the breast or give anything else to eat. This last condition was crucial, for if the mother had breast-fed the child she would have been considered crazy, her otherwise-excusable crime monstrous.[27] This fits with the nineteenth-century medical and popular understanding of maternity as both gestation *and* lactation.

Fertility

Fertility was higher among sharecroppers than artisans, the upper classes, and certain working-class elites not only because of economic differences but also because of differences in marriage relationship and worldview. The latter's higher literacy rates, exposure to ideas circulating around Europe and America, and contact with urban medical and social-welfare institutions increased receptivity to expert advice and intervention in contraception. They saw having too many children as the brute state of nature, or the lack of human agency in controlling fate, and they did not respect the taboo against talking about sex and reproduction. They were also likely to be anticlerical or at least less faithful to Church teachings than farmers, as fascist writers would later point out.[28]

This is not to say that farm couples did not use any method of family limitation, for abstinence and *coito interrotto* had been in use since time immemorial, and so had prolonged breast-feeding. Nonetheless, they were much less likely to use some of the newer methods. These included the counterproductive *amplesso intermestruale* (rhythm method), which meant abstinence for three days before and eight days after the menstrual period. There were also the more or less effective methods of condoms of rubber or animal gut for men and women; sponges, diaphragms, infusions of acid or powders blown on the vaginal walls; intrauterine devices; and balls made of vegetable and/or animal fat and spermicidal acids to block the cervix.[29]

There is a common assumption about fertility in our culture, scholarship, and even foreign policy. It is that fertility trends depend only upon women's willingness or ability to control births, but I did not find much evidence for this in Italy. The writer of a turn-of-the-century book on birth control described how women wanted to limit the number of children by any possible means, since a large family brought them material and moral misery. It was the men who impeded progress through their obstinance, ignorance, and contrariness to new things, particularly regarding sex.[30]

People now in their eighties and nineties agree that a large family meant greater miseria, and this association remains strong in the cultural memory. Many of them explicitly link their limited family size to the conscious decision to adopt a simple family structure and work a small farm. They describe a different kind of conjugal relationship thanks to being removed from the controlling atmosphere of the sharecropping system. One woman was born in 1914 to a family with eleven children, her husband a few years earlier to a family with seven, and they were both put into service before the age of ten. They had one child in order to spare others the miseria they had known. A woman born in 1898 who had two children explained to me that it was her husband who informed himself about birth control.

With the economic changes of the late nineteenth century, the multiple-family households dissolved or changed. The shift to wage work away from the farm and the rise in schooling among children brought a decrease in the time families spent together, while the older generations were economically marginalized. The complementary activities of wives and husbands became distinct and unequal as work and leisure time were separated and compensation was based on time rather than annual production. Women were left with the unpaid domestic labor in addition to their income-producing work, while men began to spend their evenings in the inns and coffee shops. For a time, field and factory workers stayed together in the dilapidated farmhouses because rural rents were cheaper, but soon this attraction disappeared and families split further.

These changes brought an erosion of the old ways of maintaining authority and distance within families, including a progressive decline in linguistic formality. The meaning of children changed when they no longer increased their parents' standing within the multifamily household or contributed labor and domestic help. Cultural ideals began to emphasize women's sexual attractiveness as opposed to their domestic authority and productive and procreative capacities, focusing more upon conjugal intimacy than the "fruit" of the relationship. Outside the tight network of family relations in the old system, parents in simple families were much more open to cultural influences and came to seek expert intervention in place of traditional knowledge. State and medical authorities would encourage them to disregard their mothers-in-law in regulating reproduction and child rearing, for complex families were impediments to the industrial-agricultural economy and resistant to state intervention and authority.

A Culture of Resignation and Fatalism

Changing Beliefs about Fertility and Infant Mortality

Beginning in the late nineteenth century, writers lamented the resignation and fatalism of traditional culture—attitudes which older people continue to express today. Even social and economic inequalities were considered immutable, for they reflected the will of God.[31] Rasponi (1914:17) describes a childhood memory of meeting a relative who presented her two children to her and explained with astonishing indifference that her other 12 had been sent to wet nurses in the mountains and died. She only complained that almost all of them died after she had paid the whole year's wet-nursing fee. So many infants were in such poor health that suffering almost seemed normal, so that "*se uno muore, è quasi un pò meno morto*" (if one dies, he is almost a little less dead).

In Santa Lucia, many families lost large numbers of children well into the twentieth century. For example, over a 14-year period early this century, one couple lost six infants in addition to two grown children; over nine years, another lost five infants before the age of one month, and one at a year and a half. It was a lucky couple that did not see any of its children die. There was little recourse to medical intervention, which was not expected to thwart fate or God's will and could even make matters worse. An old expression said that "the earth covers the errors of the physicians." When patients entered the tuberculosis hospital outside Santa Lucia, they were greeted by Dante's words from the *Inferno*, "*lasciate ogni speranza voi ch'entrate*" (leave all hope behind, you who enter).

The Church taught that couples should "grow and multiply." The burdens of a large family and the pain of seeing children die would be compensated by the mystic comfort of resignation in life and Paradise after death. Childbirth was surrounded by negative images. Woman was the origin of sin, for which all humanity paid with death; she paid with *maternità per sempre maledetta* (eternally cursed maternity) or painful, dangerous, and impure birth. There was a purification ritual in church 40 days afterward, in which the woman was not permitted to enter through the main door but had to go through the sacristy, carrying a candle, her head covered. Priests bristle with irritation when asked about this, knowing that old women continue to talk about it this way rather than as a benediction or rite of thanks only remotely based on an ancient purification ritual.

In popular tradition, sexual contact with a woman implied pollution. Even today, such contact is considered defiling or debilitating to male athletes, many of whom will abstain during the season or before competitions. On the other hand, pregnancy and childbirth had positive associations with the fertility of the earth in a cyclical conception of life, death, and rebirth, and children added to women's status and authority within the family. Yet, childbirth was also a polluting event that exposed the woman to danger, dramatically bringing life and death together. Religious ambiguities about the chastity and impurity of woman infused traditions upheld by midwives and the public such as having a virgin hold the woman's hand during a difficult childbirth, lighting candles to saints such as Sant'Anna (who looks after women during childbirth), and ensuring a safe birth by giving the woman torn-up illustrations of the Virgin Mary to eat.

The cultural value of femininity was certainly not enhanced by the preference for male children. Even medical texts affirmed that parents hoped all through pregnancy for a male child, and there were innumerable popular and medical prescriptions for influencing or guessing the child's sex. When the woman's mother came to visit after the birth, she would bring more gifts for a boy than a girl. At the baptism, the godmother would wear no ribbon or a plain one over her left shoulder for a girl, but a brightly colored one over her right shoulder to express the special joy that a boy brought.

Over the nineteenth century, sentimental attitudes about infants and children arose alongside the harsher ones we have discussed. A new conception of the role of the mother in shaping the child's health and destiny was expressed in poems about well-off urban women's attachment to their children. Mothers who were not able to find an acceptable wet nurse were strongly affected by guilt and remorse. Those who abandoned a child to the ruota left it with handmade, personalized garments and linens prepared beforehand, which were recorded in detail in the birth registers.

Some included a half medallion in the hope of reuniting later and kept the other half to confirm their identity.

Physicians and social reformers in Italy and elsewhere in Europe appealed to public authorities to increase state and scientific interest in infancy, particularly maternal breast-feeding and the teaching of hygiene. Instead of castigating the newborn, they maintained that society should recognize its cultural value and natural goodness, even if illegitimate. Rousseau's words spread: *"Tutto è perfetto uscendo dalle mani di Dio . . . Tutto degenera nelle mani dell'uomo"* (All is perfect leaving the hands of God . . . All degenerates in the hands of man). It was no longer necessary to be resigned to suffering and death.

It was easier to propagate this message than act upon it. The medical fields devoted to women and children were not popular ones. The children's institutions needed reform. Mothers and wet nurses very rarely submitted themselves for medical examination, and many child-rearing norms such as not swaddling were making little headway among the common people. In farm households there was still a great emotional distance between parents and children, and many children continued to work rather than attend school well into the present century. There were still many infanticides, illegitimate births, and cases of infant abandonment. Fatalistic attitudes about procreation, health, and mortality persisted in spite of the emergence of a hopeful, active conception of the effectiveness of medicine and the ability of physicians to control infant health and survival.

Turn-of-the-century discussions of fertility emphasized the effectiveness of human agency in shaping vital processes, while expressing frustration over the persistence of traditional attitudes among the poor and undereducated.[32] Although the relationship between population growth and economic well-being was a hot topic in political debates all over Europe, and had been for more than a century already, there was no clear agreement about it. Contemporary economic theory equated population increase with economic potential and prosperity, making the opposite view a minority one. Neomalthusianists came up against Christian moralists in their criticism of cultural attitudes of resignation regarding sex and procreation, and of traditional birth control methods such as abstinence.

The belief in moderate, planned, but not forsaken reproduction that neomalthusianists shared with the "new" feminists also put them into conflict with reactionaries opposed to any form of feminism. In Italy and all over the Continent, conservatives associated feminism with women's work and, in turn, low birthrates and an antiprocreative, antifamily morality. Ironically, many ideas of the fascist period were expressed first by the new feminists in the early decades of this century. They sought to go beyond traditional feminist goals such as obtaining women's suffrage by improving women's lives and social standing through a rationalization and elevation of maternity. This would bring women and maternity into the sphere of state interests and make maternity the moral basis of the nation-state. Men had been endowed with the exalted spiritual values of the Great War, but women had been either left in the ignorance of rural life or consumed by industrial labor that ruined their health and procreative capacities and propensities.

Yet, paid labor itself gave women the self-will that new feminists advocated. Like the popular notion of rationalization, this quality, *volontà*, was to be applied to procreation so that it would no longer be left to chance. Women were inevitably affected by the new international ideas of the early twentieth century, including those that challenged values such as female virginity, sexual abstinence, chastity, or sex as a means to reproduction rather than an end in itself. At the same time, new cultural values exalted the female body as an object of sexual attention. This was a thin, nubile body type that was the opposite of the "inevitable" maternal shape.

New magazines, fashions, and industries such as cosmetics directed women's volontà toward pleasing men through their appearance, a shift in line with changes in household organization. In cross-cultural perspective, societies composed mostly of simple families tend to uphold women's attractiveness and sexual duty to husbands as strong cultural values. In Italy, stable relationships of interdependence and social class difference gave way to social mobility and flux in professions and economic opportunities as simple families became the norm. Though no longer balanced economically, the relationship between spouses allowed for cooperative fertility control between spouses, while contributing to their dependence upon outside experts.

A contradiction was in place that would soon confound fascist leaders: their hoped-for "return" to a traditional patriarchal family morality and ideal female body type and role ran counter to the goal of rationalizing women's domestic activities. This would frustrate the effort to increase fertility rates and modernize child rearing at the same time, since the old social structure favored the former but the new favored the latter.

Governmental Intervention in Women's Work and the
Care of Infants

In the late nineteenth century, there were movements all over Europe to protect women from dangerous work and long hours, particularly after childbirth.[33] Beyond moral motives having to do with unwelcome ideologies such as feminism, there were health reasons for doing so. Industrial labor was thought to directly harm women's procreative functions and to have negative health consequences for infants such as low birth weight, irregular growth, and higher mortality rates. Consequently, it was alarming that most female industrial and commercial workers were young, almost half were married, and almost a quarter were under the age of 18. There was less concern for agricultural workers, since rural people were thought to have a healthier morality and life-style expressed in higher birth and lower infant mortality rates. There was an exception to this in the area of rice production, which was known to be damaging to the health.

Between 1873 and 1879, laws were passed to prohibit women from working in laborious jobs for at least 15 days after childbirth. In 1890, a conference of 14 nations held in Berlin set up laws to outlaw women's work in factories and workshops during the first month after childbirth, but they were not passed in Italy until 1902 (with modification in 1907). In 1917, maternity insurance was instituted, but the fund was not created until 1923, by a law that also prohibited employers from firing women during pregnancy or the obligatory period of maternity leave. Before these provisions, only workers in certain industries had been protected. For example, a 1907 law instituted leave for one month before and one month after childbirth for rice workers and required pregnant women seeking work in the winnowing of rice to present a medical certificate specifying the estimated due date. In 1913, these protections were extended to all workers, who were now required to stop working one month before the due date as well as after.

In 1916, nursing rooms and two paid half-hour breaks per day in establishments with over 50 workers were instituted. In smaller firms or in the absence of nursing rooms, workers could take two one-hour breaks a day to nurse at home. Large establishments were further expected to provide on-site day care. Laws in 1918 and 1919 regulated the wet-nursing industry; one in 1919 (with modification in 1923) unified provisions pertaining to women's and children's labor; and another in 1921 addressed prevention of infectious diseases in the schools. These were some of the precedents for fascist legislation we will discuss later.

In the late nineteenth century, governmental intervention in the institutions for infants also increased, particularly with legislation in 1890. This was to regulate all charitable institutions, favoring medical and social welfare assistance rather than traditional religious concerns such as retreats or hospices for pilgrims. It excluded priests from membership in the *congregazioni di carità* (local philanthropic organizations) that ran most of the existing charities. The congregazioni had operated independently, but with some supervision by provincial governments. Institutions for infants had had further contacts with public authorities, especially in their dealings with unmarried mothers. For the most part, the charitable institutions carried on as they had before the law, remaining tied to local initiatives and resources until the middle of the fascist period, when state control greatly increased.

Beginning in the second half of the nineteenth century, there was a shift in the character of the institutions for infants, from foundling hospitals (*brefotrofi*) to day-care centers (*asili*), which reflected the changing needs of an industrializing society.[34] Although the foster care system was still in place in some towns, economic conditions were improving enough that wages for institutional wet nursing no longer seemed attractive. Moreover, the laws requiring medical examinations to protect against transmission of syphilis and tuberculosis decreased the supply of wet nurses.

The decline in the need for foundling homes was compensated by a rise in the need for small children to be cared for while their mothers, most of whom were married, worked for low wages in the fields, factories, and households. In fact, children were better fed at the asili than at home, and diet alone was often a primary motivation for their foundation. Philanthropists and community leaders also set out to open modern preschools, but to ensure that they had a "maternal and social" character to replace the mother and family. To this day, preschools are called *scuole materne.*

The number of institutions rose rapidly. In 1846, there had been 178 asili in the Italian kingdom; by 1893 there were 2,572. In 1915, there were 4,587, increasing to 5,229 within five years and 7,069 by 1927. These institutions were almost all in the central and northern regions, which also hosted 85 percent of all medical facilities for infants.[35] This may be more a reflection of need than better infant care, for the institutions were notoriously ill-equipped and poorly operated, and continued to show high mortality rates through the early twentieth century. Today, the institutional care of young children in Italy is thought to be among the best in the world. This is a radical departure from a century ago, and part of an overall change in the treatment of the young that includes assiduous care by parents and health professionals.

Demographic and Epidemiologic Transition

Decline in Birthrates

We have discussed some of the factors that contributed to the decline in birthrates in Italy, but no one really knows exactly what caused the demographic transition in any place or time. Different social classes went through the transition at different times, as did ethnic or religious groups, geographical areas, and occupational classes.[36] In contrast to past centuries, when changes in marriage rates, age at marriage, or the proportion of permanent celibates influenced birthrates in Europe, the fertility transition of the last century in Italy did not depend upon these factors. Marriage rates have changed only imperceptibly compared to natality rates, and so has the average age at marriage.

Most of the fall in birthrates took place *before* the appearance of modern contraceptive methods such as the pill. Likewise, most of the fall in overall and infant mortality rates took place well before the intervention of professional medicine in the fascist period and afterward: *before* modern medical therapies such as immunization or antibiotics. Yet, while medical treatment did not have much effect early in the transition, compared to hygiene, sanitation, housing, ecological changes, or nutrition, it did (and does) seem to play an important role in later stages of the transition. It is difficult to assign relative weights to these factors, as they have been at work independently and together over a long span of time.[37]

As we noted in chapter 1, until the Neolithic Revolution human population growth was very slow. Then, fertility rates rose rapidly, along with mortality rates. Since the latter remained lower, population growth was rapid. By now, birth and death rates have been reset in equilibrium in the Western societies, but at very low levels compared to preagricultural times. The declines in fertility and mortality rates began later in Italy and other southern European countries than those to the north or the United States, but today their demographic patterns are all very similar.

Figure 2 shows that mortality rates began to fall precipitously in the 1870s in Italy, declining by one-half within a half century. Instead of falling with them, fertility rates rose a bit and began to decline only in the 1890s. This time lag meant that the rate of natural population growth rose in the late nineteenth century and remained around 10 per 1,000 through the 1930s (except during the First World War). It was not until the middle 1980s that fertility rates fell to below 10 per 1,000, as mortality rates had done by 1950.

In recent years, Italy has had the lowest birthrate in the world, around 9 live births per 1,000 population. In Emilia-Romagna, it is even lower, at 7 to 7.5, among the lowest of all the regions. This means that the average number of children a woman is expected to have over her lifetime is under 1.0 in Emilia-Romagna, as opposed to under 1.2 in the nation. Birthrates were higher than the national average in the nineteenth century, but passed below it in the early decades of this century. They have been consistently lower since then, the lowest in the country since the 1950s.

While birthrates in Emilia-Romagna and other industrializing regions were falling rapidly early this century, those of the southern and island regions remained high. Of the northern regions, only Veneto retained high birthrates, and it was the only one that remained predominantly agricultural. The central regions fell between the extremes. In the cities, the upper classes had the lowest birthrates, the lower classes the highest.

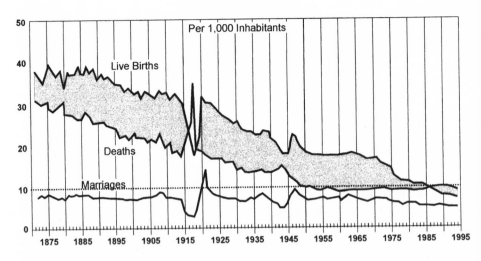

FIG. 2.   Live births, deaths, and marriages in Italy, 1872–1994. (From ISTAT 1962:12, fig. 1; 1992:12, fig. 1; 1996:107, tab. 8.3; 1997:43, tab. 2.7.)

In the rural areas, sharecroppers and other farmers had the largest families, while landowners and other proprietors had the smallest. For example, in the nine provinces around Milan, the former fell between 5.0 and 7.8 family members in 1933, the latter between 2.2 and 3.3.[38] Similar numbers were found in the national census in 1931, with laborers and workers in the professions, military, and commerce falling in between.[39] In contrast to the complex families in the central and northern regions, there was never a large proportion of nonnuclear families in the south, where the latifondi favored day labor. This difference persisted until after the Second World War, when nonnuclear families were about one-third of the total in the former but less than one-fifth in the latter. By now, almost all families are simple or minimally extended, with one to two children, rather than two to eight.

Epidemiologic Transition

Like natality rates, mortality rates fell later in Italy than in the countries to the north. Within Italy, they fell sooner and faster in the central and northern regions than the southern and island regions. By the early 1930s, death rates were 12 or 13 per 1,000 inhabitants in the former, but 15 to 20 in the latter. Today, death rates tend to be higher than the national average of 9.5 in regions such as Emilia-Romagna, with their aging populations, whereas southern and island regions tend to have lower death but higher birthrates.

There were people who lived into their nineties a century ago, and this maximum has not changed. What has changed is that almost all deaths now take place in the older age groups, thanks above all to the decline in infant mortality rates. If it were possible to survive infancy, one could expect to live into the sixties or seventies a century ago. This seems to have been the case even in 1300, when Dante considered 35 the peak and mid-point of life, as in the first line of the *Inferno* (*"Nel mezzo del cammin di nostra vita"*).[40]

As in other Western societies, the epidemiologic transition had the greatest impact on the health and disease patterns of women and children. At all life expectancy levels, women have a lower risk of dying in the postreproductive period than men, but at low life expectancy levels like those of Italy until the early twentieth century they have a higher risk of death throughout childhood and the reproductive years. As survival rates for the reproductive period improved, fertility rose early in the transition, but this did not significantly affect population growth because mortality rates were still high.[41] Then, as infant mortality rates declined, interbirth intervals increased and contributed to the decline in fertility rates.

The death rate per 100,000 women from complications of pregnancy, childbirth, and the postpartum period declined only a little between the turn of the century and the early 1920s (from 14 to 12). By the mid-1950s, it was down to 3 and currently is below 0.1. In other terms, in the late 1880s, 6,600 women died each year during childbirth and the postpartum period, 4,500 of puerperal infections. By the 1930s the number fell below 3,000. By the 1970s it was around 500, and by the 1990s around 20, all in spite of increases in population size. While puerperal fever still accounted for one-third of maternal deaths in the early 1930s, it had nearly been eliminated two decades later.[42]

Overall, there has been a qualitative shift in mortality patterns, from infectious diseases to chronic diseases as the major causes of death. In the process, diseases of malnutrition have been replaced by diseases of over-nutrition. The major causes of death have shifted from infectious and parasitic diseases, respiratory and gastrointestinal disease, and psychical disturbances and diseases of the nervous system and senses, to diseases of the circulatory system and cancer.[43] The last two account for over 70 percent of all mortality today. In the intervening years, both kinds of disease were common.

Although infant mortality rates were still relatively high early this century, young people made up a much larger proportion of the population than they do today. As recently as the 1950s, more than 35 percent of the population was under the age of 16, but only 15 percent was over 55.

Today the proportions are reversed. Nationally, more people are 65 or older than under 15. In Emilia-Romagna, there are twice as many in the older age group.

The rapid population growth in the early twentieth century led to a maximum population of around 6,000 in the 1940s and 1950s in Santa Lucia. Within a few years after 1960, the population had dropped by one-fourth because of both demographic changes and emigration. It has since stabilized at 3,000 through balances between emigration and immigration, and among marriages, births, and deaths.

These changes have had a profound impact upon marriage and family life. A century ago, only one-half of parents in Santa Lucia were alive at the time of their children's wedding, and one-fourth of all couples already had children when they married. Today, there is no shortage of grandparents, but there is a shortage of children for them to look after! Fewer than half as many infants are born to unwed mothers in the nation and region, and infant abandonment is virtually unknown. Maternal deaths are rare indeed, and so are infant deaths. We will now look more closely at the fall in infant mortality rates, to try to understand life in the past and certain ideas and fears that have persisted into present times.

The Fall in Infant Mortality Rates

A century ago, 25 percent of all infants died within a year of birth, and in some areas the proportion reached 40 percent.[44] Today, the percentage is around 0.7, as shown in figure 3. Nineteenth-century infant mortality rates were higher than they had been in the eighteenth century and remained higher in the industrializing northern regions than elsewhere in the nation. Childhood mortality rates fell sooner and faster than infant mortality rates, as the latter are more sensitive to living conditions. Between 1880 and 1940, deaths per 100 live births in the first year of life fell from 20 to 10; in the second year, from 11 to 3; and in the third year, from 5 to 1.[45]

Once again, the timing was later in Italy than other Western societies. Italy's infant and child mortality rates were already higher in the late nineteenth century, but the difference grew in the twentieth as other countries experienced much more rapid improvements. In 1950, the infant mortality rate was twice as high as in countries such as England, the United States, or Sweden. There was no longer any difference by the 1990s, giving some indication of how rapidly material conditions improved with the postwar economic boom.

Within Italy, there was strong regional variation in infant mortality rates. In Emilia-Romagna, infant mortality rates were higher than the national average from the 1860s until around 1910. Beginning in the 1920s, they fell away, to less than three-quarters of the national average by

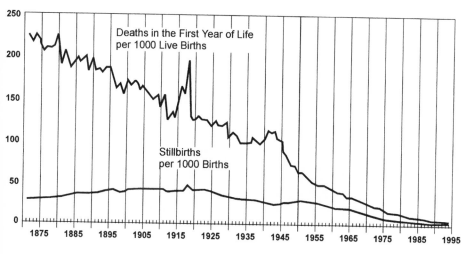

FIG. 3.   Infant deaths and stillbirths in Italy, 1872–1994. (From ISTAT 1962:12, fig. 2; 1992:12, fig. 2; 1996:107, tab. 8.3; 1997:46, tab. 2.11.)

the mid-1950s. Some southern regions like Campania took an opposite course, going from lower-than-average to above-average rates. From the 1970s on, the regional differences began to even out, but have not disappeared. In 1993, the infant mortality rate was 5.5 in Emilia-Romagna, but 8.8 in Campania.

A century ago, the number of infants who died in the first week of life matched the number who died in the second and third years together. Deaths in these older infants were the first to be reduced, both as a percentage of births and as a percentage of all deaths—in step with overall mortality rates. The mortality rate of infants under one year fell more slowly, and as a percentage of all deaths it actually increased. This was noted by fascist demographers, who observed that infant deaths had remained at the level of 30 percent of all deaths into the 1930s. The same thing happened in Santa Lucia (see appendix).

While infant mortality rates declined beginning in the 1880s and 1890s, stillbirth rates nearly doubled from 2.09 to over 4 per 100 births between the early 1860s and the turn of the century. They remained at this level until the 1920s and then declined toward today's figure of 0.46. Emilia-Romagna had a higher-than-average rate at the turn of the century, but it is now below the national average. In Santa Lucia, there were as many as 8 or 9 stillbirths for every 100 births a century ago, but in general 4 to 7 until the 1920s. Thereafter, they fell close to zero.

Variation in Infant Mortality Rates

Using the population registers in Santa Lucia, I was able to study some 100 stillbirths and 300 infant deaths out of more than 1,700 births over scattered years from the 1860s to the present (see appendix). Since I had already analyzed changes in the frequencies of various professions over that time, I was able to determine whether there were more deaths than expected in each of five occupational groups. In addition, there was another set of data that allowed me to tabulate the causes of 1,100 infant deaths over the decades from 1900 to 1960.

Comparing the results against historical writings showed that not only has there been a quantitative change in infant mortality, but there has been an equally dramatic qualitative change. There has been a transition from high mortality from infectious diseases and complications of gestation and childbirth distributed through the first years, to low mortality from congenital disorders mostly concentrated in the first days and weeks. At the same time, there has been an evening-out of differences in susceptibility by social class, season, sex, or parental marital status and occupation. This shift reflects the increasing uniformity of conditions of life in Santa Lucia and the nation, including homogenization of infant feeding practices.

One of the most striking differences a century ago was between legitimate and illegitimate infants. Nationally, the latter were much more likely to be stillborn or die as infants than the former for the entire time between 1861 and 1960; by now, there is virtually no difference. Infant mortality rates were twice as high for illegitimate infants as recently as the 1920s, especially in regions such as Sicily where infant mortality rates were high. The difference was much more narrow in low-mortality regions like Emilia-Romagna. In Santa Lucia, it had nearly disappeared by the 1920s.

In the late nineteenth century, there were notable sex differences in infant death rates in Santa Lucia. Three times as many males as females were stillborn, while more girls than boys died in the 2-month to 1-year age group. I am wary of interpreting these phenomena, but traditional preferences for males may have translated into better care and nutrition of boys and a greater likelihood that stillborn males would be reported.

Seasonality was a very important factor widely recognized by health professionals and the public.[46] Infants who died in winter were often newborns and younger babies affected by respiratory infections. Those who died in summer and early fall were older infants and small children exposed to gastrointestinal diseases upon weaning or supplemental feeding. In the nineteenth century, more infants died in winter and spring, but in the first few decades of the twentieth century more died in summer and fall. In the colder regions, the tradition of baptizing infants immediately or within a day or two of birth was and is blamed for wintertime neonatal deaths. In anticlerical Emilia-Romagna, the rejection of the baptismal rite in the early decades of this century may have contributed to the decline in infant mortality rates.

In late-nineteenth-century Santa Lucia, the average age of infants who died was around 7 months in winter, 6 months in spring, 13 months in summer, and 7 months in fall. There were almost three times as many deaths in winter and spring as in summer and fall. These patterns began to falter in the first decades of the twentieth century and no longer held by the interwar period. After the Second World War, there were few infant deaths, most of which occurred soon after birth, so that seasonal averages were all under one or two months.

Another factor was parental occupational or social class. Most notably, the children of wet nurses had a high mortality rate, as did children fed by wet nurses. A report on the Naples foundling home showed that only 2 of 2,000 babies sent to wet nurses survived.[47] In Santa Lucia, throughout the late nineteenth and early twentieth centuries there were notable differences among five principal occupational groups. Most significantly, children of the farming population were stillborn less often and died in numbers much lower than expected in all three age groups (0 to 2 months, 2 months to 1 year, 1 to 3 years). Children of day laborers had the opposite fate. Children of landowners and professionals fared better than expected in the two earlier age groups, but worse in the 1-to-3-year category. Children of artisans died more often than expected in the neonatal period, but less often thereafter. There were more deaths than expected among infants who did not fit in these categories, undoubtedly because most of them had been sent to town from Ferrara or Florence for wet nursing.

Maternal breast-feeding was most common in the farm population, which probably explains much of that group's better-than-expected mortality rates. Breast-feeding continued to protect farm children (2 months to 3 years) in the interwar period, but the higher-than-expected mortality of children under 2 months may reflect lesser access to or acceptance of medical care among farmers. This was the most notable disparity, for by this time the differences in infant susceptibility among occupational categories were much smaller. By the postwar period, infant feeding methods ceased to be a notable influence, for wet nursing had disappeared, and the artificial feeding used by day laborers, artisans, and some upper-class women had become much safer.

Causes and Interpretations of Infant Mortality

Another shift in infant mortality patterns was a change in disease frequencies. Until the Second World War, almost all infant deaths were attributed to three main causes: stillbirth, premature birth, or complications of birth; congenital weakness; and gastrointestinal and respiratory diseases. As recently as 1934, diseases of the digestive apparatus and neonatal diseases (congenital weakness, prematurity, etc.) accounted for 60 percent of all infant deaths. Well over half of the other 40 percent were caused by respiratory diseases such as bronchitis and pneumonia. The others were divided among diseases such as measles, diphtheria, and tuberculosis; diseases of the circulatory system, skin, blood, and other systems; and nervous system diseases such as encephalitis and meningitis.[48]

Infant and early childhood mortality from gastrointestinal disease did not decline much between the 1890s and the 1920s, and it remained a major killer through mid-century. Also beginning in the 1920s, deaths from influenza, scarlet fever, and stomach and duodenal diseases fell along with diseases that had begun their decline earlier, such as tuberculosis, malaria, diphtheria, or measles. Presently, congenital and perinatal disorders (prematurity, congenital malformations, asphyxia, obstetrical lesions) account for 85 percent of all infant deaths, four-fifths of which are concentrated in the first month (and the vast majority of these in the first week). The remainder are caused by respiratory tract diseases, infectious and parasitic diseases, and other causes. After the first month, SIDS is the major cause of infant death.

The same patterns held in Santa Lucia, where gastrointestinal and respiratory system diseases declined as major killers, leaving the other two main causes of infant death. By the 1950s, three-quarters of all infant deaths were attributed to congenital weakness (or "insufficient organic development" or "weak constitution") together with stillbirth, premature birth, and complications of labor. The others were attributed to infectious diseases; accidents and injuries; and other causes. Accidents and injuries in the early twentieth century often involved burns (and later firearms), and there were a few homicides recorded in the registers.

One of the most striking things about the town registers was a cause of death called *insufficiente allattamento* (insufficient breast-feeding or insufficient feeding), which was used even when the infant died within hours or days of birth. It appeared many times in the first decade of the century, but disappeared over the following two decades, and highlights the fact that the quality and quantity of infant nutrition were considered absolutely crucial to infant health and survival.

However, there are problems of interpretation regarding the role of nutrition in the past. The relationship between infection and nutrition is not at all straightforward, for even if most infections do worse in a well-nourished host, some do better. Also, not enough is known about historical patterns of infant feeding to warrant any definitive judgment of their impact on infant mortality rates.[49] What we can know is that contemporaries in Italy blamed infant deaths on defects in feeding, even when gas-trointestinal or respiratory infections were involved. It was not simply the method, but the entire life-style and hygienic conditions associated with it that were thought to influence infant health. These included the early wean-ing of wet nurses' infants and the poor hygienic environment and inade-quate care of infants sent away for wet nursing. In artificial feeding, they included constitutional incompatibility or contamination of animal milk.

The study by Rasponi (1914:44–46) illustrates the degree to which contemporaries linked infant survival and lifelong health to differences in infant feeding methods. Although the prevailing wisdom was that breast-feeding was safer than wet nursing or artificial feeding, she set out to demonstrate that artificial feeding was the best method of all. She found that the most common cause of 870 infant deaths was gastroenteritis and emphasized that the infants kept by a balia outside the home were partic-ularly susceptible to this disease. She blamed either the balia or weaning for many other infectious diseases, including meningitis and scarlet fever. The cause was too ill-defined for categorization in 15 percent of the cases, but the attending physician said that half of these infants died because they were too fat . . . and Rasponi hastened to add that they had been breast-fed. The others died because of accidents, suffocation in bed with the nurse, or burns from a bath given by a "thermometer-phobic wet nurse."

Rasponi grouped the infants in her study into two social classes (wealthy and poor), four age-groups (nursling, up to three years, up to seven years, and adolescent), and nine infant feeding methods. She found that bottle-feeding gave the lowest mortality rates for both well-off and poor infants, allowing those of the latter to approach those of the former. In both social groups, bottle-fed infants (even if after breast-feeding or in mixed feeding) were much less likely to have a mediocre development and much more likely to have a good one than breast-fed infants. Bottle-feed-ing gave the lowest death rates from tuberculosis throughout childhood and adolescence for both the wealthy and poor.

By the fascist period, wet nursing was no longer a common form of infant feeding, and the interpretation of infant mortality changed. Experts no longer associated infant mortality patterns with social class or the con-ditions of infant feeding methods, but instead connected them to women's errors and lack of a rational method in breast-feeding. All improvements in infant mortality rates were said to be the result of success in the dissem-ination of this method, rather than any improvement in the miserable liv-ing conditions of mothers and wet nurses. This was in spite of the fact that infant mortality rates had already shrunk to almost half their peak levels *before* the interventions of fascist political and medical leaders.

The fascist-era belief that women were responsible for infant death through their ignorant resistance to modern medicine finds many parallels in current interpretations of historical and present-day infant mortality patterns. Women's work and the use of formula or supplementary foods in poor countries are widely blamed for infant disease and death, almost as though infectious disease and poverty did not exist. Historical studies take it for granted that reductions in infant mortality rates in Europe were an achievement of professional medicine in teaching women the importance of breast-feeding and the necessity of a rational method.[50]

This was not the case, at least in Italy, where the adoption of wet nursing and bottle-feeding was itself promoted and demanded by the professional medical community. Women's "errors" were more often than not rooted in a readiness, not reluctance, to accept expert advice. Where there was reluctance, women did not need to be taught the importance of breast-feeding. Ironically, there is now near-universal compliance with medical knowledge and practice, which interfere with lactation. Meanwhile, compared to the past, contemporary society seems to have come to the counterevolutionary conclusion that infant feeding has little impact on either infant health or survival.

CHAPTER 4

Fascist Biological Politics
Efforts to Control Fertility and Infant Care
in the Interwar Period

One of the central preoccupations of the fascist government was the quantity and quality of the population. The decline in birthrates was feared because it foreshadowed the biological death of the nation, the descendant of a great civilization now geared up for war and territorial conquest. Population growth was rapid throughout the interwar period, but only because mortality rates were falling faster than fertility rates. Even though there were already problems of overpopulation, leaders argued that Italy faced a moment of national-cultural *necessità* (necessity) to expand and improve. This would require battles against both fertility decline and embarrassingly high levels of infant disease and death. It would increase the country's cultural, military, and economic might and make the fascist nation's influence felt through the world and history.

The heart of the program to politicize marriage and family as central obligations to the nation-state was symbolically represented in the image of the breast-feeding mother. This image exalted not the kind of unregulated, overly prolonged breast-feeding of popular tradition, but one year of breast-feeding according to a rationalized method. Breast-feeding was both a traditional "natural" function and an instrument of science. It represented not only the major weapon against infant mortality, but also the arrival of modern, medicalized maternity and the rejection of antiprocreative materialist or feminist ideologies. It proved one's dedication to procreation and mothering as opposed to work outside the home, for it continued to be very difficult indeed for working women to breast-feed. The mother-child relationship in breast-feeding not only was a central unifying concept of fascist domestic politics, but also became a powerful symbol of fascism, as in figure 4.

Two things converged in fascism to enable leaders to intervene domestically as no one had before: an unprecedented assumption of moral authority by the state; and an unbounded mixing of biology with politics. In essence, domestic politics meant demographic politics, based upon the concept of *politica biologica.* That is, there was thought to be no distinction between culture and biology, morality and physiology. Individuals

95

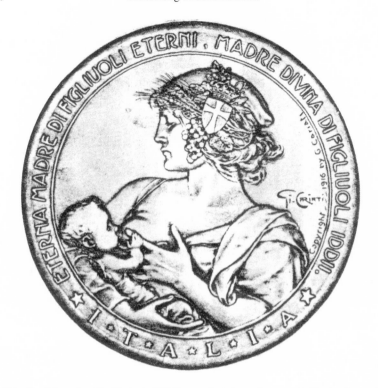

FIG. 4. Plate by G. Cariati (1916), reprinted as the cover illustration of *La Preparazione Materna* (1939).

were to identify with the nation as cells to an organism, with families forming the bridge between them. Families constituted the nation in a biological and moral sense, so that urbanism and depraved political ideologies harmed reproduction directly through both biology and morality.

Biological politics aimed to rationalize and unify production and reproduction, fusing biology with economics. This meant ruralizing the population and preventing urbanization, reconciling with the Church, maximizing agricultural and industrial production, and retaining the population within its borders. Other measures included regulating women's work, providing inducements to marriage and procreation, overseeing children's upbringing, and increasing medical intervention in maternity, with the primary goal of promoting regimented breast-feeding.

Fascism claimed to be a regenerative movement that moved forward by looking backward. This aphorism encapsulated the deepest contradictions and tensions of a rapidly transforming society caught between traditionalism and an ideology of progress. Modern bourgeois ideals held that women should be not only extremely devoted to housekeeping and child rearing, but also sexually attractive to their husbands, in a rather antimaternal way. Fascist leaders approved of the former, so long as it was guided by reason and rational method, and the latter so long as the ideal body image conformed to the "maternal" one. The politicization of parenthood was to lead both men and women away from self-indulgent ideologies and toward self-sacrifice for the good of the family and nation. Yet, by emphasizing that women should do this for the glorification of their husbands and the state, fascism effaced the personhood of mothers.

The contrast between the insularity of large farm families and the openness of small simple families to cultural influences was a particularly thorny issue. The latter were more receptive to both new ideas about maternity and breast-feeding, *and* antiprocreative and antimaternal fashions and attitudes. Those not caught up in trends and fashions were more likely to reproduce and breast-feed, but they were from traditional families more isolated from and resistant to the intervention of experts. As we shall see, this discordance affected the rate at which medicalized breast-feeding practices spread through the population, during and after the fascist period.

Responses to Demographic Transition and Modernization

Phases of Fascism

The fascist movement formed soon after the Great War.[1] The party took over at the national level in October 1922 after the March on Rome, although fascists had won local elections before then. It remained in power for two decades, a period known as the *ventennio*. Historians divide this period into at least two major phases: fascism of the movement (1910s and 1920s) and fascism of the regime (1930s and the war years). The first phase was characterized by ideological heterogeneity and relative lack of organization, with administrative power concentrated at the provincial and local levels. In fact, in the early 1920s, there were still more than a dozen opposition parties. In the second phase, government power was focused at the center, while dissenting factions and individuals were silenced and excluded in favor of mandatory party affiliation and consent. Party politics and repressive violence gave way to the leadership and normalizing interventions of the state.

In practice, the appearance of popular consensus was achieved, and not just because of the influence of coercion. Most people complied with

or supported the regime until the middle 1930s, if not for ideological conviction, then out of a sober sense of resignation to political change that
had been cultivated over centuries of foreign and Church conquest and
rule. There were also practical motives, for many people had to enroll in
the party not to lose their jobs. Even among the many who complied out
of conviction, there remained a more permanent notion of the primacy of
individual and family self-interest.[2]

The regime's relationship with the Church also underwent a change in
the 1930s. Until then, fascist ideology regarding the family and morality
had run parallel to Catholic beliefs about procreation and the roles of the
spouses. Over time, the encroachment of the state on the Church's
influence over family life and social services caused increasing discord
between them. Fascism taught that mothers gave life and raised children in
glorification of Mussolini, the nation, and the country's grandiose past
and present civilization; fathers gave life, but also took it or sacrificed their
own as warriors. This mission transcended the individual's own identity,
but, unlike the Church's calling toward procreation and life for the glory
of God, it venerated war and death in service to the state. The Church also
did not share fascism's emphasis on the body, expressed in the participation of both boys and girls in sports and military exercises in school and
the youth organizations. The Church saw the attempt to create a national
health and social welfare service as a direct encroachment on its activities,
motivated by political expedience rather than Christian charity. In the latter half of the 1930s, the distance between the Church and the regime grew
as the country moved toward war on the side of an anti-Catholic country.[3]

While there was some intellectual and political opposition to fascism,
Italy's organized resistance came late. Nevertheless, it has become the
dominant paradigm for historiography as well as politics in the postwar
period, tending to reduce awareness or recognition of the widespread com-
plicity in fascist politics and culture. This has also obscured the continuity
in institutions and personnel between the fascist and postwar governments, and covered the roots of present-day conceptions of the relationship between the individual and the state. As we will see, the fascist intervention in infant health had significant, if localized, effects on disease and
death. On the level of culture, fascist propaganda and policy had a lasting,
if largely unacknowledged, impact.

Biological Politics

Italy was not alone in fearing for the decline of the "white" races. All over
Europe and the United States, scholars and politicians were concerned
about falling birthrates and the death they portended of peoples and
nations.[4] To countries like Italy, Spain, and France, the numbers of Ger-

mans, Russians, and British subjects at home and in the colonies were frightfully large. Causes of reduced procreation were sought in the rationalizing and hedonistic mentality that had emerged with urbanism, industrial society, and the French Revolution.

With the defeat of socialism and industrial bourgeois society in the First World War, fascism proclaimed itself the voice against materialism and neomalthusianism, using awareness of the possibility of manipulating birthrates to ends opposite those envisioned by Malthus and his followers. Fascist leaders called for a rebirth of Italian society through holistic biological and moral improvement of the land and population. This would bring population growth, colonial expansion, and a return to the Roman unity after centuries of political differentiation in Europe. Large population size meant economic and cultural improvement, not to mention political and military might. A decrease brought a reduction in discoveries and inventions, spiritual improvement, material well-being, and civilization in general. As Mussolini was fond of saying, *"il numero è forza"* (number is strength, the title of an essay he first published in 1928).

But there was a problem. Even many fascists acknowledged that the country was already overcrowded, for it was growing by a surplus of half a million births over deaths per year. The "tragedy of the Italian life" lay in the formidable "antithesis" between its social and political problems: "we are many for our territory and our resources, few for our necessary task."[5] Mussolini (1928:15) insisted that the standard of living of the 42 million Italians in 1928 was far superior to that of the 27 million in 1871, or the 18 million in 1816. There would be room and bread for 60 million "in an Italy all reclaimed, cultivated, irrigated, disciplined: that is, fascist" (1928:15). A high natality rate was a measure of the strength of the *Patria* (Fatherland) and would distinguish the Italian populace from other European societies, "in that it will bespeak its vitality and its will to pass on this vitality through the centuries" (1928:23).

Fascist Italy would avoid the fate of Rome, which had been doomed by insufficient numbers to "defend its history and reaffirm its right to life and universal dominion."[6] The fecund and morally sound patriarchal family of the Roman Republic, not the declining Empire of later years, would be the model for contemporary society. The measures used by Caesar and his successors to bolster population size would be a start: land grants to fathers; subsidies and distinctions for prolific fathers and mothers; punishments against bachelorhood, childless marriages, adultery, and induced abortion; and institutions for children, where the imposition of a rational diet promised to reduce infant mortality rates. The "demographic battle" was launched with Mussolini's 1927 Ascension Day Speech to the Camera dei Deputati. By the 1937 meeting of the Gran Consiglio, the "demographic matter" was the *"problema dei problemi."*

Since just about everything affected the population, most domestic interventions were said to have demographic aims or consequences. As the nationalist politician and professor of "general doctrine of the state" at the University of Rome, Sergio Panunzio, explained, all of the laws of fascism, "not just the technically demographic laws, regard and discipline among us the fact of the population in relation to the state" (1933:135). For example, control of internal migration together with land reclamation would slow urbanization and promote rural values associated with higher fertility. Emigration had to be stopped not because it reflected poverty, but because it was motivated by "demoliberal individualism" and brought the social imitation of Western ultramaterialist beliefs. By retaining and reproducing the population, the nation would follow its natural, necessary capacity to expand outside its own boundaries. This was Italy's "historic necessity." Failure to act would make it fall among nations "without physiognomy and without history."[7]

But how could a political movement based upon pragmatic individual action justify intrusive autarchic government? The answer was to make the interests of the people coincide with those of the nation-state. Fascism styled itself as an anti-idealist response to nineteenth-century liberalism and materialism grounded in a totalitarian concept of action. At its heart was the fascist aesthetic, an understanding of the human spirit which was at once biological and political. In the words of the endocrinologist-eugenicist Nicola Pende, fascism rejected abstract and metaphysical concepts contrary to "biological reality," in favor of an "eminently practical science of pure Italian mark, which aims on the one hand at rational human reclamation, on the other at the construction of a state which is perfectly harmonious and robust morally and materially" (1933a:8).

The nation was said to be more than the sum of individuals or political parties. As in the Roman conception, it was civilization and spiritual elaboration. The nation was the supreme synthesis of all of the biological and cultural values of the *stirpe* (stock), an entity with its own individuality, history, and destiny. The state was power and action, the guardian or *allevatore* (breeder) of these values. It was charged both with improving material conditions by combating poverty and disease and with helping each person and the collective to reach their biological potency.

The distinctions among individual, state, and nation, which the liberal state had presupposed and maintained, were collapsed along with the liberal distinction between politics and public morality. Individuals were thought of as harmonious cells of a collective organism, institutions as organs. No individual could be permitted to damage the state, as the cell of a malignant tumor damaged the stability and vitality of the body. Of all of the organs, the institution charged with caring for mothers and infants,

ONMI, was hailed as one of the most active and indispensable organs contributing to the healthy, blooming life of the great organism.

Through the perfect identification of the individual with the collective body, consent became a virtue of the whole being and dissent a theoretical impossibility. This justified the elimination of contrary political factions, as heresy had been rooted out from the Church. The state's organization of work, leisure time, political activity, and family life would make opposition meaningless as individuals conformed to their biological destiny and identified organically with the goals and necessities of the nation-state.

Infant and child nutrition were said to be the foundation of "human breeding," which was rooted in rational maternal breast-feeding. Nutrition directly affected survival and shaped the child's lifelong health and development. Even if a child not "nourished according to the rules of physiologic upbringing" did not die, it would never grow to be healthy and instead would always bear "a physical or psychical deficiency which, even if not apparent, will not permit that fullness of physical vigor and willful energy which determine, in the individual, the character."[8]

The central place of controlled breast-feeding and hygienic management of childhood in "state breeding" meant that not just men, but also women had to be brought to understand the national necessities. These included intervening in current generations through control of gestation and child rearing, as well as future generations through shaping the earliest upbringing of girls. The "preparation of future mothers" would prepare them to desire maternity and undergo it rationally, as opposed to following antinatural fashions or occupations.

Modern breast-feeding was not only biologically predestined and sound, but also recalled the glory of Rome, for that civilization had understood its fundamental importance. Further, it implied commitment to the notion of women's proper place in the home and helping professions rather than the workplace or the soft bourgeois life-style, imbued as the latter were in the antiprocreative individualistic hedonism and sensualism of urban life. The application of modern scientific approaches to the improvement of an ancient biological process was a celebration of the backward- and forward-looking faces of fascism.

Integral Reclamation of Land and Population

Since the demographic problem was a biosocial one, it required a biosocial solution: the rationalization of production and reproduction through the *bonifica integrale* or *bonifica umana razionale*. These terms united the notion of *bonitica umana* (human improvement) to the traditional concept of *bonifica terriera* (land reclamation for cultivation and settlement). The word *integrale* expressed wholeness or completeness in the improvement of land and population, while *razionale* suggested modernity and rationality. One of the central proponents of this program was Pende, who established an Istituto Biotipologico-ortogenico at the University of Genoa, where he was director of the medical clinic in the early 1930s. He later chaired the surgery and medicine department at the University of Rome and the board of the thermal clinics at Salsomaggiore. Pende introduced many new terms such as "educational social prophylaxis," "Fascist Hygiene," "biological assistance and improvement of human life," "political anthropotechnics," and "politics of rational state human breeding" (see 1933a, 1933b). The legitimacy of timelessness and the glory of Rome were emphasized in the often-repeated Latin phrase that the mind is healthy when in a healthy body: *mens sana in corpore sano.*

By favoring ruralization and agricultural self-sufficiency, the regime would promote the farmers' inherited Roman military and moral virtues of austerity, moderation, and family patriarchalism behind their better health and higher birthrates—solving, simultaneously, the demographic and economic problems of the new century. The rural morality and family organization were defined as the antidote to the moral corruption of urban industrial capitalism. Accordingly, fascist agrarian politics supported smallholding, but disfavored sharecropping because the large, complex households were traditionalists about farming and diffident with regard to modernizing behavior.

The ruralization program sought to transform day laborers and sharecroppers into independent farmers, and primitive farmers into modern, robust, technically competent agricultural experts using mechanized, intensive farming methods. State support of a mixed economy based on agriculture emphasized particular industries such as food processing and the production of fertilizer and agricultural equipment. This was complemented by land reclamation and resettlement programs, together with infrastructural development of the rural areas. There was meanwhile a "politics of frugality" and a program for the "rational" feeding of the populace. Finally, institutions such as ONMI, together with the "battles" against sterility, tuberculosis, malaria, and other diseases, aimed to influence health and fertility more directly.

The central concept behind all of this was rationalization, a term welcomed everywhere except in the area of fertility decision making. The Italian version of the concept was said to be a spiritual-aesthetic notion, not just a technical one. This meant "economy of time and means, such that it is a factor of wealth [and] progress and therefore power," in the words of the multitalented lawyer, journalist, expert at fencing, and head of ONMI, Sileno Fabbri (1933a:35). Fascism proposed a "third way" between bourgeois capitalism and socialism, upholding private property but justifying significant state intervention in the economy. This involved the rationalized, holistic direction of the economy, labor and management, and the relationship between work and family. As Panunzio said, the "greatness and originality" of fascism was its rejection of bolshevism, Fordism, and German industrial rationalism. Fascism disemboweled the large factories, projecting workers into the happy countryside, for the factories were truly, in America as much as in Russia, the "*delirium tremens,* the great human prisons of capitalism" (1933:139).

The Italian state began to organize the economy in the 1930s through umbrella "corporations," complemented by the *sindacati* (labor-management organizations under fascism, unions otherwise). In theory at least, they oversaw but did not interfere with private initiative, and assured equidistribution of product while keeping purchasing power in proportion with production. This was to prevent the uncontrolled accumulation of wealth in a few hands, for those at the top of the social scale were the least prolific. The Sindacato not only overcame class struggle between owners and workers, but acted as an "organ of associative life and collective moral education, having distinct supereconomic and educative ends," that allowed it to go even beyond the Church in watching over and penetrating the "intimate enclosure of family life" (Panunzio 1933:137). The after-work organization, or Opera Nazionale Dopolavoro (OND), favored the harmonious moral and economic integration of the individual in work through recreational activities that relaxed and regenerated the spirit. This was the "new Italy," renewed in work, culture, and the purity of the family.[9]

Aesthetics, Not Eugenics

The agricultural and moral emphasis of economic interventions infused the "great politics" centered upon new institutions for mothers and children. Very commonly, children were spoken of as agricultural products and women as agricultural inputs or fields for state intervention. As Pende continually reiterated, state action aimed to produce healthy and robust agricultural goods and children (1933a). Children were conduits of the excellent, ancient, national stirpe, defenders against the enemy, and efficacious instruments of the state. They had to be actively cultivated through a politics of natality and conserved through a politics of rationalized protection, education, and surveillance of health and sexual development from gestation through adolescence. "These young and robust little plants, dear wards of the Regime, growing up in this way will modify the face of the current society and present to the new century a new and fascist society which will reproduce and hand down through the centuries the style and spirit of the Revolution of the *Camicie Nere* [blackshirts]."[10]

The agricultural orientation was also at the heart of differences with German racism. Italian biological politics aimed at improvement and increase of the stock and could ill afford to define large numbers of people as biologically undesirable—as the German health minister did when he proclaimed that one-third of the population should not reproduce. Until the late 1930s, Italian writers spoke about stirpe rather than *razza* (race), a holistic concept expressing both biological and spiritual elements handed down through the ages. Italians were proud of the historical coexistence and mixing of Etruscans, Romans, Normans, and other groups throughout the peninsula. At least five different races (Mediterranean, Nordic, Alpine, Dinaric or Adriatic, and Baltic-Oriental) were said to be present in every part of Italy and Europe, every local area, and indeed most individuals. Now that science understood that the mechanism of heredity was not the blending of elements in the blood, Italian theorists affirmed that it would be useless to try to distill one race from the others: better to mix them and try to understand the useful qualities of each.

As the head of the state statistics bureau, Professor Corrado Gini, pointed out, historical rebirths of the Italian population during the Middle Ages, Renaissance, and Unification took place during periods of healthy crosses between people of different regions, bringing prolific reproduction and hybrid vigor (1930:78). This would be repeated now in integral reclamation: the stock would be improved through "fertile crosses" between farmers of different regions in the reclaimed areas. Such "happy mixings" were the source of a nation's strength and beauty, according to Mussolini, who did not believe that a biologically pure race could ever exist: "Race, that is sentiment, not reality" (in DeNapoli 1934a:258). Panunzio argued that fascism was an active pedagogic politics, not a "testimony to out-of-date positivism and biological naturalism." It was aesthetics, not eugenics: fascism, not racism (1933:136).

The German laws for compulsory preventive sterilization were scorned by Italian scholars, politicians, and religious leaders, who rejected them on biological and humanitarian grounds. Although some negative eugenic ideas circulated in Italy, most leaders argued that Italy shared neither Germany's impossible conception of racial purity nor its popular affection for vulgarized science—in this case, the dubious results of studies on heredity. Lacking a sound biological basis, German racism could only be the product of an intellectual abstraction. It was the super-illumination, the too-dazzling light that Germany projected upon the world that justified racism. Mandatory sterilization was a "typical expression of enlightenment and internationalistic science, of the most arid bolshevik conception of humanity forever removed from the mystery of its divine origin."[11] Germany's false eugenics simply gave pseudoscientific backing to policies which were in reality about political predominance.

Italy's racial legislation came late in the fascist period, in 1938, after years of resistance to German pressure and soon after the formation of the Rome-Berlin axis in 1937. The term *razza* began to appear in official writings, including the birth registers of Santa Lucia, around this same time. Like everyone else, Italian Jews had joined the fascist party in large numbers, and there had been Jewish *squadristi* in the fascist squads early in the movement. Internal exile to the south or islands had been instituted in the 1920s for political opponents, some of whom were Jewish, but systematic policies against Jews were not instituted until just before the war.[12] Although it cannot be said that Italian culture was devoid of racism, racism was not a fundamental part of rational integral reclamation or biological politics—although it did find an outlet in the colonization attempts in East Africa beginning in 1935. Yet even there, alongside brutal attempts to physically eliminate the opposition on racial grounds and the creation of laws proscribing sexual contact with the native population, there was a high degree of immersion in local life together with many mixed romantic relationships and marriages.[13]

Italy's lesser concern for safeguarding the "racial" characteristics of the population may have been due in part to a relative lack of immigrants and ethnic differences, as well as the slow growth of the working class considered so decrepit and deviant in other countries. The science of eugenics was late to organize in Italy and was strongly influenced by Catholicism. It would have been unthinkable to alienate the Church and the public by suggesting that some people should not reproduce. Nevertheless, the biological essentialism infusing the natural and social sciences since Spencer's and Darwin's time did find expression in Italian ideas about procreation and gender roles. The ideas of nineteenth-century anthropologists such as Cesare Lombroso and philosophers including the Romagnan Alfredo Oriani established a "natural" separation between maternity as an altruistic, instinctive function, and paternity as a sentiment that strongly affected fascist pronatalist rhetoric and policy.[14]

The Politicization of Marriage and Procreation

Reactions to Materialism, Neomalthusianism, and Feminism

We have seen that the simple, arduous life of the countryside—that "human breeding ground"—was considered healthier both physically and morally than the life of the city. The low natality rates in the urban areas were alarming not only because of demographic consequences but also because they reflected the spread of undesirable values. Fabbri was one of many who criticized urbanites for having deserted the countryside in search of stimulation, comfort, and economic gain in the city (see 1933b, 1933c). Even if Italy retained higher birthrates now (due to its greater attachment to the earth than other European countries), it was headed for imminent decline as other empires had in the past—thanks to the decadence of city life, which extinguished the individual's sense of responsibility in the perpetuation of the nation.

Women were considered both the primary cause of the dissolution of the family, and its salvation. The feminine spirit and degree of moral elevation were the "barometer" of civilization, which now signaled decay, and were the root of all society's moral and economic hardships.[15] Throughout history, women's refusal to remain within the limits assigned to them by nature had caused children to be raised in disordered and corrupt environments, and nations to perish. Now, women were thought to be corrupted by egoistic sentiments, their maternal instinct suffocated, thanks to the "social homosexuality" resulting from the nineteenth-century tendency to grant women equality with men.

This equality in the intellectual, social, and legal fields, as well as work, science, public life, and sports, created an "antibiological" and neo-malthusianist femininity leading women away from their historic mission. The odious "nineteenth-century mother," unfortunately seen often in everyday life, considered her responsibility finished once the umbilical cord was cut; she was "so-called emancipated, Americanized," and "very probably even holds some record or is fairly popular in her social circle."[16] This kind of self-indulgence was contrary to the ideology of sacrifice at the basis of the "true" female spirit, with its sentiments of the family, religion, and patria.

A most disturbing distortion arising from "social homosexuality" was a challenge to the position of the husband as the head of the family and marriage. Federico Marconcini, economics professor at the University of Turin and the Catholic University of Milan, and winner of the Royal Prize of the Italian Academy for his book *Culle vuote* (Empty cribs), explained that this destroyed unity in a "dispersion of spirits" that created a mutilated form of paternity. Cohabitation was transformed into a "banal and, in final analysis, tedious relationship of sexuality as an end in itself, no longer stretched toward the offspring which is the sole source of its only nobility" (1935:330). It was the woman who paid the "most immediate and painful price" for this contract-type marriage and calculated reproduction, in few or no pregnancies and the loss of that "singularly hers and highly noble function of vestal of her husband's dignity" (1935:321).

When women deviated from their destiny of giving life, not making a living, they formed a "third sex: true monstrosity . . . which, beyond making nature deviate, destroys the womanly fascination, which is the most potent incentive and stimulus which the eternal feminine can exercise upon all of humanity."[17] The figure of woman had defined Italian life since Roman times and was now the most potent means for the rebirth of the nation. It was time to return woman to her mission, reconsecrating the cult of the civic virtues and giving her a modern upbringing and practical education in the art of governing the house. This was the base of the new civilization.

The state would lead the way, in contrast to the liberal individualistic nineteenth-century European state. The latter had been indifferent to ethics, morality, and religion. It was therefore an accomplice in the demise of the institution of the family through rapid industrialization, urbanization, and the hedonistic social conception of liberalism and socialism. By constructing nationalism, economics, and politics as the only sources of individual influence in social life, the state had failed to honor parenthood and the family as the cell of the nation and its social concerns. Marconcini explained that materialist individualism, the "dominant formula of the nineteenth century," poisoned marriage with the "excessive pathogens of calculation and rationalized artifice" (1935:278, 321).

Now, fascism had burst out of the sacrifice and heroic virtues of the First World War, as a reaction to individualism and materialism that revived the sentiment of the family. Panunzio described it as the "philosophy of discipline, of morality and of the spirit; against every affirmation of individualism, anarchy, egoism, immorality and philosophical and social materialism" (1933:135). The institution of the family, that primordial nucleus of the nation and its continuation in history, was the "bridge of passage" crossing the liberal distinction between individual and society, politics and morality. This bridge allowed the individual to become "an element of society and therefore at the same time factor and instrument of the state—means and end of the state" (Fabbri 1933b:141).

Fascism was the opposite of both bourgeois mercantile liberalism and materialistic democratic socialism, both of which shared the same spiritual foundation in individualism. This was why neomalthusianism appealed to the wealthy and the socialist and working classes alike. The family was attacked on both sides, as a bundle of social and economic interests independent of the state and also as an institution to be destroyed together with private property and the Church; and the Roman concept of marriage was denied in favor of free love, state marriage, divorce, and promiscuity. Fascism instead upheld indissoluble marriage, as the natural destiny of Rome and the fulfillment of divine law: it protected women and gave their lives meaning, elevated the spouses spiritually, and connected the individual to the state through the formation of the family.

According to fascist thinkers, the false individualism of bourgeois and materialist thinking brought a loss of true liberty, justice, and individuality. The fascist concept of indissoluble marriage did the opposite, for matrimony, family, and paternity represented the true, ethical individuality. Fascism provided the spiritual and moral conditions that strengthened the family and honored the mother and child as the supreme values of the national stock. As the Romagnan journalist and later Minister of Propaganda Giorgio Pini explained, liberty meant consciousness of necessity, not some individualistic, physical concept. The body was imprisoned to liberate the spirit, protecting indissoluble marriage: this was the spiritual democracy of true civilization (1923:6–7).

Justice, the "essential ethic of our national state," was realized through the natural, individual fact of love applied toward the organization of society. Marriage was "the most ancient manifestation of justice," while divorce represented revolt. Where divorce, free love, and the contractual conception of marriage were common, the woman lost her individuality and lust replaced chastity as the spouses worked toward their own interest and enjoyment. "Then everything considered the woman, wife, concubine, or prostitute, reduced instrument of the senses and article of fashion, loses any superior destination" (Pini 1923:31).

Fascist ideology upheld private property and indissoluble marriage by claiming to purify and renovate bourgeois capitalist civilization and its odious individualistic democratic spirit. That is, "it is exactly the quality of corrective of nature that legitimizes matrimony and makes it noble, inasmuch as, as in work and property, love must subject itself to justice" (Pini 1923:29). This conception justified unprecedented intervention in individual and family life. Unlike liberal theory and practice, by nature fascism tended to subject the needs of the individual to the state, "even certain private needs. . . . As the single individual must frame himself in the family, so the family frames itself in the state which interferes in it from its origin, matrimony, just as the family interferes in the individual from birth" (37).

Paternal Fulfillment and Maternal Sacrifice in the Fruit
and Scope of Marriage

Beyond intervention in marriage, the state had a duty to intervene in procreation and child rearing, for the nation depended upon regeneration. All of fascist political action was premised upon a "moral atmosphere of faith and passion" that reconducted individuals and families back to their God-given mission and historic function of procreating and raising children for the state. "The fascist accepts, loves life . . . understands life as duty, elevation, conquest; life must be high and full: lived for itself, but above all for others, near and far, present and future" (Mussolini, in Fabbri 1933b:141).

This implied different things for women and men. For men, procreation was a natural right and religious and patriotic duty that fortified and immortalized their personality. A man who sought only immediate material pleasures and comforts or avoided sacrifice by forgoing reproduction "not only limits every possibility of descendence, but proscribes to himself every reason for being: and he fades away in the shadows of nothingness."[18] As Mussolini said, paternity represented the "joy and pride of being 'continued' as individual, as family and as populace" (1928:22). Mussolini added a new twist to Hegel's statement that he is not a man who is not a father (*"non è uomo chi non è padre"*) by saying that he is also not a fascist if not a father: *"non è fascista chi non è padre."* Recalling a Roman expression, he argued that paternity made man an effective member of the family and society: *"terra proles valida gens."*[19]

While man was a whole and complete (*integrale*) person—political, economic, religious, holy, and a warrior—woman was a mother, pure and simple. Man's glory depended upon her self-sacrifice and self-effacement through productive housework, withdrawal from the labor force, and denial of cerebral or physical pleasure. Woman's main responsibility was to keep her place as his constant, silent, hidden support and companion, the light or flame stimulating and directing him in his daily struggles and most arduous and noble conquests. She must absent herself from the struggle for existence made of toil, efforts, and movement, for she had neither the temperament nor the physical capacities for it.

Woman's heroism came not from being able to excel at sports or drinking contests, or working for emancipation. Instead, it was "feeling herself tear at the spasm of the live fleshes, to give birth to a new life," accepting the humility and tedium of domestic life, and contenting herself with her station rather than striving for material improvement. It meant raising her children to high moral standards and "with serene and conscious acceptance" submitting herself and her mind to he who, "accepted one day by her, became from that day and forever the leader of her and her house."[20] She and her children were the "continuous and living bridge" between man and his future.[21] Woman "sheds, universally, the sublime joy of paternity."[22]

The woman who renounced motherhood or performed her duties badly would lose her right to dignity and legitimate pride in the national strength. She could be a genius, but she would not be a woman, and she would be plagued by intimate, unconfessed regrets and unhappiness in proportion to the distance by which she removed herself from sacrifice. One extreme view was that, instead of admiring the beautiful Lesbia of Catulla, it would be better to idolize the chaste Alcesti of Euripedes, the veiled wife who guarded the hearth and was devoted to her husband and children to the point of self-immolation.[23] Pende said that the principles of the fascist revolution would be reached, the reconstructive power of its values completely successful, when the newly germinated Italian woman brought up fascistically "will know how to assume her true place of responsibility in the important office which nature assigns her as one of the most delicate and most fruitful motors of the state machine" (1933a:97).

Predictably, agricultural metaphors were brought to bear in the assertion that paternity made the father a man through the complete possession of the mother implied in fertilization. Man dropped the seed in the furrow he had plowed. Woman held the fertilized seed and organized its sprouting, keeping the sower attached to the earth through the fruit of the union. Beyond this, woman was said to have a centralizing hereditary role in altruistically conserving the biological characteristics and useful variations of the species. Through procreation, she meanwhile contributed to the development of the husband's personality, served as the socializer of children and men, and perfected her own body, making it more beautiful and pleasing to man. She united herself to her husband in a single flesh, in both physiological and psychological terms, as in the Indian proverb: "Man is a half man, the woman also half. Only father and mother with their child form a whole man."[24]

In return for his sacrifice in becoming a father, man deserved by natural right not only to relive and continue in time through the child, but also to possess it spiritually, etching the imprint of his own personality on its spirit. The mother must not obstruct him, for, in Marconcini's words, "where the woman denies and subtracts herself from the personality of the man, paternity conserves prickly or few charms" (1935:330). Yet, as Fabbri pointed out, man should appreciate the gift woman makes of herself, feeling the religion and respect of maternity, of "she who gave birth to him loving him in the pain . . . of she who would every minute give to him her life which she has already offered him being born, of she who will present herself comforter to his dying spirit together with the divine light of mercy and forgiveness" (1933a:94).

Pende was more revealing of contemporary men's frustrations and desires when he complained that, regrettably, modern women were nothing like his own mother (1933a:211). He explained that woman should always be maternal with man, for man always needed to feel the "warm and strong heart of a mother" by his side, "even when the winter of life has brought white snow upon his tired head" (1933a:122). As we will see, this yearning for a generation that was turning toward the sunset contradicted the effort to make women approach mothering with a forward-looking scientific rationality. The rigid sexual division of rights and duties in the family contradicted the reality that it was women who mainly directed the household, and it was through them that the state sought to reach into family life.

Scientific Mothering

In keeping with the emphasis on procreation and the protection and improvement of children—now viewed as highly valuable to the future of the nation—fascist public assistance programs reached out to mothers not for their own benefit but for the good of their children. It was better to help an undernourished or otherwise physically compromised mother obtain a "healthy product of conception" today than provide for a deficient or sickly child tomorrow.[25] In Fabbri's words, "the 'mother' is not assisted inasmuch as she is such, but in that the child must be assisted through her person" (1933c:68).

By accepting state intervention, mothers not only demonstrated that their lives aimed to a higher end, the national interest, but also produced healthy and robust offspring that would be useful to the Patria. Public assistance had new meaning now that the state assumed an obligation to assist the poor and disadvantaged, but this was done less out of charity than to protect society against passive and parasitic people. Assistance would produce morally conscious and physically robust citizens who would be useful and productive in the rebirth of the nation.[26]

For example, ONMI was considered an institution not of charity but prevention. Its primary duty was the coordination of the "obligations incumbent upon families," in the context of vigilance and propaganda working toward the physical and moral improvement of the population. ONMI was absolutely central to demographic increase, for it aimed to form in mothers a hygienic-sanitary consciousness that reinforced the nation's vital force and brought to the Patria numerous, healthy, and robust children.

The assumptions behind the moral and physical education of girls and boys reflected the ideas discussed above. The "total man of tomorrow" would be raised as an active worker and potential soldier on the rational, practical base that Pende called "orthogenetic harmony of muscles, hearts, and brains" (1939:2). The orthogenetic formation of the total woman, that is, the "woman mother or maternal woman," was its complement. Woman's part of sharing in the work of the social machine meant being full of abnegation and altruism in the family and society. Her development aimed for a "complete and harmonic" woman who was prepared for the demands of the feminine aesthetic and vanity and also her domestic and procreative functions.

Girls should no longer learn abstract or sublime subjects such as complicated poems at school, but instead be taught practical skills for motherhood. From the first days of childhood, the true meaning of the attributes of their sex should be instilled in their "ingenuous and inexpert spirit"

(Pende 1933a:210). This would teach them that they cannot turn over their psychology and physiology to egoistic ends without moral and physical damage. In middle and high school, they would study the "triple science" of woman, child, and house, and Pende even envisioned college degrees in these subjects to force women to abandon "masculine" studies and professions (1939:4).

For already grown women, it was necessary to teach courses on infant care, childhood education, and domestic economics. Courses were directed at young industrial workers and farm women. They approached housekeeping and child rearing as scientific subjects based on the disciplines of hygiene, industrial chemistry, technology of commerce, and educational science. Women were taught to observe simplicity, order, and precision in their duties, making themselves an *orario* (schedule). According to the Fascist Confederation of Industrial Workers (CFLI), "this means to know the exact time required for every operation and to always do them in the same succession" (1940:300). In this way, fascist women demonstrated that they were well-informed and capable mothers.

Here too there was a contradiction, for the foundation of the domestic economy was said to be women's natural good sense and spirit of sacrifice and dedication, but they had to be directed in their activities and taught how to go about them. They were to make do with whatever they had, but at the same time they were exposed to new domestic implements and standards of order and cleanliness. Further, although women were elevated in their role in the achievement of national goals as producers and educators of children, their social worth did not emerge from their own person but from their association with children and men. They were to be exalted, but at the same time effaced. For their part, men were to command within the hierarchy of the family, but submit to lifelong service in the military hierarchy of the state.

Biopolitical Interpretations of Hyponatality, Defeminization, and Work

Causes of Hyponatality

The most widely blamed cause of low birthrates or "hyponatality" was urbanization. The great modern cities were compared to malignant tumors that initially exalted the functions of the body but finished by irradiating outward and killing it. As Mussolini observed, the city drew the country population into itself and rendered it infecund like the preexisting population, presaging the demise of all society. "The fields are deserted, but when the desert extends its abandoned folds, the metropolis is taken by the throat: neither its commercial enterprises, nor its industries, nor its oceans of rock and reinforced concrete can restabilize the equilibrium by now irreparably broken: it is the catastrophe." The city dies, and since the nation no longer has the "vital saps of youth of the new generations" but is composed of "vile and aged people," it cannot resist the younger populations of rapidly multiplying "races of color" pressing at its borders (1928:9–10).

The mechanism by which urbanization reduced fertility was, to many experts, above all biological and medical. Pende called the past half-century of declining natality a "progressive disease" (1933a:191). Since marriage rates were not declining, but the fertility rate in the first year after marriage was, it seemed to them that the "white" races were undergoing a biological weakening of procreative capacity. At the core of this was the concept of gracility we met in the last chapter. In the strictest sense, gracility referred to the appearance and apparently low physical resistance of people suffering from or predisposed to tuberculosis, but it came to apply to anyone with an anemic weakness or thin or waifish form. There was a frequent contrast made between gracile urban women and robust country women. The former were moving ever farther from the higher birthrates and healthier life-styles, values, and reproductive systems of rural women.

Urban social diseases such as tuberculosis, syphilis, malnutrition, exposure to toxic fumes in industry, and alcoholism were blamed for sterility, loss of pregnancy, and birth defects. Both sexes were said to be affected, causing huge differences in family size across current generations. In addition, women's behavior contributed to biological change. Homemakers suffered from a "poverty" of menstrual blood, due to the fact that because of electricity they had the habit of making night into day and day into night, causing a defect in ultraviolet radiation leading to anemia and chlorosis. Working women's labor and work environment lowered their resistance, allowing for the establishment of diseases such as tuberculosis. They had lower stature and body weight, less muscular strength, poorer menstrual flow, and puberty delayed by one to one and a half years. Finally, urban life brought nervous disorders, from hysterism to impotence from sexual neurasthenia. The noises, "hyper-excitations," continuous stimulation, and excesses of pleasure of urban life affected the nervous system of city dwellers, with their "unreal dreamy ideals" and artificial way of life.[27]

Gini proposed another theory for fertility decline. He argued that individuals, like the cells of an organism, had variable reproductiveness, in strict negative relationship with social class (which he defined as wealth, position, and residence in the city) (1930:21).[28] As races, groups, and nations moved through the parabola of evolution with variable velocity, so families that elevated themselves above the others and became the germ of the leading classes presented the "organic characteristics of decadence" in advance (1930:26). The force of their genetic instincts waned, bending the mind to the persuasive arguments of reason and rendering it satisfied with a scanty family size. They were left with the "illusion of not wanting that which, without forcing nature, they could not obtain" (1930:27). It was decidedly *not* birth control practices—whose ineffectiveness reached as high as 84 percent—that caused fertility decline, but physiological change.

Gini cited international scientific literature proving that the intellectual or "cerebral" classes were weakened in their "genetic instincts" and procreative capacities. Studies of British and American women found them inadequate with respect to sexual desire and plagued by "disgust or repulsion for sexual relations." Cerebral women used birth control methods much more often than the general population, proving that those who resorted to them were the same ones who were most frigid and abnormal anyway. They were found to have a "strongly acidic" vaginal fluid and inadequately alkaline cervical secretions. Their fecundity was limited to a part of the menstrual cycle, and their passivity or particular body position during coitis independently interfered with fertilization. Cerebral men's fertilizing "power" was likewise reduced through weak sexual excitement in coitis and a diminution in the quantity of alkaline prostatic liquid needed for the stimulation of spermatocytes. These physiological effects were to be feared because they could work at the population level through a generalized increase in cerebralism (1930:37–38).

An alternative view of fertility decline inculpated social forces directly. Marconcini attributed the discrepancy between a stable impulse to marry and a declining desire to have children to economic decline, women's work, and the demise of religious and traditional values. The prominent demographer Giorgio Mortara pointed out that marital fertility rates had fallen too swiftly to be accounted for by physiological factors. The 21 percent reduction in a quarter century must be due to voluntary limitation of births, which had already existed at the turn of the century (1933:37). The abominable neomalthusianist propaganda and practices such as repeat abortions were most common in cities near the borders with northern Europe such as Trieste, whereas cities like Venice that were not in communication with other centers retained higher natality rates.[29]

More commonly, social forces were thought to interact with biological ones, for changes in morality and behavior manifested themselves in biological defects of female development and maternal aptitudes. Urban sterility was fundamentally the result of late marriage, the egoism of the spouses and the estrangement of woman from the hearth, pursuit of material pleasures, and the dissolution of the family through adultery, separation, celibacy, libertinism, and neomalthusianism. The "stupidity of very

many feminine souls unconsciously imbued with feminist theories" made
women aspire to a job permitting independence and personal gain, but this
conducted them away from the womanly spirit of sacrifice and acceptance
of the responsibilities inherent in parenthood.[30]

Indeed, the odious agglomeration of women for factory or office
employment brought the maximum of "feminine delinquency" compared
to homemaking or work in the fields. It fostered "shameless discourse"
and "reciprocal sexual excitement," and it opened the way to neomalthusianism, prostitution, and diseases of vice.[31] "One woman alone, can be an
angel: two women together, are less than two angels: many women
together, with daily contact, for a long period of time, in the hangars of a
factory . . . are material in a state of permanent demoralizing fermenta-
tion."[32] Some jobs such as tobacco processing exacerbated the problem
through their abortifacient and sterilizing effect, or by introducing toxins
into the body. Echoing the word of the day, Pende concluded that factory
labor could not be compatible with "the conservation of good aptitudes of
the body and spirit for maternity and the rational rearing of offspring"
(1933a:135).

Defeminization

The biological consequences of urbanization, women's work, and ideologies such as materialism, feminism, and neomalthusianism were thought
to arise from women's different "biological reality." This reality was
rooted in women's role as conservator of the biological characteristics of
the species and in their particular physiological and psychological composition. As Pende said, it was a "biological truth" that men and women were
"born to complete one another, not to equal one another" (1933a:102).
The physician Gelli—rather an extremist, but one with a respectable position as professor at the obstetrics clinic at the University of Florence—
argued that evidence from modern anatomy, physiology, anthropology,
and psychology confirmed the "natural, primitive, innate, and therefore
instinctive concept" shared by religious belief that the role of woman was
as complement and companion of man (1931:4). To him, the difference
between the male and female destinies explained all morphological and
behavioral differences between women and men, from fetal heart rates to
skin color, from sleep patterns to tolerance of pain.

By emphasizing women's "proper place" and "first and fundamental
nature" in maternity, fascist medical writers pointed out the futility and
"absurdity" of international arguments for gender equality. Women did
not share men's somatic and psychical aptitudes and were justifiably to be
excluded from equal social duties, including work and civic responsibilities. Woman lacked man's robustness and was not adapted for the domi-

nation and exploitation of the world. Like a child, she had less strength and speed, and a lesser respiratory and cardiac capacity.[33]

Indeed, the size, shape, weight, and functioning of the brain were said to be of absolutely lesser value in woman, making her a being intermediate between a boy and a man.[34] Moreover, her endocrine system influenced her in a preponderant way, activating her "natural" functions at a loss to her cerebral ones. This explained both the negative consequences of intellectualism and women's lack of success in the arts and sciences—even if there had always been individual women capable of exercising all of the male professions very well. Modern environment, upbringing, and training may be changing woman's tendencies, but could never transcend the "insurmountable obstacles" of her organic constitution and the natural laws regulating all female functions (Gelli 1931:31). Once she appreciated her true nature compared to man, and her place and duties in the nation-state, she would comprehend the necessity of procreation and breast-feeding for her happiness and physical well-being.

Women's participation in sports, bourgeois leisure activities and fashions, work, and "male" behaviors such as smoking and drinking was inebriating them with an idea of their own independence and will, but this caused a woeful *sfemminilizzazione* (defeminization) or masculinization that made them less attractive and useful to society. Gelli went so far as to suggest that women who espoused feminist ideas were like lesbians, or indeed were lesbians, often being ugly aged-looking girls and badly married women liked by neither men nor women (1931:31, 35). Further, women who renounced breast-feeding caused homosexuality in the next generation. That is, since the mother's body adapted itself to the sex of the child, to deny it her milk or to give it milk from the mother of an opposite-sex child was to create a "state of physical and psychical neutrality," an indifference to the satisfaction of sexual desire (1931:944).

Given their particular essence, women should seek to develop their bodies in ways different from men, as Pende explained. Men were destined to intellectual, artistic, and muscular effort, causing greater development above the waist. By contrast, the "normal woman" should be more developed between the waist and knees, and have a much more delicate face, neck, shoulders, thorax, arms, and lower legs. Her thyroid kept her upper half in check while her ovary stimulated the bottom half: the "strength" of the latter determined fecundity and the degree to which the width of the hips predominated over the shoulders. Through successive rounds of gestation and breast-feeding, the body approached the maternal shape ever more, except that during breast-feeding the upper body was favored so that the child could be nourished, cradled, and carried. The reign of femininity then extended from the region of the ovary to the heart, from instinct to altruism: and the woman truly became a mother (1933a: 111–14).

These arguments were a reaction to the "cult of the *maschietta*"—the mania for a boyish figure—which fascist writers blamed upon the "perverse" antinationalistic fashion, art, and literature coming from cities to the north.[35] Whatever their origins, new cultural ideals showed up all over women's magazines (such as *Cordelia, Rassegna Femminile,* or *Vita Femminile*). They were embraced by bourgeois women whose economic well-being allowed them to live up to rising standards of female attractiveness as well as maternal devotion to home and children. Fascist policies even contributed to new attitudes and activities, for sports were heavily promoted in the schools, military, after-work organizations, and professional and amateur competitions, and became more popular among both men and women.

To reconcile the apparent opposition between maternity and desirability, it was necessary to make the ideal body type the "inevitable" maternal shape seen in great Renaissance art exalting mothers with "potent thighs" and babies at their breasts, and in sacred images of nursing mothers "irradiated with sweetness." To try to remain attractive, including attenuating the effects of childbearing on the figure, was considered a worthy activity, so long as women emphasized maternal attributes and avoided becoming costly and parasitic to their husbands.[36] Women were reminded that they could not defy the laws of nature, for almost every part of the body, external and internal, was irreparably changed by maternity. One female writer comforted pregnant women by saying that their husbands would "like you better like this, with the figure which gets a little heavier . . . with all of that shadow of suffering and tiredness that falls every bit more to veil that triumphant splendor of youth which fascinated him until yesterday, and whose passing eclipse renders you still more tenderly dear and sacred to him."[37]

Given their persistence to the present day, we will make note of a couple of ideas about women's athletics. One was that an athletic or trim figure with long or muscular "disharmonic" legs was biologically contrary to reproduction, for the insufficient and abnormal ovarian function at its base also caused deficient development of the uterus. The other idea was that participation in sports and other "masculine" activities rendered women involuntarily sterile. Their participation in abusive, competitive, irrational exercise, whether before or after marriage, invariably caused "aesthetic deformation," particularly muscle-tendon enlargement, and defective sexual and reproductive functioning. Like literature, theater, and radio, it also tended to cause harmful erotic feelings in women, due to their greater "physiological absorption" in the sexual life. Cycling and equitation were singled out as giving particular stimulus to the genitals and provoking harmful nervous disorders.

However, women should not be completely inactive, either. Some physical activity such as walking was highly useful to women, as to all people, so long as it was not done to the point of tiredness—much less exhaustion. To suit their body type and abilities, women's exercise aimed for agility, rhythmic coordination, and development of the lower body. Some experts such as Pende preferred light stretching exercises in place of all sports, but most allowed a measure of exertion in activities such as dance, swimming, skiing, skating, racquet sports, or fencing. A new term arose in the medical literature, *ginnastica medica* (medical exercise), which became a favorite topic of physicians writing about maternity. ONMI training courses for physicians and surgeons included a section on the topic. The idea was that exercise, like so many other things, should be supervised by physicians. It could be used as a treatment for gracility or other conditions, but must never be entrusted to women's caprice or personal pleasure.

The "Antithesis" between Maternity and Work

Like sports, work outside the home or family farm was considered harmful to fertility and maternal functions. Political demography sought to channel female labor into a few acceptable fields, but mostly homemaking, child care, and volunteer work. This was said to respect women's reproductive physiology and genetically endowed character, especially the traits of altruism and self-sacrifice. It was a step toward the "preparation of future mothers," with biological, economic, and moral components and consequences. That is, the "protection" of working women through maternity insurance, breaks for nursing, and exclusion from dangerous jobs was a response to truly harmful working conditions, but also an explicit attempt to remove them from the workplace.

Women were refusing to be the "angels of the hearth" demanded by religious and political ideals. It was undeniable that many women worked out of economic necessity, that industrialization had been accomplished through female labor, and that during the war women had admirably performed every possible kind of profession. They were now employed throughout government, the professions, and industry and commerce. Yet, reactionaries argued that this was no longer in the national interest. Women were trying to suppress the predominance of man and invade his field without restriction, out of sheer vanity. It was time to root out this "cancer," for it was the direct cause of male unemployment and insufficient male salaries.

Interestingly, some writers found it necessary to argue for wage parity, in spite of themselves. The discrepancy between male and female wages reached a maximum during the interwar period, and everyone knew that women were a main element of low production cost.[38] As a result, to remove the financial incentive to employ women, it would be necessary to increase the cost of their labor.

As in other times and places in the Western world, postwar labor competition corresponded with a flood of studies demonstrating that maternity, or femininity itself, was incompatible with work.[39] As a result, the most commonly cited reason for excluding women from most jobs was that they were both ill-suited for them and gravely harmed by them. Work weakened and broke women's "organism" physically, morally, and spiritually, at a great cost to their sentimental and reproductive capacities. Conception took place under serious physiological alterations, and the offspring was always sickly, deteriorating if not assisted in time and subject to a high mortality rate. Moreover, poor working women left their children all day with inexpert persons or in day-care centers or schools, or else abandoned in the streets to gather all possible moral and physical contagions.

Reform of the labor legislation to safeguard women's reproductive functions was considered an essential complement to land reclamation in the bonifica integrale. It was especially important to protect young women, married or unmarried, who made up the majority of the female work force in industry and commerce. The ideal was to limit women's work to a minimum, severely restrict it in difficult and unhealthy jobs, and entirely prohibit it for pregnant and nursing women and mothers with children under two years of age.

Scientific interest in the dangers of women's work emerged not only in the context of postwar labor competition but also an expanding role for physicians in the workplace. Physicians were instrumental in the "scientific" rationalization of work hailed by industrialists and government leaders. This did not simply mean industrial standardization, but instead the maximization of worker efficiency through understanding the effects of fatigue, providing technical instruction to young people, and matching workers to jobs appropriate to their constitution, temperament, and health. This would keep *ogni uomo al suo giusto posto* (every man in his proper place). Pende pointed out that in bee society, "that most perfect animal organization," the female that procreated was exempted from work, while female workers were not fit to be fertilized (in Lorenzoni 1933:71).

Women's work, whether manual or intellectual, combined with domestic labor, gestation, and breast-feeding, was said to cause exhaustion and excessive, early wear and tear of the maternal organism. This led to organic weakness, constitutional gracility, lymphatism, chloroanemia, hypergenitalism, and skeletal anomalies, as well as disturbances in the off-spring's development and constitution. Menstrual periods had an effect on workplace performance, while work in turn had a deleterious effect on menstruation, especially if the work involved standing, sitting, or moving all day. Industrial areas had higher rates of gonorrhea and syphilis, which were the leading causes of sterility and of perinatal mortality and stillbirth, respectively. Syphilis was also a factor in a large proportion of premature births and spontaneous abortions. Studies grouped cases of infection according to women's professions, showing the number "caused" by prostitutes, laborers, typists, or shopkeepers.[40]

Urban women were found to be more susceptible to reproductive failures and deficiencies than rural women, including sterility, spontaneous abortion, premature birth, "pathological childbirth," stillbirth, and infant death. In an essay on urbanism and sterility, Cesare Coruzzi attributed these outcomes to "hyper-excitation of the uterine musculature," as well as a "hedonistic sentiment" toward a desired limitation of births (1933:67).

Women's work more than doubled diseases in pregnancy, increased the number of spontaneous abortions by seven times, and raised the number of premature births by four or five times.[41] It also increased the rates of stillbirth and infant death. Industrial workers weighed less than house-wives, and their infants weighed less too. Yet, these infants were also more likely to be overly large and therefore prone to disease. The industrial work environment itself created a predisposition to tuberculosis, which contended with the venereal infections for first place in causing sterility. During both pregnancy and breast-feeding, not only work in itself but also work-related behaviors such as sweating, thinking, or experiencing emotions were said to threaten the health and life of the fetus or nursling.

Working women even had narrower hips. This was considered an aspect of their gracile constitution, causing abnormal pregnancies and frequent spontaneous abortions and premature births.[42] One study found twice as many "*bacini ristretti*" (narrow pelvises) in working city women than other women. Only one-fourth of the former experienced a normal childbirth, which was followed by a difficult and dangerous puerperium because of the "excessive tiredness" of uterine musculature.[43] Women who started working in adolescence were particularly affected, for the work "struck" their physical and mental development as well as maternal functions, delaying development and the onset of puberty.

Certain industries were particularly dangerous for women. The female organism was considered much more susceptible than the male to the action of toxins such as lead, which caused sterility and infant death. The birthrate of women in the mining and textile industries was three times lower than that of the general population. In addition, compulsory work position could cause pelvic distortions. Less than a third of textile workers had a normal birth because of the narrowness of their hips, which was alarming because two-thirds of the workers in this industry were women 14 to 20 years old. Textile workers who began at the age of 14 had higher rates of caesarean section, forceps birth, and surgical intervention in childbirth than women in general or women who worked in either a sitting or standing position. The pedal-driven sewing machine was extremely damaging to the organism, especially during menstruation and the postpartum period, while a prolonged standing position caused uterine deviations and blocked the return circulation of the lower extremities and lower trunk in pregnancy.

If this were not enough to prove that women were ill-adapted for work, studies showed that women were less productive workers in agriculture, industry, commerce, and the professions. The rhythms of industrial machines were not adapted to the "female organism," for which reason women had more workplace accidents. They had higher disease rates and longer sick leave, even in certain intellectual jobs such as teaching and office work. Studies from the United States were cited to show that, even though they were younger, women died in notably greater numbers than men doing the same work.

What these studies did not take account of was that women were more often employed as unskilled laborers and worked in much worse safety, hygienic, salary, dietary, and housing conditions than men. They were almost entirely denied exposure to fresh air, sunlight, and exercise. Mussolini had this to say about female factory workers: "entering in this enterprise, I am invaded by a wave of disdain in seeing the pitiless machine suck the life out of our girls and young women like a vampire. . . . Their tired aspect, from which is exiled the flower of health, speaks in words not doubts all of the evil which industrialism has worked upon woman" (in DeNapoli 1934b:400).

Rural women's working and living conditions were hardly better. Contemporaries observed that the cost of moving to a cash economy was the physical degradation of and inhuman hardship imposed on farm women and children.[44] Clearly, women continued to do strenuous domestic and extradomestic labor in insalubrious and harmful conditions, irrespective of whatever politicians had to say about the "absolute incompatibility" between maternity and work.

Appropriate Women's Work

We have seen that some politicians and scientists advocated eliminating women's work altogether, for the sake of producing more numerous and healthy children and better wages for men. They believed that women's work (together with increased literacy and education) was the cause of the deplorable feminine ignorance in housekeeping and maternal functions behind the higher infant mortality rates of the industrialized areas. They succeeded in passing laws that severely limited women's employment in upper-level schools and the national government, although they had little practical effect.

Most people recognized the economic reasons why women had to work, and why employers often preferred them. Fabbri even argued that it was wrong to see women only as housewives, when instead the widening of their horizons should be welcomed—so long as they do not act the suffragette and renounce their femininity (1933a:93). What was needed was to make work less dangerous in the immediate term and more appropriate to the characteristics of women's "organism" in the long term. This would liberate women from the depersonalization of the large industries, which overwhelmed their "harmonic and sentimental mental tendencies" and damaged their maternal instincts and functions.[45] The "civil mobilization of women" would reconduct them into agriculture, artisanry, homemaking, and volunteer work, respecting their natural destiny and allowing them to be productive, not parasitic.

According to Pende, all experts in feminine biopsychology and psychotechnics knew that, because they gave their thoughts and actions a "bath of sentiment," it was difficult for women to work in jobs requiring "cold logic and complete objectivity" or a "creative effort in abstract or theoretical thought." These included most intellectual professions, with the exception of teaching young children. Women could equal or better men in jobs requiring "meticulousness, veneration for detail, analytic spirit, patience, [and] rather automatic repetition of movements, ideas, commands" (1933a:131). They should be preferred for certain positions in public and private administration, not just because they were paid less but because these jobs matched their aptitudes and were free of harmful occupational conditions. The best jobs were manual and artisan, especially those of the needle. "Here is the true and narrow field of women's work, where the woman can reign sovereign and is truly in her proper place" (1933a:134).

Even if it were possible to remove women from the work force, it would be wrong to make them idle housewives. They must become active and productive citizens, working just as hard at housework and child care. As Pende put it, woman should be a little sister and intelligent adviser to man, not a parasite on him (1933a:106). This meant that bourgeois women who neither engaged in productive labor nor reproduced were the worst of parasites, on their husbands and society. Those who denied the "sole function" for which they were created, even if only by renouncing breast-feeding, would suffer in every way for their unnatural behavior (1933a:129,

208). Well-off women who had servants were to make themselves useful in charity work and the direction of the house, both of which required the "intelligence and heart and spirit of sacrifice and abnegation, which only a woman, above all if well-born and well-formed, can reunite in a harmonic synthesis of human virtue" (1933a:136).

Women, especially well-off women, were invited to carry out much of the political demographic program, continuing the tradition of wartime volunteers. The regime would compensate them for all that had apparently been lost in political life by providing them a sense of dignity and value in the family, schools, organizations, and entire society. The fine white hand that would otherwise be playing tennis, bridge, or the piano would now be engaged in laudable activities such as providing hospital assistance to pregnant women, helping workers obtain paid rest before and after childbirth, and assisting women living abroad to return for childbirth. They would sew clothes for children, provide food and clothing to the poor, and work in day-care centers, youth organizations, evening schools for illiterate adults, after-work programs for adolescents, and sanatoriums, outdoor schools, and camps for convalescent and sick children.

The very heart of maternal activity was participation in the *fasci femminili* (women's leagues). These were the theoretical complement of the men's *fasci di combattimento*, but by the mid-1920s they had already been stripped of any political dimension. Instead, they were to focus upon social and moral concerns. Much of their work was related to ONMI, whose moral and material assistance was "naturally" provided by female committee members and social workers. Women from the fasci staffed ONMI maternal refectories serving meals and snacks to pregnant and nursing women, and organized local "obstetrical guards" of midwives and physicians. They volunteered to visit pregnant and needy women in their homes. The fascist woman's role as conduit between state ideology and the families was considered the purest expression of Italian womanhood and the outcome of Mussolini's call for her to "go toward the populace." In fact, professional midwives who were not registered in the fasci could be excluded from competition for a posting, as Santandrea (1992:28) describes from her own experience in 1927.

Women's volunteer and technical participation in the fasci and other organizations was directed, however, by paid, mostly male, political, governmental, and medical officials. The female element was considered the most efficacious in the practical field, while the male element represented the intellectual, political, and moral force of the nation. It was the male side that gave women a military-like training in volunteerism and professionalism for their civic, educational, and domestic duties. Charity work and homemaking thereby became regimented, productive, precise, and orderly, much like the paid labor women were urged to renounce. This naturally extended to breast-feeding and infant care, as we shall see.

Institutions and Legislation of Fascist Political Demography

Legislating Morality

The reconciliation of the state and Church in the Concordato or Lateran Pacts was considered a "masterpiece" or "stronghold" of fascist politics. It felicitously solved the "Roman question" of the balance of power between the two and removed one of the historical relics—antireligiosity—that weighed most on Italian life. The Concordato was described as the logical outcome of the reawakening of religious sentiment brought about by the war and fascism, and the merging of politics with morality. It was the expression and elevation of the traditions and values of the populace toward a single moral-spiritual end and at the same time would allow education and religion to reach where the law could not or was insufficient. Together with the bonifica integrale, it was a demographic law per eccellenza and ushered in a new phase of the fascist revolution.[46]

In practical terms, the Concordato reaffirmed the indissolubility of marriage by reuniting religious and state marriage through a change to the civil code. This meant that couples no longer had to go through two different ceremonies if they wished to have a church wedding. Morality was policed or coaxed in many other ways as well. As early as 1926, a commission was formed to protect the family against the dangers of neomalthusianism. One of its products was a public security law that outlawed publication of statements in newspapers or other periodicals about how to prevent fertilization or interrupt pregnancy. This was subsequently incorporated into the penal code drafted by Justice Minister Alfredo Rocco. Early in the 1930s, the Rocco Code, together with new public security legislation and a new civil code, provided both punitive and repressive measures protecting the morality of the family and infancy, and the health and integrity of the stirpe.[47] This included suppression of modern literature, the seed of out-of-control proliferation of the feminist mentality.

Crimes against family morality were divided into four categories: sterilization; promotion of birth control methods; willful spreading of syphilis and gonorrhea; and procured abortion. These crimes carried prison sentences and fines, which were higher for health professionals and for particular circumstances. For example, punishment for abortion reached up to 20 years imprisonment if the woman was under 14, persuaded by violence or deceit, or died or suffered a bodily lesion. On the other hand, the sentence could be reduced by half or one-third if the abortion was procured to save the honor of the woman or her family. The Church further punished abortion by having bishops excommunicate women and those who helped them if they reached their desired effect and by denying church burial to any woman who died as a result.

Other provisions that protected indissoluble marriage and patriarchal authority included prison sentences for the crimes of bigamy, adultery of the wife, and the husband's keeping a concubine in the family house or notoriously elsewhere. "Crimes against family morality" such as incest or the publication of offensive materials were punished with imprisonment and fines, respectively. In addition, there were crimes against family status (failure to report or misreporting of births or their civil status) and crimes against family assistance (abuse of disciplinary methods, failure to provide for children).

Through social and economic incentives, the regime sought to favor large families tended by dutiful and informed mothers and reduce women's need to earn an income. There were financial awards for engagements, marriages (with a free honeymoon in Rome), and births. Married men and men with children were favored in housing, transportation, taxation, employment, and government job competitions and promotions. The most directly punitive measure was the annual tax on unmarried men. Births were honored with a white ribbon attached to the main door of the house, and there were prizes for good mothering. An annual "Day of the Mother and Child" on Christmas eve brought prizes to the largest families in every city, while the mother of the largest family of each province was brought to Rome the previous day to be received by Mussolini.

Although the prevailing postwar idea is that these measures involved small sums of money and were ineffective, many people remember otherwise. In fact, the cash award for the largest families each year was greater than the average annual salary of a skilled worker. Townspeople in Santa Lucia often point out that one of the wealthiest families today used to be one of the poorest. They stopped the Duce on his way through town to show him their many children, and thanks to his gift of cash they have prospered ever since.

Ruralization and "Rational Human Reclamation"

Fascist moral legislation was complemented by economic support of simple patriarchal families through inheritance laws, credit, and other measures supporting the trades, crafts, and agriculture. For example, the De Stefani law of 1923 protected small farms by abolishing inheritance taxes for relatives of the first two degrees. The enlargement of the National

Organization of Veterans promoted internal colonization, while new territory was opened up for settlement and cultivation by the completion of centuries-old land reclamation projects (*bonifiche*). These included the draining of wetlands and the clearing or reforestation of land throughout the country. Electricity and water systems were extended into the rural areas, together with roads, bridges, and new or renovated buildings, with the goal of diverting people from overly dense areas to new population centers.

The elimination of urbanization and emigration aimed toward the same ends of promoting ruralism and natality. In 1928, prefects were granted the power to create ordinances limiting the growth of urban areas, and emigration was outlawed soon after. This quickly ended an exodus that had reached high numbers since the late nineteenth century and had been encouraged through state financial assistance and rapid passport processing. Within five years of 1930, the emigration rate had dropped by five times. However, the return migration rate also fell by more than three times, in spite of provisions favoring the repatriation of emigrants.

While these measures did not stop internal migration, they did make it difficult for people to find jobs in the cities, as the world-renowned Italian novelist Ignazio Silone shows in the first of two books he wrote while in exile. In *Fontamara,* two country men are unable to find work due to laws prohibiting train travel without a permit, the difficulty in gaining access to the employment office without the proper paperwork, and their misfortune of having been declared ideological enemies of the state.

Although in the larger picture the extent of resettlement was not great, its cultural impact as a propaganda tool was significant. In addition, many people were materially affected, including large numbers of Romagnans. They went to work and settle the Pontine marshes near Rome, but many died from malaria—the scourge of the *bonifiche* and a major public health problem. Others pushed wheelbarrows of dirt from the hills to fill the wetlands in the Po River Valley, and people still sing folk songs about them.

Land reclamation, together with mechanization and agricultural intensification, aimed to maximize the exploitation of the soil and bring agricultural self-sufficiency, symbolized in the "battle for wheat." It was said that since the Italian diet was based upon bread, self-sufficiency in grain production both symbolically and in fact equaled meeting the dietary needs of the population. Annual production of wheat per hectare nearly doubled over the quarter century leading up to 1933, when the battle was won and there were no imports of wheat.

Alongside the *bonifica terriera* of the land, there was the *bonifica umana* of the people. It began with conception, emphasizing the education and surveillance of mothers and small children. The education of young people would prepare them for parenthood in their turn. ONMI, as the central institution of political demography, played an essential role in both of these areas. Its complement was the youth organization created a year later in 1926, the Opera Nazionale Balilla (ONB). Together, the two were widely considered the greatest works of fascist action, though this was said about many initiatives.

The ONB was a military and recreational youth organization charged with the physical and moral education of young people from 6 to 18 years old. Members were divided into subgroups by age and gender. Within two years of its creation, there were one million members in the ONB—a number that grew to 3.5 million by 1933, organized in some 900 leagues. By the early 1940s, nearly the entire population of children and adolescents was involved in the youth organizations. Boys and young men were taught sports, military, and agricultural skills, while girls were taught to become future fascist mothers. The rural focus of the regime was emphasized along with the moral virtues cultivated by bucolic settings.

The ONB provided not only physical education and moral guidance, but also health and work-related insurance as well as scholastic assistance including books, medicine, clothing, and hot meals. There were buildings for youth activities, campgrounds, sports fields, pools, and gymnasiums, numbering in the thousands and serving millions of children each year. The ONB hired physicians, teachers, and physical education instructors, and it organized athletic events and demonstrations. "Intellectual" services included libraries, courses of "culture," theater and choral groups, orchestras, rural schools, schools of domestic economics, and evening schools. These activities permeated the public schools, for children were forced to wear their uniforms in order to participate in sports and extracurricular activities. Health services were provided to millions of children each year through several thousand medical facilities including mountain, riverside, lakeside, and seaside spas. There were thousands of outpatient clinics and emergency medical teams, and hundreds of courses on hygiene.

The Dopolavoro extended the work of ONMI and ONB to adults. The OND was said to provide a moral, social, practical education that would bring adults culturally and professionally up to date and in line with the training of the new generations. Already in the first quarter of 1929, there were more than 1.25 million workers registered in the OND (a number that rose to over 4 million in 1940), and 4.5 million workers participated in OND-sponsored sports, outdoor recreation, arts, and educational events. These activities were part of a larger picture of mass involvement in excursions, sports, and the celebration of *Italianità* through fashion and cuisine that had once been the province of the upper classes and had a significant effect on family life.

Women's Work

As we noted earlier, there was growing consciousness throughout the Continent of the need to protect female workers from dangerous or laborious jobs, especially just after childbirth, and the first reforms of this kind were instituted in Italy in the 1870s. In 1923, night work was outlawed for women in industry, the maternity fund instituted six years earlier was created, and public assistance to infants was reorganized. Employment or "placement offices" were created in 1928. Legislation passed in 1929 and 1930 established maternity leave of one month before and one month after childbirth for workers and office employees, a protection extended to all nonfarm workers in 1934 and to agricultural workers in 1936.[48]

However celebrated these reforms were, the reality was that they did not cover most working women, such as farmers, artisans, and domestics. Compensation for mandatory maternity leave was only a portion of women's normal salary and, moreover, came from a fund made up of contributions from employers and female workers only. The prohibition against work during pregnancy and the postpartum period was constructed not as a right, but as a duty in the public interest. The regime intervened above all to protect children through their mothers, not women in their own right. For those working outside the home, excluding agriculture, family enterprises, or government or public assistance, this abstinence from work was obligatory, as it was for public employees, except that it was compensated as sick leave rather than out of the maternity fund.

A 1927 law (as well as others in 1929, 1930, and 1934) updated the 1916 one that had required nursing rooms and breaks in firms with over 50 female workers between the ages of 15 and 50 (although the rooms were not required if there was a nursery nearby). Women were ensured two paid half-hour breaks for nursing in the morning and afternoon, or two one-hour breaks to nurse at home if they worked in a smaller business. The employer, not the mother, set the schedule. It was subsequently ruled that in enterprises with over 100 women the Corporativist Inspectorate could order that nursing rooms be transformed into day-care centers run by trained staff. However, these laws were often simply ignored. Compliance with the nursing rooms, breaks, and day-care centers was rare from their earliest beginnings, and very few of these places existed even in the late 1930s.

Women were also regulated in their activities at work, particularly in industry. The law dictated how much weight they could lift and prohibited them from carrying weights during the last three months of pregnancy. Women aged 15 to 21 (and children under 15) were excluded from 70 "dangerous, fatiguing, and insalubrious" types of work, although 24 of them were permissible if special precautions and conditions were respected. Yet, like the nursing rooms, there was little compliance with these laws. For example, women were excluded from working with phosphorus, arsenic, mercury, sulphur, and rubber, given that contact with them had noxious effects on the organism and especially the reproductive system. Nevertheless, as Lorenzoni observed, young women were used almost exclusively in the industrial production and commercial processing of these very substances (1933:71).

Indeed, there was little compliance with any of the maternity and work legislation. For example, the 1938 provision requiring public administration to cut its female staff to 10 percent was not followed in any other economic sector. The lack of compliance was due at least in part to confusion over the specifications of the laws, such as how long maternity leave lasted. Yet, in spite of all of this, the legislation had a profound long-term impact, for it laid the groundwork for the ideas and laws that continue to regulate women's work today.

State Medicine

Given that the protection and improvement of the physical and moral qualities of the stock was now a function of the state in its role as *allevatore* (breeder), there was a much greater intervention in public health. By the early 1930s, the state had passed comprehensive health and social legislation, including reform of the sanitary regulations, the battle against malaria and tuberculosis, and regulation of the hygienic conditions of the workplace. The state statistics bureau (ISTAT) had been in place since 1926, with an aggressive program of data gathering on demography and health. Since 1923, all workers had been obligated to pay into the national insurance against infirmity and old age, and local and provincial governments had been required to institute new health services. The Istituto Nazionale Fascista per la Previdenza Sociale (INPS) was created in 1933 to provide maternity, pension, and disability funds paid through obligatory insurance. A 1937 law instituted a local public assistance organization in every commune.

Health services fell under the Ministero dell'Interno (Ministry of the Interior), which was known toward the end of the period as the Istituzione di Sanità Pubblica e Direzione Generale della Razza (Institute of Public Health and General Direction of the Race) (unlike in the United States, the interior ministry was concerned with people rather than lands and parks). There was not a separate institution for health services until the 1970s. This meant that they were directly tied to the state, including the military, which had been mutually involved ever since Unification in health-related activities such as registration of vital statistics and control of sanitary conditions. Broader health services would now be organized on a military model, the system of district health officers oriented toward "educational prophylaxis" and transformed into a "National Militia for the Health of the Race."[49]

Physicians were consequently endowed with new authority in vast fields of public and private life, including the workplace. The "hygienic surveillance of work" provided by "fascist medicine" or "fascist medical politics" involved periodic visits by ONMI physicians with the scope of reducing injuries, diseases, and poisonings. Medical examinations and certificates were required to extend or shorten mandatory maternity leave or receive the cash benefit for the birth of a child (or for loss of the fetus during the third trimester). They were needed for employment in dangerous industries and could be demanded by the Corporativist Inspectorate if there were unhealthy workplace conditions such as excessive humidity or temperature, or sudden changes in temperature. Wet nurses, and eventually all domestics, were required to undergo physical examination and blood tests before presenting a pre-employment medical certificate to the local health officer. No woman could become a wet nurse until her own child was several months old, unless a physician judged her capable of breast-feeding both infants at once.

Another field of state medical control was the surveillance of infancy and youth. ONMI's charter required local offices to report to Public Security or the Public Prosecutor any cases of abuse of family property, crimes of abandonment or mistreatment, or other abuses and crimes toward minors. Physicians increasingly oversaw hygienic conditions and made medical visits at nursery and elementary schools, helping orient children toward certain professions or sports according to their abilities, temperament, and "biotype." This was a step toward the realization of "every man in his proper place" and was said to prevent disease, infirmity, and injury.

Abnormal children were to be weeded out through "medical-pedagogic selection" and tracked through "biotypologic" charts begun in preschool. "Biographical files" and "family leaflets" were proposed, by which each communal medical service could record the health status of the individual and family as a form of "biosocial" documentation for use in clinical study and the science of prevention. This would include obligatory reporting of deformities or lesions in newborns prefiguring a future inability to work. Some experts wanted to require medical certification of "healthy and robust constitution" for entry into job competitions such as those for academic and governmental positions.

According to the penal code, physicians were required to report cases of sexually transmitted disease to the government. Hospitals had to treat these patients, while provincial capitals and larger towns and cities were obligated to provide free clinics for prevention and treatment—often staffed by ONMI physicians. Physicians were required to report all abortions, whether spontaneous or procured, to the provincial medical officer.

Midwives had to request the physician's intervention whenever they noted anything unusual in a pregnancy, birth, or puerperium and report deformed infants to the mayor and local health official within two days of birth. In these and many other ways, the authority of physicians was affirmed and increased, while medical professionals were formally linked to the administrative apparatus of the state.

Through their participation in political demographic action, women were expected to be instruments of state-medical intervention in maternity and infancy. This required the spirit of abnegation and sacrifice said to be associated with maternity and implied rejection of contemporary feminist and liberal individualist thought. Yet, the historical romanticism regarding women's place in the family and society contrasted sharply against the rejection of history regarding health concepts. That is, participation in the new state medicine meant embracing modern medical thought, while also remaining loyal to the traditional family and its ideas about the body and health.

There was a further contradiction between state investment in children's development and the sacrifice of the young to war and colonization. Moreover, the naturalistic emphasis on maternal (and more generally feminine) love and devotion to children conflicted with the rejection of indulgence toward infants incorporated in the fascist exaltation of farm values such as austerity and hard work. While breast-feeding was a fundamental demonstration of basic, natural, motherly love, it was to be performed in a mechanistic, rationalized, controlled manner. While the virtues of rural families were extolled by the regime, the manner of breast-feeding actually practiced by them was considered erroneous and life-threatening to children. As we will see, a vast program of policies and propaganda emerged to correct women's mistakes by regimenting breast-feeding, but the political and medical emphasis on the infant as distinct from the mother was counterproductive to fascist demographic goals.

CHAPTER 5

Schedules and Scales
Fascist Discipline Applied to Maternity and Child Care

The politicization of maternity discussed in the last chapter was part of the process of medicalization that has transformed the experience of gestation and lactation. At its heart was the conceptual and practical separation of mothers and infants at birth rather than after weaning. The emphasis on the value of infants to the family and nation meant that mothers were seen mainly as intermediaries between children and the state. It was through expert intervention in their behavior that infants would be protected. That is, the other side of the belief that erroneous maternal behaviors directly caused infant disease and death, was that improvements in infant mortality rates were the result of medical intervention, especially in the area of dietary practices.

Breast-feeding was regarded as a discrete stage in the mother-infant relationship, and one that primarily served the infant. The direct blood-milk relationship that had formerly interlinked mothers and infants gave way to a new understanding that all biological functions, including lactation and digestion, were governed by an immutable "natural periodicity." Breast-feeding came to be seen in terms of the product rather than process, and method became more important than the constitution or other individual health factors. One outcome was a weakening of the ancient belief in the incompatibility between lactation and menstruation. Another was that the benefits of maternity to mothers derived more from the generative and sexual powers of male secretions in completing their organism, than the humoral interactions between mother and child.

New medical beliefs, together with cultural values such as industrial notions of work and time, led to a heavy emphasis on the regimentation of life-style—and infant feeding practices in particular—because this was thought to provide a lifelong benefit to children. Regimentation was also favored by the growing concern for digestion as the central determinant of health and well-being, and by enduring beliefs in the potentially noxious or fatal effects of germs, humors, and atmospheric influences. Together with the infant's presumed need for regular growth, these beliefs determined the need to schedule meals and measure the quantity of milk produced and consumed. Until this time, experts had argued that infants should be breast-fed at least one year; now, all mothers were to breast-feed one year, but not a day longer.

To promote the idea of breast-feeding as a natural and sacred obligation of all mothers, it was important to highlight women's universal capacity for it and reduce the number of contraindications. However, this was undermined by the suppositions that women tended to make mistakes in parenting, that physicians were the best judges of women's suitability for breast-feeding, and that breast-feeding was destined to last only a short time. While imposing a method that interfered with lactation, medical ideas juxtaposed the conflicting assumptions that all women can and must breast-feed, but that most women cannot or must not breast-feed.

Scientific mothering exalted the worthy rural values promoted by political demography with respect to fertility and homemaking. At the same time, the reality of women's participation in the labor force, and its recognized benefits in the assumption of rationalized attitudes and time schedules, called for the cultivation of urban industrial values. These included submission to medical examination and intervention.

The idea that the proper technique had to be taught to mothers was an expression of the contradiction between the traditional and modern faces of fascism. Historical romanticism was juxtaposed against delight in futurism in the construction of breast-feeding as an eternal, instinctual feminine duty, but one which must now be informed by progress in science and industry. Medicalized breast-feeding expressed, at one and the same time, the glorification of the "traditional" natural functions of maternity and the deliberate renunciation of past or popular methods and knowledge of breast-feeding.

Reshaping the Fluid Link between Mothers and Infants

From Blood and Milk to Mutual Periodicity of Functions

The blood-milk unity was shaken in the interwar period by the idea that the maternal-infant symbiosis was interrupted anatomically at birth. Breast-feeding helped to keep the bond close compared to later in life, but no longer implied a subtle interplay of substance and spirit between two people. Instead, it represented the continuation of mammalian "maternal activity in favor of the child" that began with the mother's giving of herself with an egg and then nourishing the fetus with her own blood. Her breasts' secretory activity was itself stimulated by enzymes and hormones produced by the embryo. Angiola Borrino, a female physician and director of public medical clinics for children, explained that, "according to the biologists," breast-feeding was the "last stage of a progressive adaptation of the organism of the mother to the nutritive needs of her creature" (1937:72).

The work of the placenta was continued by the breast, so that the milk was homogeneous with the blood that had organized fetal development. The milk therefore belonged "by right" to the neonate. The 1930 midwifery legislation reminded midwives that the child was entitled to its mother's milk and would be more likely to fall ill and die without it. Midwives were to persuade mothers, and their families if necessary, of the "great utility of maternal breast-feeding for the neonate," provided there were no contraindications noted by the physician.[1]

Older understandings of the relationships among secretions continued to resurface in ideas such as the belief that suppression or diversion of mother's milk brought increased secretion of urine and postpartum blood (lochia) or that frequent and abundant menstruation—characteristic of weak women—caused a notable decline in milk quantity. In addition, it was said that a breast-feeding woman with "abundant and insistent" lochia lost too much humor and became "weak, pallid, and a bad *nutrice,*" and that milk production was rapidly and considerably diminished by any other type of lost humor.[2]

In general, however, the stress was now on toxic materials rather than fluid relations. "Milk fever" was no longer considered a manifestation of humoral transformations, but rather the result of mechanical damage from the crushing and bruising of tissue in the genital tract during childbirth. When the ensuing highly toxic "juices" coagulated with stagnant lochia, they were absorbed by the uterus and gave rise to fever.[3] It was only by coincidence that this occurred contemporaneously with the arrival of the milk. Likewise, a rise in temperature resulted from retention of fecal materials, which were more altered and encumbering than usual. Unblocking the intestine with a purgative produced a more abundant elimination of lochia and altered uterine residues, favoring the involution of the womb. Breast-feeding also helped by utilizing the organic materials left available by the regression of the genital apparatus.

The most decisive blow to the mother-infant unity came from interpretation of studies showing that there were materials in the milk, such as casein and lactose, that were not in the blood. As Bumm's obstetrics text said, one "had to admit" that the milk was not a simple transudate of the capillary vessels surrounding the alveoli, but a particular product of the glandular epithelium (1923a:286). Meanwhile, studies of infant stomach capacity and rates of assimilation showed that lactation and digestion also followed the "fundamental law" of the "natural periodicity" of all organic functions. Both the mother's milk glands and the infant's secretory epithelia and absorptive structures required discrete intervals of rest time between active phases.

Arguments for the feeding schedule (and also the double weighings) were sustained by measurement of infant stomach capacity. This was defined as 30 cubic centimeters initially, with an increase to 160 at six months and 300 at one year. The stomach's mucosa secreted the same gastric juices as in later age, plus a special ferment found in young animals which coagulated the casein in milk in ten minutes. The serum passed on to the intestine, while the block of casein, "like a piece of cheese," was digested little by little.[4] The intestine was slow, lacking in musculature, and long compared to the adult. This favored the stagnation of liquids and gas and explained the appearance of those "children with bloated bellies which make fools smile and physicians shudder."[5]

After 2 to 2½ hours, the stomach of a healthy, robust breast-fed infant was clear of milk residues, but this took 2½ to 3 hours for other kinds of milk. Given that rest must follow activity, an additional, "necessary" pause of at least one hour was required, to maintain the motor-secretory and bactericidal activity of the stomach and intestine at the highest level. Further, there was no reason to exempt the infant from the "physiological rhythm" of six, seven, or more hours of night rest, which was necessary also for the mother and especially the father, whose own daily occupations must not be compromised by drowsiness.

This led to a standard interval of at least 3½ and commonly 4 hours between meals (*poppate*). In special cases, somewhat closer intervals were allowed, but almost never under 2 hours. Infants might be permitted to feed a few times during the night in the first weeks or months, but thereafter only once or twice, and preferably not at all. In all cases, experts were very precise about the number of feedings and the intervals between them.

The possibility of transmitting moral values in mother's milk was not dismissed entirely with this mechanistic understanding of lactation. Instead, the focus was shifted to the *act* of giving the milk, which was said to double maternal love and raise and educate the child. The breast was the organ of spiritual maternity, transmitting a "true spiritual food" fitted to the child's psychic constitution. Through this "true, great and human" maternity the image of the mother and the sentiment of the family were imprinted on "the heart and mind of the child, of the adult and old man, until death."[6]

Women's anatomy and physiology proved their natural adaptedness and biological need for breast-feeding. This began with conception, which stimulated the undeveloped, dormant, prepregnant breast with a "breath of new life."[7] This brought active epithelial and glandular proliferation and the development of a network of dilated and bluish veins. Already from the second month of pregnancy, the breast could express colostrum, demonstrating how providentially the mother's organism adapted itself to the feeding of the child, before and after birth. Further proof came from the harmful physiological consequences of abstention from breast-feeding. The penetration of germs favored by the retention of milk and irregular emptying of the gland caused infection of the mammary glands. Retained milk also caused excessive distension of the areolar epithelium and mucosa, which increased susceptibility to lacerations, infections, and the drying up of the gland. The cure was the periodic suckling of the infant, or, if he were lazy or weak, the use of a breast pump at scheduled intervals.

This last example illustrates the transformation of old ideas about the stagnation of secretions to emphasize the harmful properties of the fluids themselves, rather than their flow. Its treatment also incorporates the rising emphasis on the need to schedule and ration infant meals.

Lactation, Menstruation, and Fertility

Now that lactation was seen as a discrete phase in the mother-infant relationship, and milk as a product rather than the outcome of a process, postpartum amenorrhea was no longer the logical result of physiological incompatibility between the secretions of the uterus and breast. The influence of lactation was said to be mediated hormonally, but weakly and only for a short time. This explained why early capoparto and new pregnancy (even before the return of menstruation) occurred most often in women who did not breast-feed. That half of all mothers saw the return of menstruation after the fifth or sixth month and many became pregnant beforehand was taken as proof that reproductive function was not generally suspended during breast-feeding. The "glands of maternity" (ovary, hypophysis, thyroid) resumed their cycle within a couple of months, without signaling themselves through menstruation.[8]

Oddly enough, while denying the effect of lactation on fecundity, professional medicine upheld certain beliefs about the powerful influence of the menstrual cycle on other bodily functions. During pregnancy, there were bothersome uterine contractions sometimes accompanied by blood-stained material or pure menstrual blood corresponding to the usual time for menstrual periods. Before and during this time, the internal genital organs were more sensitive to disturbances, including those that influenced the psyche and nervous system. This meant that pregnant women must follow the hygienic norms for menstruation with even greater attention.

After childbirth, the capoparto at 40 days produced a physiological change that temporarily affected the mother's milk, whether or not menstruation had resumed. Sexual relations were said to hasten the return of menstruation, even in the healthiest women, especially if forced by an "intemperate, debauched, and brutal husband."[9] Sexual relations led to a transitory decrease in milk quantity or alteration in quality. This was also the reason for prohibiting sexual relations toward the end of pregnancy and for the first few months afterward, and making sure they were always moderate.

Most experts and laypeople thought that mother's milk became unpleasant or noxious to the child during menstrual periods or, in their absence, the days corresponding to the usual menstrual period. The public's fears were fueled by physicians' claims to have found dyspepsia, insomnia, agitation, diarrhea, weight loss, fever, and eczema in the infant, due to toxic substances and alterations in the composition of the milk. Some experts tried to calm parents by saying that the disturbances were transitory and easily overcome, that the return of menstruation was not a contraindication to breast-feeding, or that, so long as the child was fed in an orderly way, it would suffer no harm.

Similarly, the "old prejudice" that a new pregnancy required immediate termination of breast-feeding was both sustained and rejected by modern medicine. For example, it was said that the nausea and vomiting that signaled new pregnancy caused reduced milk production; that breast-feeding during pregnancy damaged the maternal organism; and that lactation drew nourishment away from the fetus. In gracile, poorly nourished, or exhausted women, a new pregnancy would alter the quality and quantity of the milk. In healthy women, the effect on the milk was said to be minor during the first three to five months of pregnancy. To avoid a dangerous sudden weaning of the infant, the woman should stop breast-feeding after waiting three to four weeks.

Like other organs, the milk glands required regular exercise of their physiological functions. Normal use caused proper functioning and even an increase in the size of the breasts, while disuse or disease caused atrophy. The breasts atrophied if a woman did not breast-feed, or when she stopped breast-feeding, and in any case between the tenth and twelfth month in primiparous or the twentieth in multiparous women. This supported the limit of one year of breast-feeding, which was further justified by the presumed biological consequences of prolonged lactation. For example, protracted mammary activity was believed to cause pathological amenorrhea through inhibition of ovarian and uterine function, leading to uterine lesions, deficient ovarian function, atrophy of the organs, and sterility.[10]

Although breast-feeding could no longer be counted upon to prevent subsequent pregnancy, if carried on too long it could be blamed for reproductive disorders. Such contradictory notions were a disincentive to breast-feeding, for they justified setting a limit on its duration while denying the existence of one of its primary benefits to women. The same attitudes continue to affect medical advice and women's propensity to breast-feed to the current day.

Germs, Humors, Atmospheric Influences

We will now pause a moment to consider changes in general health beliefs that modified traditional understandings of the constitutions. The concept of rationalization gave a modern aspect to classical hygienic principles concerning the importance of moderation in biological functions, exposure to the elements, and behaviors and experiences of all kinds. There was room in this conception for microscopic disease agents, for they interacted with environmental, behavioral, and physiological factors to cause disease. For example, while all people were advised to take a bath at least once a week in order to eliminate microorganisms and stimulate the body's organic reactions, children were to take a bath every day at exactly the same time, for the added reason that they needed an orderly regimen.

The importance of sunlight and fresh air in the suppression of infectious agents added new appeal to ancient rules about the design of buildings. These rules had been transgressed in the construction of airless, dark buildings over the past centuries, including foundling homes. As a nun who has been providing day care for decades says, in the interwar period there was an expression: *dove c'è il sole non c'è il medico* (where there is sun there is not the doctor)—or, in the words of a contemporary, *dove non entra il sole, entra il medico* (where the sun does not enter, the physician does).[11] Sun and air were the primary enemies of tuberculosis, explaining why life in the mountains and near the sea were protective for children— as were sports done with moderation. Exercise and walks outdoors were particularly indicated for children of "morally dangerous heredity."[12]

While classical health principles were still considered valid, experts noted that the public exaggerated in its obsessive fears of cold air, drafts, and other imbalances. They urged people never to close the windows at night, even in winter, and to learn not to be afraid of air or cold, but of people who have a cold.

The regularization of nutrition and digestion was becoming a dominant theme in the medical literature of the interwar period, for a disorderly diet was considered the root cause of disease, including infectious disease. "Diet is the most important phenomenon of life; it is decisive for the health of the individual and for the full efficiency of the collective."[13] Even sterility was blamed upon dietary deficits, deviations, or excesses. Similarly, tuberculosis could be prevented by fortifying the body with good and sober nutrition, taken on a precise schedule as part of a regular, normal, hygienic life-style free of excesses in work, rest, dress, or exercise. Institutions such as schools, hospitals, and the army led the way by rationalizing food intake according to scientifically studied nutritional standards and caloric values.

To regenerate modern society—that mechanical, quintessentially affected civilization–fascist writers argued for a rationalization of the natural medicine of the classical Romans. These ancients had understood disease as a perturbation of life, itself containing the principle of recovery. Their only treatments had been movement, sun, air, water, massage, diet, and will (*volontà*), which would now be employed through promotion of the clean, active country life and a greater sense of responsibility toward children.

One particularly grievous effect of modern civilization was a loss of maternal attributes through individualism, cerebralism, inactivity, and indoor life lacking in fresh air and sunlight. Zanelli, a specialist in women's reproductive disorders and head of the thermal clinic at Salsomaggiore, argued that a rational physical regimen would correct women's bad habits and environmental conditions, and also normalize the circulation, digestion, and nutrition. Together with air and sun, moderate sports activity—suspended during puberty, pregnancy, and breast-feeding, however—prepared women for maternity and favored fecundity, as seen in farm women. "Well more than work and physical efforts and sport, it is sloth which obstructs maternity, creating and feeding the need for unproductive pleasure and corrosive and destructive cerebralism" (1939:29).

This statement brings together several threads from the medical and political themes touched upon so far. It unites modern and ancient health concepts to the notion that women's participation in work and intellectual and leisure activities had precise negative consequences, including disorders of reproduction and parenting.

Homology and Utility in Sex and Reproduction

Breast-feeding was now set apart from other stages of maternal-infant interactions. Its importance for infants took the spotlight, shading past conceptions of lactation as an essential reproductive function for women. This function had been dictated by the universal need for regular exercise of sexual and reproductive functions to avoid suppression or retropulsion of secretions. The reciprocal humoral effects between mother and child were now relatively ignored, the utility of maternity described mainly in directional terms from men to women. Maternity was a biopolitical duty because it fulfilled evolutionary and social needs, completed women's organisms through the transfer of male properties, and defended against the antiprocreative ideas and biological effects of modern civilization.

Maternity was a "perfectly physiological state," which completed or "integrated" the woman according to natural law. Indeed, women were not thought to reach complete development and full health until the third child. The aptitudes and dispositions for the conservation and perpetuation of the species were imprinted upon all of women's organs and cells,

particularly in the nervous and reproductive systems, by genital and systemic substances that followed the path of the humors. That is, maternity
was both physiologically necessary for woman and determined by her role
as repository of the moral and biological characteristics of the species.
This message was literally written upon her biological essence, motivating
her body and mind for reproduction.[14]

Menstruation was no longer seen as a useful physiological process for
maintaining fluid balance, as the ancients had thought, but as failed reproduction—the "abortion of an unfertilized egg," or an "empty" cycle.[15] The
same rejection of humoral relations caused medical experts to ignore the
link between forsaken breast-feeding and breast cancer, even though they
noted that the frequency of malignant tumors seemed to be increasing on
a daily basis. Nevertheless, it was still observed that women who had given
birth to and breast-fed many children enjoyed a survival advantage over
men in later life, and better physical and psychical health than women who
had not. "The gynecologists will discover one day that pregnancy is the
best means for avoiding a great quantity of feminine affections."[16]

To postpone or forsake maternity was to provoke physiological as
well as psychological damages. This was a widespread problem given that
marriage was delayed to around age 30, but women became sexually
mature at 12 to 15. Postponing procreation devastated the organism and
spirit of young, chaste women, causing "suffering without end and without equal," including grave and tortuous neurohormonal disturbances
such as hysterism.[17]

Failure to reproduce altogether led to misgivings, remorse, and innumerable, unnamed miseries falling under the general term *neurasthenia.*
The childless woman might remain more beautiful and well-preserved
than her friends, but she excluded herself from the essence of feminine life
and always suffered from a "chest which has not breast-fed, a womb which
has not shaken in the spasm of childbirth."[18] In fact, by disobeying natural
laws governing women's "congenital organic need" for maternity, modern
women themselves were held responsible for the discomforts, sufferings,
and risks of pregnancy, childbirth, and breast-feeding. The only women to
escape the damages of modern civilization, in spite of their greater physical labors, were the "common women" and others who had many pregnancies.

While normal procreation brought health benefits, "perverse uses of
sexuality," such as birth control, abortion, homosexual behavior, and
masturbation, did the opposite. The "antiprocreative maneuvers" caused
pelvic disturbances, menstrual irregularities, congestions, displacements,
and *nevraglie* (pains from nerve inflammation). Prostitution and homosexual behavior compromised reproductive capacity, while masturbation
caused women (and men) of all ages to become ugly and repugnant, with

more developed and sometimes excessively large external genitals. Health problems included nervous disorders, sterility, early menarche, and menstrual dysfunction. If a woman did not breast-feed and in general conduct a regular and chaste life, after menopause her atrophied glands were replaced by fat, leaving the breast sacklike, withered, and of "unpleasant and repulsive aspect."[19]

In contrast to the old concepts of homology and humoral balance, maternity was now said to benefit women through the transfer of valuable properties and attributes from the man by way of conception and "spermatic impregnation." Ferdinando DeNapoli, of the University of Bologna, explained this in his two-volume treatise *From Malthus to Mussolini*. The maternal-fetal symbiosis initiated with conception brought the mother "paternal hereditary elements" that changed her blood, organs, and general conditions and rendered the shared blood homogeneous through at least the first few years of the child's life. This "infection," "imprint," or "inoculation" of the mother was verified by observation of dogs, horses, and widowed but remarried women who had given birth to offspring resembling a deceased mate. The first male to fertilize the female had such a strong effect on her that his "hereditary mass" would be transmitted for many generations and in successive couplings with other males, "sometimes in an indelible manner" (1934b:331–32).

Regular "spermatic impregnation" through conjugal relations brought "profound humoral modifications" in women. The spermatic liquid was mixed and absorbed with the female secretions, acting as a *ricostituente* (tonic) to reinvigorate and complement the feminine organism and contribute to its physiological equilibrium. Without it, the woman suffered nervous, circulatory, and digestive disturbances which could, in turn, be cured by spermatic *opoterapia* (replacement therapy). Widows and married women who used contraception suffered from autoabsorption of their own secretions, even more than if they had been chaste. These secretions normally stimulated the body, spirit, and personality, but when retained caused possibly incurable nervous and visceral disturbances leading to "physical and psychical ruin and . . . the loss of the gift of maternity" (DeNapoli 1934b:367).

Breast-feeding was also advised on the basis of women's physical and spiritual health, as it related to the larger picture of morality and the future of the species. Gestation and lactation brought hypertrophy of the woman's organs, causing an "exaltation of functions" evident in her healthy appearance and making the mother more physically and spiritually beautiful, robust, vigorous, and moral. Breast-feeding was useful and pleasant, for it stimulated the appetite, optimized the metabolism, and improved the assimilation of food. It elevated maternity and was an index of morality. "The more a mother has of the prostitute, that much less will she want to breast-feed the offspring herself; that much worse will she know how."[20]

Abstention from breast-feeding was described as a crime not yet written into law. This reflects both the growing political emphasis on infants and the new medical understanding of lactation—which centered upon milk as a product (to which property rights pertained) and minimized attention to mothers. DeNapoli argued that, just as it was illegal to interrupt the uterine-fetal relationship with abortion, so it ought be illegal to interrupt the infant-breast relationship, to "defraud the child of *his* milk." This was a "grave sin" that made a mother who could, but would not, breast-feed more guilty than one who procured an abortion. The state should intervene with laws and punishments against women who obtained false medical certificates allowing them to bottle-feed (1934b:423–24).

In this global biopolitical and moral understanding of maternal functions, women needed to reproduce and avoid birth control practices in order to maintain and complete their organisms, conserve the species, and provide moral stability to men and children. The work of reproduction was continued by breast-feeding, but no longer because it was thought that the milk was made from the same blood that had fed the fetus. Instead, breast-feeding was a natural right of the infant that incidentally contributed to the mother's physical and moral health, but more importantly showed that she took part in the glorious rebirth of the new fascist nation.

Ideas about Maternity and Infancy

Health Outcomes of Incorrect Maternal Behaviors

The general health concepts of the interwar period melded the old with the new, the political with the medical. The avoidance of excess through control of behavior and exposure incorporated both modern ideas about microbial agents of disease and fascist principles of discipline and order. This meant that not only could immoderate maternal conduct cause loss of pregnancy and other negative, often fatal outcomes, but so could imprudent or uninformed behavior. The obstetrician Vicarelli expressed this in his observation that women arrived at childbirth completely ignorant or only vaguely or erroneously informed with respect to their own and their child's health, relying instead upon instinct, or the "sentiment" of maternity. For her ignorance, "the young mother very often pays with her own health, sometimes with her own life, other times with that of her child" (1926a:2).

Even a "little imprudence" was said to cause spontaneous abortion.[21]

Medical writers admonished the modern woman to understand all of the factors that led to pregnancy loss, because, "in the majority of cases, she can, if she wants to, avoid abortion and premature birth."[22] The most susceptible women were those who worked in the factories, fields, and sweatshops; the overburdened mothers of large families; women who were constantly emotional, excitable, or apprehensive; and women who refused to renounce sports, outings, and trips using modern, rapid transportation.

The equation of maternal misbehavior with untimely birth justified many medical, governmental, and popular restrictions on women's behavior. Working women were singled out for expert scrutiny, and the legal requirement for women to stop working before and after childbirth was proudly noted in most medical and political texts. Midwives were prohibited by law from treating or caring for dangerous pathological cases including, by definition, every abortion, for it was presumed that physicians better recognized the importance of preventing abortion. ONMI sought to prevent abortion by providing assistance to poor mothers and deceived and seduced girls.

Most, if not all, causes of abortion were considered maternal, even though there were a few fetal or paternal causes described in the literature, such as weakness of semen or the sexual excesses of young husbands.[23] Most paternal factors were considered fundamentally "maternal" causes, anyway. For example, paternal syphilis had once been considered a direct cause, but now it was said that the father transmitted syphilis to the mother and she, even if asymptomatic, passed the disease to the fetus. Many fetal causes also depended upon maternal causes, such as death of the embryo from poisoning, autogenous toxemia, or infection transmitted by the mother. While repeat abortions were of unknown cause, careful investigation promised to reveal a morbose maternal condition (most commonly syphilis or chronic nephritis) that was latent, ignored, or missed due to incomplete observation.

Many of the more frequent and important maternal causes were described as predisposing influences or conditions, such as reproductive system abnormalities or heredity from a mother who had often aborted. Other causes of abortion included a nervous temperament; too young or advanced age; poor general health due to anemia, deficient nutrition, obesity, or infectious disease; and displacement of the uterus (either extroflexion caused by wearing very high heels and constricting the abdomen, or retroflexion due to inflammation). Circulatory disturbances and uterine contractions could be provoked by frequent sexual relations in very excitable or predisposed women; nervous shock or vivid emotions such as pain, pleasure, fright, or surprise; and diseases such as pneumonia, typhoid, or chronic nephritis.

Direct and indirect traumas of every kind were believed to cause abortion, including blows to the abdomen; jumps or falls; travel by train, automobile, boat, bicycle, or horse; and any kind of excessive sport or muscular exertion at home or work. They also included rough vaginal examination by the midwife or physician; sexual abuses; overly hot or cold showers; and hot, cold, or high-pressure vaginal irrigations. Some uteri were so excitable that a simple gynecological exam or small trauma such as the rapid descent of stairs was enough to provoke detachment of the ovum and uterine contractions.

Oddly, medical texts describing these many pathways to abortion often contained statements concerning how difficult it was to provoke abortion and the observation that wars, disasters, and earthquakes had not increased the number of abortions. Modern women's continual state of emotion due to excessive movement and the struggle for existence should have caused abortion and premature birth to occur with greater frequency than they did. In certain women, violent traumas, the roughest gynecological examinations, or even the exam with the probe did not provoke abortion. Indeed, unless the pregnant woman was very excitable, she could tolerate "even the gravest operative acts."[24] These included amputation or incision of the breasts, extraction of teeth, ovariotomy, appendectomy, operations on the liver, stomach, or intestines, and even aspiration of cysts or tumors from the uterus and ovaries. Prolonged anesthesia did not harm pregnancy unless it caused strong circulatory disturbances, and neither did many drugs unless taken in toxic doses.

These contradictory statements about women's responsibility for loss of pregnancy reflect the growing belief that medical interventions were harmless to women and children, but that women's misbehavior could have grave and fatal consequences. As we will see, this message pervaded expert discussions of child rearing, in which medical intrusion was said to promote proper breast-feeding while maternal ignorance and imprudence threatened it.

Digestion and Nutrition in Maternity and Infancy

The emerging idea that digestion and nutrition were the foundation of health and well-being was central to contemporary conceptions of gestation and lactation. Human milk was the "obligatory nutriment" in early life—the best guarantee of health, normal development, high intellectual capacity, and mental and moral equilibrium—but it required careful regulation. Modernized breast-feeding respected biological laws about periodicity, balance, and moderation and served sociopolitical ends in the transmission of values, health, and life itself. The protection of babies from nutritional disturbances "raises the nation and determines the true human progress, with the formation of beings [who are] intellectually whole, gifted with the best mental and moral equilibrium."[25]

Since successful breast-feeding depended upon a proper pregnancy and childbirth, it was necessary to rigidly control behavior and exposure to noxious influences throughout the period from conception to weaning. In the child, nutrition was said to act synergistically with other factors of development, so that anything that disturbed it damaged the entire organism. Contrariwise, a proper living environment, exposure to the sun and fresh air, and protection against infection and sudden atmospheric changes maintained the normality of processes of nutrition and therefore skeletal and nervous system development. For women, moderate physical activity such as walking outdoors was part of the "tranquil and methodical life" prescribed during pregnancy and breast-feeding because, among other things, it favored the processes of digestion.

The relationship between nutrition and intestinal function had two sides. The "administration" of colostrum and milk from the mother influenced the infant's digestion, while milk production was, in turn, shaped by maternal nutrition and digestion. This affected the timing of breast-feeding after childbirth, in a departure from the popular practice of waiting until the milk arrived (and the lochia diminished or stopped). Instead, physicians were recommending "early" initiation at 20 hours, or on the second day (a norm written into the 1930 midwifery legislation). Although this delay conflicted with the observation that the suckling reflex was so strong that the child would suck the obstetrician's finger while still in the womb, it was maintained for the sake of the mother's and child's rest. It was also necessary to wait for the expulsion of material clogging the newborn's digestive pathways, even though experts knew that this was facilitated by ingestion of colostrum. The mother meanwhile kept herself "light" until her intestine was well-emptied upon administration of a laxative or purgative on the second or third day. Once both of their digestive pathways were clear, regular breast-feeding was permitted.

To ensure proper milk production, the mother's diet had to be moderate and orderly. The pregnant and nursing mother's meals were to be taken at "fixed hours" and consist of simple, unseasoned, and mixed foods—with the possibility of a precise quantity of wine—for indigestion and excessively stimulating foods or drinks were believed to cause grave harm to the regular course of pregnancy and lactation. After childbirth, the diet would be bland and liquid or semiliquid, reflecting women's "instinctive" aversion to solid foods and compensating her loss of fluid. During lactation, which represented a "heavy burden" that occupied the mother day and night, the nutritious diet would consist of bland, substantial, easily digested foods and abundant liquids to address the increased thirst.

The complement to careful nutrition was scrupulous, daily regulation of the intestine. Women were "habitually and obstinately constipated" anyway, but especially prone to digestive irregularities in pregnancy and after childbirth.[26] They were advised to use purgatives and enemas when necessary, but under medical supervision (particularly in pregnancy, since some provoked contractions). After childbirth, the abdomen must be tightly wrapped for a month, not only because it offended the aesthetic but also because otherwise the woman would develop obstinate intestinal and abdominal disorders. Milk production was to be regularized by purging the intestines at least every day or two. This could be done with cooked fruit, herbs, or pharmaceutical products. The latter had to be chosen carefully to avoid disturbing digestion and urinary function, which could deviate the formation of the milk and render it poisonous and purgative for the nursling.

Constipation in the child was a main preoccupation of parents and medical experts, often blamed upon abnormal health conditions in the mother or child. Medical texts detailed the number of evacuations the normal infant should have each day, depending upon its age, and gave thorough instructions regarding purging through the mother's milk, mechanical stimulation, enemas, or oral purgatives. It is little wonder that, as experts complained, families were more preoccupied with children's constipation than the more dangerous diarrhea and tried every means to remedy it, sometimes causing more damage than the condition itself. This contradiction in medical advice has left its legacy in current concerns about intestinal function in breast-feeding mothers and infants.

General Norms for Maintaining Maternal and
Infant Health

The emphasis on digestion gave force to precautions about avoiding atmospheric imbalances, for events such as exposure to immoderate temperature or humidity were thought to cause circulatory problems, respiratory ailments, and diseases of the internal organs, including the intestines. In newborns, abrupt exposure to cold, as in immediate baptism or transport to a wet nurse, was said to directly cause fatal infantile diseases, inability to suckle, and prostration from lack of breath and livid skin. On the other hand, children should not be covered excessively, their circulation impeded and their skin prevented from respiring, as in the outmoded practice of swaddling. Children should be kept in an environment free of crowding, with good illumination and ventilation and sufficient but not excessive humidity and heat. To alleviate pain in the digestive or other organs caused by dietary irregularities, a uniformly hot and moderately humid atmosphere was best.

Excessive stimulation was said to threaten cerebral and motor development, as well as digestion and nutrition, leading to norms that limited physical contact between parents and infants. Mothers were told not to pick up their infants except to wash or breast-feed them, and to make their arms and bodies felt as little as possible when they did so. After the poppata, infants were not to be shaken, laid on their stomachs, rocked to sleep, or bothered by the tightening of their clothes, for these disturbances could bring regurgitations of air and milk, if not vomit of the entire meal. For the first year, children were not to be given any kind of excitement, including cuddling and songs or lullabies, as this was superfluous if not damaging indeed. Parents harmed their brain and nervous system by rocking them in their arms or a crib, or helping them to sleep by carrying them, telling stories, or keeping company at the bedside.

The avoidance of stimulation was necessary for the added reason that infant bones were pliable, especially in the early months. Parents were advised to limit their infants' movements, take them out in a stroller rather than their arms, and keep them from sitting up or crawling until it was time to walk. Pacifiers of any kind, including the fingers, were harmful because they produced excessive saliva, tiring the digestive functions and provoking a damaging "nervous excitation" and exhaustion. If necessary, the child's arms were to be restrained with cardboard sleeves or pinned to a sash so they would not reach the mouth.

Expectant and nursing mothers too must avoid cerebral or emotional stimulation, for changes in their nervous and mental system rendered them ever more emotional, sensitive, and excitable. Excesses would have grave consequences, including loss of the fetus or gracile newborn. Pregnant women were to avoid all emotions, joys, and pains, including those aroused by cinematographic shows. After childbirth, they were to be left in bed in solitude and quiet for a week or two, given their "instinctive" need for tranquillity and rest, with relatives and friends exercising moderation in their displays of emotion. During this time, the mother should remain lying down, even for bodily functions, but move the limbs and back to favor digestion and the elimination of bodily secretions.

Medical writers imposed many behavioral restrictions designed to avoid stagnations and "congestions" that upset the balance among physiological functions. Babies and pregnant and nursing mothers were to take baths according to precise time limits and temperature ranges for women's and children's baths, to avoid extremes of heat or cold as well as unsuitable times such as just after meals. Healthy pregnant women could go swimming after the third month, so long as the water was not too hot, cold, or agitated, but abortion and premature birth could result from the striking of waves against the body, the gulping of salt water, and the light asphyxia and internal organ tension caused by dives and swimming under water.

Because pregnant women's nervous and muscular capacities were thought to diminish in step with their intellectual capacity, they were encouraged to do light domestic chores and brief, not tiring walks, but prohibited from all sudden, disorganized, and excessive movements and emotions. These included maintaining a prolonged standing or curved position; sewing with a pedal-driven machine, washing, and ironing; and traveling by animal or mechanical means. These things disturbed the movements of the heart and lungs, affecting the general and uterine blood circulation and the nutritional relations between mother and fetus. They caused external pressures on the uterus that could provoke contractions. During train and other rapid travel, fast movement and sudden and strong shakes caused anemia of the brain, with violent rushing of the blood to the uterus and possible loss of pregnancy.

All of these considerations pointed in one direction: the mother must govern her own behavior and impulses, and in this way shape the behavior of the child toward discipline and order.

Correcting Errors of Governo

Rationalization and regimentation were core values incorporated into the notion of the just *governo* (direction) or upbringing of children. Much of this revolved around infant nutrition, that "most difficult affair" given the rules to be followed as well as the influence of persistent prejudices and ignorance. Bad and irrational maternal conduct was said to provoke gastroenteritis and cause a "slaughter of innocents"—more than 50,000 each year, by Borrino's reckoning (1937:649).[27] She explained that maternal errors, together with congenital malformations, represented the dominant pathology of the first month. For the entire first year, and into the second, maternal errors of diet (quantity, quality, preparation) and governo (such as exposure to cold and infection) played a predominant role in infant disease and death, for this was when the child grew most rapidly and nutrition was of primary importance. Weaning very often brought disturbances due to the "real difficulties of upbringing in this age [beginning at 6 months] and the innumerable errors which are committed in both the diet and governo of the infant" (1937:43).

The notion of governo hinged upon the unquestionable importance of time scheduling. The infant was said to be "naturally" methodical and a "creature of habit," with an intrinsic need for the "systematic" ordering of all activities, including meals, baths, play, and outings. The shrewd mother habituated her newborn to the "fundamental rhythm" between eating and napping by day, and to sleeping 8 hours in a row by night—increasing to 10 by the end of the first month and 12 by the second. This paved the way for a standard schedule for naps and evening bedtime as the child grew older, as part of a life structured by "fixed and regular hours" that facilitated early development and education. Even diapers should be changed according to an orario so the child would learn to relieve itself at regular hours. Toilet training could begin within the first six months—using a daily suppository of cocoa butter if necessary—to create the "habits and capacities of autodominion, and regularity of life, which form the base of physical, organic equilibrium and personal dignity."[28]

The child had rights to his mother's milk and attentions, but also had duties: "duties that one must teach him!" "Above all *discipline:* not to sleep in the maternal bed, not to ask to be picked up for nocturnal breast-feeding, not to stay during the day in the mother's arms except when purely necessary, not to develop 'bad habits.'"[29] By respecting children's "fundamental need" for their own bed, and indeed their own room, parents ensured that children learned their place in the family and contributed to their development. To sleep in the parents' bed was dangerous and "unhygienic," besides. The most deplorable habit of all was to allow the child to fall asleep breast-feeding in the mother's arms or lap, or worse, in bed with her, as working women were prone to do. Instead, the mother should sit in a chair and immediately deposit the child in the crib afterward, "far away from herself," ignoring his cries or whimperings.[30]

Mothers were exhorted to learn to combine love and knowledge with order and method, disciplining their children for their mutual benefit. They were urged to discourage, from the very first days, the newborn's tendency to disorder in feedings and sleep and to continual attachment to the breast. The mother must remain unmoved by her child's tantrums, whims, and screams. After being left to cry for two or three days, "not seeing himself satisfied, the little rebel will calm himself."[31] He will sleep and digest regularly, without excessively tiring and disturbing his caretakers, grow and prosper, and develop his senses and intelligence according to the laws of nature. Even a child brought up badly out of inexperience or misplaced compassion could be put in order in a few days if placed under a rigorous method.

The infant's presumed need for a feeding schedule was supported by the notion that overly frequent meals were harmful to the body and spirit. Experts warned mothers not to offer the breast when the infant cried, arguing that, provided they were not capricious, infants rarely cried out of hunger—and never cried if healthy, clean and dry, dressed properly, positioned comfortably, and free of disturbances such as noise, light, or insects. If they did cry, it was because they had eaten too much: the stomach was too full and the digestion disturbed and difficult. By exactly regulating the child's activities, the mother could prevent it from crying when

it ought to be sleeping, for insomnia was "none other than the most evident sign of too copious or too closely spaced meals." The remedy was to
"correct the error committed."[32]

Nothing was considered more harmful to the health and life of the
child than to feed it irregularly or excessively. To give milk too often or too
much was to create a "damaging supernutrition," by which the tiny stomach and intestines expanded little by little and became diseased. This led to
too-rapid growth, agitation, restlessness, unsatisfied hunger and thirst,
and crying. It caused chronic indigestion, with flatulence, burping, vomiting, excessive salivation, diarrhea, inflammation of the diaper area, and
obesity together with scarce vitality and skin ailments such as eczema.
Together with underfeeding, overfeeding caused intestinal disorders with
arrested bone and muscle development, and it delayed walking by as much
as two years. Accordingly, to treat abdominal pain with additional milk
could only be damaging, so mothers should instead give water and an
enema in case of constipation lasting as little as a day.

ONMI training courses taught physicians and surgeons the "importance of method for the good success of maternal breast-feeding." This
included avoiding "overfeedings from too frequent, too abundant, too
rich meals."[33] The need for women to learn to feed their babies at the "prescribed hours" was written into many demographic laws and regulations.[34]

Not only did the poppate have to be limited in number, duration, and
frequency, but there was an upper limit on the overall length of breast-
feeding. The ideal was exclusive breast-feeding for up to six months and
continued breast-feeding through the first year—but no longer, unless the
physician granted an exception. Given the expert disdain for prolonged,
"irrational" breast-feeding, it is little wonder that mixed feeding was often
initiated after three months and weaning completed by five or six months.
As we will see, health professionals found meals of formula and other
foods easier to regulate than breast-feeding, and, however inadvertently,
promoted their use.

Ideas about Breast-Feeding

Qualities of Mother's Milk and Characteristics of Its Production

The emphasis on the product rather than process of lactation reflected
both the new understanding that mother's milk did not derive directly
from the blood and the rising cultural emphasis on infancy. Although the
method or technique of breast-feeding came to be more important than

the mother's behavior or characteristics, these too were considered to influence milk quality and quantity. Mother's milk was examined in great detail, its chemical composition and energetic value compared to cow, goat, and donkey milk to show that it was perfectly composed for infants according to the velocity of human growth, while the others were not. It was indisputably essential for the infant's first few months of life.

Scientific studies demonstrated that the quantity of mother's milk responded to infant demand, increasing as the child grew or if the mother nursed more than one child, while quality changed as breast-feeding progressed. The milk was "alive" with hormones that influenced the child's health and development, as well as special soluble ferments affecting digestion, nutrition, and vitality. It transmitted microorganisms and general and specific immunological substances, making the milk of each woman unique. The robust, well-developed mouth structures of the newborn further indicated biological adaptedness for breast-feeding, and only very rarely was a mother's milk unsuitable for her infant's constitution.

However, while mother's milk was exalted as a vivifying, whole, perfect food, it was also described as only *almost* perfect or complete. It was a not-quite-irreplaceable food, which could be scarce or have defects, such as excessive fat content obstructing the emptying of the infant's stomach.[35] Moreover, the quality of the milk of healthy and robust women was "good" for only the first 11 or 12 months, and only "passable" until 18 months.[36] The quantity was also said to decrease at 12 months, and no nutrice was good after 18 months because the insufficient milk assumed noxious qualities. Weaning was a welcome transition from a monotonous diet to the "mixed and free" diet of the adult, made inevitable by the declining quality and quantity of mother's milk.

Beyond the effect of time, mother's milk could be altered in innumerable ways. Even though science could no longer sustain the belief that psychic properties were transmitted in the milk, disturbances in the mother's emotional state were considered capable of damaging milk quality and quantity, and even inhibiting the secretion temporarily or permanently. Such disturbances included fright or any strong emotion, painful or pleasurable, or any emotion at all in a sensitive or neurotic woman. Frequent sexual relations, as well as overexertion or its opposite, laziness, would have the same effect. As Bumm explained, "the secretion is favored by a copious diet and muscular repose; the loss of humors, such as hemorrhages and diarrheas, or physical exertions, diminish it rapidly and considerably" (1923a:284).

While it was taken for granted that the mother's constitution and nutrition notably influenced milk composition, there was some ambivalence about the influence of diet on milk quality. On the one hand, the mother's diet influenced the quantity of vitamins in the milk and if deficient would bring the infant grave diseases, disorders, and even death. On the other hand, the milk retained its composition even if the diet was poor in minerals such as calcium and phosphorus, since they were extracted from the mother's reserves. Studies that tried to increase mineral content gave contradictory results, indicating that it was difficult to modify milk composition. This argued against the popular practice of overeating during lactation, for the mother who became too fat did not make a good nutrice. Even worse, it did not preclude the loss of the milk secretion since this could depend upon other causes, independent of nutrition.

In addition to the vulnerability of milk quality and quantity, medical experts made the further assumption that milk production was likely to fail in spite of women's best efforts. Women's fears of inadequacy were fueled by the chemical and microscopic analysis of their milk, which mothers and health professionals remember as a common medical practice from the 1930s through the 1970s. There were also products to improve milk production. Traditional home remedies to improve mother's milk generally involved compresses to the breasts or certain foods or drinks. Commercial products available through pharmaceutical companies and medical clinics included micronutrient supplements, devices using massage or electricity, and medicines and hormones. One product, Galattologo I.T.R., was made of extracts from functioning mammary glands, placenta, and anterior hypophysis.[37]

Given the presumed susceptibility of mother's milk to alteration, the nursing woman's daily "regime of life and diet" assumed critical importance. This involved renouncing work, all physical or mental exertions, and society life—including evenings at the theater or dancing—together with careful attention to diet, tranquillity and rest, exposure to fresh air, and personal cleanliness. The last of these was highlighted to address the popular belief that taking a full bath would make the milk diminish, in response to which Gelli remarked that "also cows if cleaned and brushed well every week, give a greater quantity of milk than those kept dirty" (1931:790). Pregnant women were told to scrub and massage the breasts every morning and evening to prepare for breast-feeding and to correct any anatomical impediments to nursing, such as introflexion of the nipple. Nursing mothers must clean and sterilize their nipples and hands as well as the child's mouth before and after every feeding, to prevent and treat lesions which could otherwise terminate breast-feeding.

Moderation in the mother's diet was achieved through the scheduling of meals, rationalization of food quality and quantity, and regularization of intestinal function. Too frequent meals were said to lead to scarce milk production, while irregular or insufficient meals led to variations in milk quantity and deficiency of milk. Tables detailing total daily caloric needs and meal plans for institutions were presented as guides for all women, who were encouraged to monitor their body weight very closely.

Regarding the choice of foods, women were strongly discouraged from taking any stimulating or excessively flavorful food or drink, as well as anything thought to pass odorous or poisonous substances in the milk. Forbidden foods included common ones such as onions and garlic, as well as almonds, strawberries, asparagus, mushrooms, aromatic herbs such as thyme, and turnips, carrots, and other roots. They also included preserved and too tender meats, and tea, coffee, or liquor if used habitually.[38] Medicines included all drugs such as opium and many common purgatives, sedatives, antipyretics, and tonics, especially if prepared from potassium iodide, salicylic acid, arsenic, or mercury. Mother's milk carried odors and fumes from stalls and domestic animals, gas, ammonia, and tobacco. Smoking was doubly harmful, causing early exhaustion of lactational function because of the effect of nicotine on women's neuropsychic equilibrium.

Proper milk production was said to depend upon the regularization of several different functions. As we have seen, intestinal function had to be controlled through moderate exercise, an appropriate diet, and the use of laxatives, enemas, and suppositories. Likewise, since nipple stimulation excited and maintained mammary activity, the infant's sucking must be periodic, regular, and of moderate frequency and duration. The gland must be emptied at consistent intervals, for it worked according to the "fundamental law of training" regulating all muscular, secretory, and digestive functions. Failure to do so over several days was the best way to dry up the gland, whereas periodic suction could reactivate milk secretion even after weeks of quiescence. The schedule was to be imposed from the outset and would lead to certain and regular sucking and stabilization of the mammary secretion.

Milk left too long in the breasts lost its good qualities, assumed noxious ones, and would vanish if the condition persisted for days. Both breasts should therefore be emptied at each feeding. Whenever the breast was not completely emptied, whether because the child took too little or the mother produced too much, the "superfluous" milk was to be expressed by pump or the hands of the mother or midwife. In another illustration of the transition from human to mechanical solutions, Gelli observed that such methods had replaced the women who used to suck new mothers' breasts to activate the secretion and empty the gland until the infant had started to eat regularly (1931:745, 764).

The need to empty the gland and stimulate the nipple was interpreted as supporting the scheduling and metering of feedings, even though, as we saw in the first chapter, to do so actually interferes with milk production.

This was only one of many contradictions. Mother's milk was described as a perfect product adapted to the needs of the child, but its production could cease or diminish for unpredictable reasons, was adequate for only a limited period of time, and was susceptible to injurious modification through maternal behaviors and deficiencies. These notions justified greater medical supervision and intervention in breast-feeding, and they generated other contradictions in their turn.

The Universal Capacity to Breast-Feed

Since errors in infant nutrition were considered the principal cause of gastroenteritis and other diseases of nutrition, and therefore of the elevated rates of infant morbidity and mortality, physicians and politicians defined the spread of rationalized child-rearing norms as a social problem of maximum importance. It was the medical experts who knew about breast-feeding and would teach mothers how it should properly be done. Their texts were now oriented more toward maternal breast-feeding than the alternative feeding methods required by the well-off women who used to be their main clients. ONMI courses on infant care taught physicians and surgeons that the possibility of maternal breast-feeding existed in the "near totality of cases."[39] Yet, in medical texts and courses, women's natural ability to breast-feed was typically discussed just before the physiology and physiopathology of breast-feeding and contraindications to it. That is, the proclamation of women's universal capacity to breast-feed was juxtaposed against elaboration of situations in which breast-feeding was inadvisable or destined to fail.

The argument that the ordinary physiological function of breast-feeding was a "fundamental general possibility" of women was the antidote to prevailing ideas about the biological decline in lactational function in Europe since the middle of the nineteenth century.[40] These ideas assumed a degeneration of the female sex due to civilization and its diseases, such as tuberculosis, nervous diseases, alcoholism, and hypoplasia or weak functioning of the mammary gland. The reason 20 percent of city women were unable to begin or continue breast-feeding was that generations of disuse had left them with deficient and atrophied glands. The inappropriate modern dress also arrested breast development, especially among upper-class women who were loath to compromise their bodily elegance by breast-feeding and who used mechanical compressive means to reduce their breast size. The suitability of these ever-smaller breasts inevitably diminished, while the nipples became introflexed and defective.

An alternative view was that the growth of the cities and the rise in women's industrial employment, together with improvements in the sterilization of animal milk and preparation of commercial foods, had meant that women could just abandon breast-feeding for no valid reason. The First World War had demonstrated that biological forces were *not* to blame since German and Austrian women had been forced to return to breast-feeding, with great success.

In contrast to the situation in Germany, where physiologists and physicians explained that only 25 to 30 percent of mothers breast-fed because of an inherited degeneration of the race—apparently not considering that this was also the time of greatest enthusiasm for artificial feeding—obstetrical clinics such as Borrino's showed that almost all mothers could breast-feed, at least for the first few weeks. Borrino argued that nearly every presumed difficulty either was not a real problem or could be overcome with the *buona volontà* of the mothers, under "good medical direction." She noted that in Monaco, almost two-thirds of the mothers did not breast-feed, but a real incapacity was found in only 13 percent of the cases (1937:58–59). In her own clinic, Borrino found an absolute necessity for mixed or artificial feeding in only 2 percent of all cases in which they were used. These few cases involved anatomical malformations of the nipple, infant incapacity to suckle, and grave maternal illness, whereas all the others were the result of "errors of judgment, unfounded fears, lack of proper medical advice" (1937:62).

Not surprisingly, physicians took credit for any increases in the popularity of breast-feeding, for they saw it as a function they permitted to women so long as the latter were suitable for it and performed it properly. While maintaining that all women were capable of breast-feeding, medical authorities immediately enumerated reasons why they should not or must not, even while claiming that the number of contraindications was smaller than in the past. They presented many circumstances in which breast-feeding could harm the child or mother, repeatedly emphasizing that the physician's judgment was necessary in all cases and might have to override the woman's naturally overwhelming desire to breast-feed.

Contraindications to Breast-Feeding

The accepted contraindications to or difficulties in breast-feeding were of many types, including maternal or infant health problems and anatomical disorders, defects in milk production, and social and behavioral factors. Many experts railed against these obstacles in order to promote breast-feeding. Borrino argued that almost all of them could be overcome, leaving only two "truly insuperable difficulties or absolute impediments to maternal breast-feeding" (1937:91). The mother could not breast-feed in the case of "unbeatable" malformation of the nipple (*mamilla inversa*), and she must not breast-feed if infected with tuberculosis or a few other grave diseases (such as heart defects, epilepsy, or serious mental disease).

Nevertheless, whether by presenting numerous contraindications or challenging them, experts advanced the authority of physicians in decisions regarding breast-feeding and its everyday practice.

Most of the contraindications listed in the literature were traced to defects in the mother, her breasts or nipples, or her milk production. These included the previously mentioned diseases, plus scarlet fever, chronic kidney disease, transitory febrile illness, malignant tumors, and weakness (a term encompassing anemia, lack of appetite, and progressive deterioration). They also included hysterism, neuropathy, psychological disorders or a predisposition to them, and predisposition to madness. In addition to nipple malformation, there were prohibitive breast lesions, including abscesses, rhagades, and mastitis, as well as imperfect nipple shape or size. If not absolute contraindications, factors such as maternal age, parity, ill health, anemia or constitutional thinness, and nervous disorders were said to interfere with breast-feeding. Syphilis was the one condition that required maternal breast-feeding (or artificial feeding if necessary), to avoid endangering uninfected nurses.

Defects in the production of milk commanded a great deal of attention in both the medical literature and the popular imagination. The rarest of these, after the first few days, was excessive milk production (*galattorea*). The overproduction of watery imperfect milk was said to be caused by excessive weakness and sensibility, especially in anemic, chlorotic, neurotic women, and would further exhaust the mother. Lack of milk (*agalattia*) was a more frequent problem affecting up to one-third of all women, and was attributed to internal conditions or hormonal anomalies. Although it was often invoked as a reason for not breast-feeding, Borrino argued that agalattia did not exist but was instead a misdiagnosis for scarce secretion and late arrival of the milk, for which the child was not put to the breast and the gland not periodically stimulated and emptied (1937:113–14).

The most common "defect" of milk production, and that which received the most attention in the literature, was insufficient milk production (*ipogalattia*). There was a widespread cultural belief that if the infant left the breast early, then the milk was scarce. Borrino criticized both health professionals and mothers, especially young first-time mothers, for their deep fear of this condition, which she found difficult to verify with quantitative methods such as the doppia pesata. The "ignorance of midwives" and "lightness of physicians" contributed to the switch to mixed or artificial feeding which women sought due to "vague unspecifiable causes" cited out of ignorance and prejudice (1937:67, 65). These included the infant's agitation; the bad advice of a neighbor, old mother, or midwife; the perception or simply the fear of inadequate milk quality or quantity; the return of menstruation; or a scare, displeasure, or misfortune. Physicians deserved a portion of the blame because they discouraged or prohibited breast-feeding on the basis of anemia, gracility, or a "certain degree of *nervosismo*" (1937:67).

The solution most often suggested was not to reduce the influence of midwives and physicians, but increase it. This would remedy both perceived contraindications and real obstacles (work, grave obstetrical operations, disease, infant difficulties in sucking), returning even those mothers who had asked for a supplement of cow's milk or already initiated mixed feeding to exclusive breast-feeding. It was up to health experts to calm hyperemotive and impatient mothers, instill a will to nurse in women, and correct the errors of judgment behind almost all cases of renounced or compromised breast-feeding. Under no circumstance should the mother's judgment be the cause of or justification for the abandonment of breast-feeding.

One of the conquerable difficulties mentioned frequently in medical texts was women's *imperizia* (lack of skill), especially with the first child. This led to the abandonment of breast-feeding because women did not know how to hold the infant properly. Mothers needed to be taught that pain, fright, indignation, or anger did not affect the milk or the infant's well-being, except for diminished production for a day or two during the most acute phase of the emotion.

Medical experts argued that even brevity of the sublingual frenum (connecting the base of the tongue to the floor of the mouth) could be overcome. There were still many parents, midwives, and physicians who considered this one of the most common infant disorders and corrected it with an incision. In Santa Lucia, it was listed as the cause of death of many infants early this century. Experts now wrote that the true disorder was very rare and, moreover, did not explain a child's difficulty in sucking. On the other hand, surgery was still indicated for harelip, oral tumors, or macroglossia, but the infant could be fed breastmilk expressed regularly according to the feeding schedule.

The administration of expressed milk, whether by spoon or dropper through the mouth or nose, was considered capable of overcoming all other accepted infant impediments as well. These included congenital weakness, prematurity, and lack of vigor in suction; obstruction of the nasal passages; and disturbances of the innervation of the musculature for suction and swallowing, arthritis of the jaw, and rigidity of the mouth walls. They also included psychic torpor from idiocy or mongolism, and lesions or disorders in the mouth or nearby parts due to stomatitis, oral thrush, syphilitic infection, otitis, or parotitis. With this method, all infants could receive mother's milk at least for the first few weeks, which was decisive for their survival and future growth.

With regard to social obstacles, Borrino assured wealthy women that they could breast-feed and still have a social life because the child could be cared for by someone else in their absence: so long as feeding was regular, "with feedings at fixed hours, [and] with a longer pause in the night" (1937:137). The elite life-style was becoming less of an issue anyway now that wet nursing was out of favor, and to feed one's own child was considered a duty and source of dignity even for women of high society. This had led to greater recourse to artificial feeding in many countries, but a return to breast-feeding in Italy and other Latin countries, although, as Borrino noted, in both cases women were responding to fashion and vanity.

Women's work, on the other hand, was thought to present more difficult, complex problems given its unfavorable conditions (excessive physical strain, antihygienic environment, toxic substances), prolonged and inconvenient orario, and inadaptedness to the nursing woman's abilities. Yet, it did teach women the importance of time scheduling and productive labor, with benefits to breast-feeding. Borrino thought that if women's work were better protected and limited mainly to white-collar jobs, it could be expected to improve infant care. She explained that infant mortality rates were lowest in countries such as Sweden, Norway, and Denmark, in which it was the norm for women to have their own economic independence, and most were educated and exercised middle-class professions or worked in industry or commerce. Within Italy, infant and childhood mortality rates were *higher* in places where women generally were housewives, such as Siena, as opposed to industrialized Turin.[41]

Work in the home, such as piecework, was unfavorable to maternal functions since it was not protected by government provisions and was disorderly, poorly compensated, and exhausting. Worst of all, the infant's continuous closeness allowed the mother to quiet it by offering the breast, forcing it to take irregular meals. Even the well-off housewife, whose domestic labor was not too physically demanding, was prone to cancel the advantage of her nearness and freedom by responding too readily to her baby's every movement or cry. By making the child her exclusive interest, she violated the necessity of periodic rather than unregulated meals, and continuously stimulated the psyche with toys, noises, and movements, and, later, her teachings. The ideal caretaker was the well-regulated housewife or working mother who followed a strict, busy schedule of productive work and mothering.

Technique of Breast-Feeding, Supplementation, and Weaning

The Feeding Schedule

Medical intervention in breast-feeding in the interwar period centered around two main techniques: the spacing of feedings (*l'orario*) with the elimination of nighttime feeding; and the double weighing of infants at each poppata (*la doppia pesata*). These methods promised to eliminate maternal errors in breast-feeding, respect natural laws, and prevent over-nutrition, thereby maximizing infant health and development.

The feeding schedule was vaunted by its proponents as both respecting and improving upon children's and women's nature. Borrino marveled at the adaptability of the infant organism, noting that it could handle many different kinds of food under various methods or no method at all. She also prescribed putting the child to the breast every hour or even every time it cried in special cases such as late arrival of the milk, noting that woman's instinct would suggest this very treatment. Yet, to her both of these natural inclinations were transitory. Maternal instinct lasted only a short time, for soon the mother learned to recognize the child's natural need for rationalized, orderly feeding. For its part, the healthy and well-kept infant soon began to take meals at fixed hours. "Many infants after the second month, *spontaneously put themselves on five meals and even only four meals in 24 hours,* making a very long pause in the night" (1937:143).

Fixed hours were not arbitrary, but suggested by experience, for they corresponded to the functionality of the digestive tract and permitted the best growth and upbringing to the greatest number of infants. To calculate the schedule, one took the minimum distance between meals and added a little extra time to yield the "rule of five feedings," or "at the most, *not habitually,*" six in 24 hours. The hours were 7:00, 11:00, 15:00, 19:00, and 23:00, or 6:00, 10:00, 14:00, 18:00, and 23:00, and possibly also 2:00 or 3:00 in the night, "*meal however not habitual,* conceded for some cases of less tranquil nights" (Borrino 1937:143).

To increase the frequency of nipple stimulation in first-time mothers with insufficient milk secretion during the first two or at most three months, the physician could prescribe a modified schedule: six poppate spaced three hours apart, at 6:00, 9:00, 12:00, 15:00, 19:00, and 23:00–24:00. For a few days, the infant could be reattached "even" after two hours or sometimes more often if the secretion had not been started well, needed to be reactivated, or had been interrupted. In the case of limited breast functionality, breast-feeding and the use of a breast pump were done every hour or two, but the infant was always to be fed on the three-hour schedule (1937:144, 145, 148).

While other experts offered slightly different feeding schedules, all agreed that a "just periodicity" between rigorously spaced meals must be respected.[42] The orario must be invariably and definitively stabilized; the child should be waked for feedings and must habituate himself to it. Gelli, claiming not to be uselessly pedantic by insisting on very precise hours, magnanimously said that "naturally fifteen minutes" in either direction would not bring any harm (1931:767). He warned mothers not to give in, even to a syphilitic or otherwise ill or uncomfortable child, for this would only increase its sufferings and complicate things (1931:765–66).

The feeding schedule not only specified the intervals between meals, but set limits on their duration. The duration was longer than in on-demand feeding, for the schedule eliminated "all those little tastes and snacks" taken by babies put to the breast at every cry (Borrino 1937:146). For the first days, feeding could last 20 to 25 minutes at both breasts, then 15 to 20 through the first month. Data from many doppie pesate showed that it could take this long for the newborn to absorb the required ration of milk because of sleepiness. But very soon the baby would spontaneously stop eating after 10 to 12 minutes. After three months, with more effective suction and full glandular activity, 5 to 6 minutes were enough to extract as much as 250 grams of milk (1937:146–47). While some experts allowed longer feedings for a month or two more, most agreed that they should last no more than 5 to 10 minutes, regardless of individual differences among mothers or infants.

More than any other aspect of the new approach to breast-feeding, the feeding schedule was thought to unequivocally represent progress and consensus in the medical care of maternity and infancy. By respecting time limits, women imposed discipline and order upon themselves, proving that they knew how to go beyond instinct and had learned to exercise will and rationality in their behavior. They displayed their modern, scientific orientation, as opposed to inexperience, lack of knowledge, or inability to resist compassion for their children.

Double Weighings

The scheduling of meals was accompanied by a mechanistic approach to assessing nutritional status, in contrast to traditional indicators such as the infant's humor, skin condition, immune response, feeding behavior (willingness to eat, absence of digestive problems, and food intolerance), and temperature, respiration, and pulse. Infants were expected to grow in a constant, regular, never excessive way. This was known through frequent measurement of weight, hailed as the index of health and well-being. Growth in stature was also expected to be regular, but since it was considered a less useful tool it required only monthly measurement.

Infants were weighed at ever-closer intervals, closing the gap from many months or years to every month, week, or day. Medical texts presented tables of average weekly weight gain for breast- and bottle-fed infants through the first year, and even standards for daily weight gain in grams. The norm, which is still roughly the same today, was to measure body weight every two to three days in the first weeks—in spite of the knowledge that infants lose weight during the first week—and then space weighings at weekly intervals. After the sixth month, they could be taken every fifteen days. The method was to always use fixed times and days for weighing the child in the same clothes (or always undressed), clear of urine and feces, and far from the last feeding time. The weights were to be recorded unfailingly by the mother in a special printed table, to make it easier for the physician to compare them with standard values.

It is not a large leap from weekly or daily assessments to double weighings at each poppata, although not everyone was completely in favor of them. Experts admitted that it was difficult to know exactly how much milk was needed at any stage of life, and impossible to establish a precise relationship between energetic needs and infant body weight or surface area. Growth patterns varied among infants, while milk consumption changed between days and feedings. Milk components such as fat oscillated over the day and within single feedings (changing from watery to dense), strongly modifying its energetic value. The two breasts could produce different quantities of milk. Moreover, the infant's need for food varied according to external and internal conditions such as temperature and season, "strength" of digestion and assimilation, motor activity, appetite, state of health and development, sex, age, and basic psychological humor. Borrino concluded that it would be "absurd to want to stabilize *fixed doses* of food and impose them on the nursling with the test of double weighings" (1937:151).

Yet, these considerations were readily swept aside in the presentation of precise data in medical and popular texts on infant care, including Borrino's. She argued that clinical observation of a large number of infants had made it possible to extract certain "fundamental norms to empirically stabilize the sufficient and suitable ration in the majority of cases" (1937:83). The most basic of these was the maximum limit of one liter of milk per day—the same amount normal women were considered capable of producing (although healthy, robust women who fed two infants at once, whether in an institution, to help another mother, or for twins, were said to yield up to 2.5 liters per day). Maternal production and infant needs rose proportionally to half a liter in the first weeks, more than three-quarters of a liter by the end of the third or fourth month, and a full liter sometime after the sixth or seventh month.

Borrino limited herself to providing standards for daily consumption each week beginning at birth (1937:84). Most other experts were much more exacting, giving standards for each meal from the very first days of life. This was done by dividing the daily ration by the number of meals permitted (based on the baby's age). Another formula developed at this time, and still in use today, was based upon the child's body weight: for every kilogram of body weight, the child needs 100 calories per day (90 in the first two weeks). Since each liter of breastmilk contains 700 calories, the ration is 140 grams of milk per kilogram per day. To save the reader trouble, Gelli provided tables indicating standard ranges (minimum and maximum intake in grams) for each of a given number of meals, the average per-meal and daily ration, and the average body weight for each day of the first week and each week or month thereafter (1931:770–72).

These specifications were typical of the narrow time frames and detailed recommendations becoming more and more popular over the interwar period. Earlier texts from the 1920s were comparatively vague, specifying per poppata rations over relatively long time periods such as the first two weeks (20 to 40 grams), the next couple of months (60 to 100), and thereafter (120 to 200). Later texts were more exacting, specifying the amounts allowed the first day (3 to 4 grams), and each of the first four weeks (30 to 40; 50 to 60; 50 to 60; and 60). Thereafter, rations were given by month: 90 in the second, 100 to 130 in the third, 120 to 150 in the fourth, 150 to 180 in the fifth to seventh, and 160 to 200 in the seventh to twelfth.

If there was any doubt, the mother was always advised to give less, not more milk, in order to avoid the maladies discussed above. That is, the rationing of meals was undertaken not as much to ensure that infants got enough to eat as to keep them from taking too much. It was not insufficient feeding, but unregulated, excessive feeding that heightened health risks for infants.

Supplementation and Weaning

The same impulse to regulate milk consumption and production was behind the imposition of an earlier weaning than was customary in tradition and popular practice, but this was still later than that to which many urban women had become accustomed. Once again, clinical experience was the justification for a new medical norm: weaning should begin at six months and be completed within the year. As recently as the early 1920s, the booklet given to newly married spouses by the state had continued to insist that breastfeeding must, as a rule, be carried out for *at least* one year.[43] Now, it was "erroneous and damaging to the mother and infant to prolong maternal breast-feeding beyond one year."[44] Indeed, the extended exclusive milk diet and disorder in child rearing among poor families were considered the main dangers to infants in the second half of the first year. The common practice of breast-feeding for 18 to 20 months or more made mothers experience precocious aging and loss of teeth, abdominal *ptosi* (sinking down or prolapse of organs), emaciation, and a tired aspect. Many women did this to prevent pregnancy, but medical opinion now denied its effectiveness while asserting that interference with resumption of the menstrual cycle caused atrophy of the sexual apparatus, very grave nervous disturbances, and sterility.

Further, experts explained that mothers were tired or needed to take up their usual occupations by the time they had breast-fed one year, when there was also considerable distance from the hormonal stimulus that had initiated the secretion. The quantity of milk spontaneously began to decline as the child, now eating other foods, suckled less at the breast. Whether or not the quality changed, it was necessary for the child's health and development to give supplemental foods in place of some milk feedings beginning at around six months. Among those who believed that the milk did indeed lose its virtues by one year, especially in first-time mothers, there was the belief that the infant would lose weight, giving rise to flaccid tissues, pallor, and restlessness, if it continued to eat the "imperfect" human milk poor in salts, minerals, and albuminous substances.

Given the arguments against prolonged breast-feeding, there was a tendency among the "most modern" specialists in infant care to favor earlier initiation and termination of weaning. This meant definitive weaning before the tenth month, but not earlier than the seventh since it was necessary to wait until the first set of several teeth had appeared. Earlier weaning was justified by the argument that the capacity to digest and assimilate foods was already developed before the half-year, and that certain conditions made precocious weaning not only desirable but imperative. These included grave maternal illness, necessities of work or family, new pregnancy, the return of too-abundant menstruation, an excessively laborious life, and infant digestive disease causing milk intolerance.

A few circumstances called for later or delayed weaning, such as illness of the child, summer season, epidemics of infection, or dentition. In particular, the high heat of summer altered foods and made infants more susceptible to gastrointestinal diseases. These were already latent in them, because poorly conducted maternal breast-feeding and artificial feeding brought damage to the nutrition, development, and digestive system. Summer dealt the final blow, for "infants get sick *by diet* and die *by infection.*"[45]

Medical experts seconded the public's awareness that weaning was a dangerous time by saying that an imperfect technique of weaning was one of the three things (the others being dietary errors and infectious diseases) that most damaged the infant's growth in the second semester and second year of life. More "highly cultivated" mothers were less likely to commit gross dietary blunders, so that the education of lower-class women in the proper method of weaning was expected to reduce the frequency of disturbances in infants. This depended upon increasing the acceptability of cow's milk or other substitutes and hastening the disappearance of wrong-headed beliefs about serving animal milk unboiled to keep the nutritional components intact.

Most experts advised gradual weaning, with new foods introduced slowly and in orderly succession. Gelli thought it should be sudden, given his belief that changing the schedule made the milk lose its good qualities since it was no longer secreted regularly. Even if weaning was gradual, he felt that breast-feeding should be suppressed suddenly once the child was used to a more substantial diet, to avoid giving bad milk secreted too rarely. Sometimes, sudden weaning was actually mandatory, as in mothers who, out of an "exaggerated, almost morbose affectivity," would not renounce breast-feeding even when it was obviously insufficient or harmful to the infant (1931:799).

The medical literature was rich with daily meal plans for use from six months until weaning and beyond, including insistent injunctions that they be prepared with the requisite precautions and thoroughness. There could be no snacks, and no exceptions. The child must sit in a "rational position" during meals, but, in contrast to common practice, not at the family table until the age of three. Children were to be kept from eating the family meals until then, or even until they were six or seven. This would prevent access to inappropriate and harmful foods and drinks, and consequently the establishment of bad habits and vices. It thereby prevented chronic indigestion, constipation or diarrhea, ill-being, *nervosismo,* and weakness: conditions that led, in turn, to anemia, rickets, scrofula, and a predisposition to tuberculosis and lethal diseases of the stomach and intestine. Evidently, well into the child's life the consequences of maternal errors and excessive affection could be severe.

Mercenary Breast-Feeding

Virtually the same norms for breast-feeding applied to wet nurses as mothers. Well into the fascist period, medical texts still devoted special sections to wet nursing and often directed general recommendations to mothers and wet nurses together. This reflected the expectation that wet nursing was fairly common, for relatives and friends continued to help each other, nurses were needed when wealthy women died in childbirth or took ill, and some foundling hospitals and working-class families still hired nurses, even if it was increasingly unpopular among the wealthy.

One point repeated in the literature was that mothers must not be allowed to choose wet nursing by their own whim or perceived need, but only out of true necessity as judged by the physician.[46] The physician would examine the prospective wet nurse, looking for some familiar characteristics listed in older medical texts, such as age between 20 and 35, parity greater than one, and absence of a number of health conditions. The latter included any nervous, infectious, or nutritional disease; weakness from difficult childbirth, hemorrhage, or infection; disease or disorder of the skin, mouth, teeth, or breast; and excessive menstruation or any discharge from the genitals.

The prospective nurse's breasts should not be too big or fat, but moderately sized and shaped, and covered by warm skin showing a rich venous network, with an unscarred club-shaped nipple of medium size. A few other qualities were mentioned, such as brown rather than blond or red hair, similar age to the mother, and parentage of a same-sex child to the nursling. The nurse should have given birth within the past three or four months, for otherwise the milk would not be appropriate. If she was a "balia of second milk" who had already fed another child, she could be used only for the balance of normal lactation (a year in first-time mothers, a half-year longer for experienced mothers).

To test the milk, one could take a sample for chemical and microscopic examination, or simply press the nipple: if it did not shoot at a distance but dripped out in large, dense drops, it was concluded that the nurse did not have milk. Another test was whether the woman's own children had perished. If not because of acute or accidental disease, their deaths were necessarily the result of "bad breast-feeding or habitual negligences of the mother for too much ignorance, bad volontà, or great miseria."[47]

For nurses who came to the city from the country—unaccustomed to closed, crowded, sunless environments—experts imposed special precautions requiring close surveillance by the family and physician. It was necessary to carefully regulate the balia's first baths, because the sensation of the first bath in a tub, or excessive heat or cold, purportedly had been known to cause a sudden arrest of the milk secretion. The nurse's diet must be especially orderly and sober, because the new life and richer food led her to eat irregularly and excessively, causing difficult digestion and making her lazy, anemic, nervous, and unhappy, and thereby altering the milk.

Otherwise, the balia was subject to the same behavioral norms as nursing mothers, such as scrupulous cleanliness and sufficient but not excessive rest, nourishment, activity, and exposure to the open air. Atmospheric imbalances, strong emotions, and intestinal disorders were to be avoided. The nurse must keep the infant very clean and give it milk at the indicated hours and in sufficient quantity, which the family could verify through frequent doppie pesate at home or in a clinic. At night, she must not feed the infant in bed, allowing it to remain attached to the breast, but get up according to the established orario and breast-feed in a low chair.

In short, wet nurses, like mothers, were expected to breast-feed methodically, without any misplaced affection. Yet, as with mothers, the wet nurses' constitution and behavior were also thought to affect the milk, mostly in a negative way.

Mixed and Artificial Feeding

With the decline of wet nursing and the earlier initiation of weaning, it came to be expected that most children would take formula or animal milk before the end of the first year. In addition to the decline in quantity and quality after the first few months, mother's milk was also said to undergo transitory alterations upon parental sexual relations, return of menstruation, or in the days corresponding to the usual menstrual period. Mothers too were said to be harmed by prolonged lactation, especially if they were weak, gracile, had abundant or frequent menstruation, or became pregnant. This was taken to mean that supplementation actually improved maternal breast-feeding and infant nutrition.

As in all other decisions regarding infant nutrition, only the physician was held to be competent to judge whether "deficiencies" in the mother (including work away from home) or her milk warranted recourse to mixed or artificial feeding. Mixed feeding could be initiated as early as the first, but preferably the second completed month. If methodical, it was said to give no disturbance to the infant and to permit a completely regular growth and development, if not results that were superior to exclusive breast-feeding. After the sixth month, mixed feeding was indispensable since infant growth slowed or even diminished under exclusive breast-feeding, especially from a primiparous, gracile, or working mother. The child could either receive alternating meals of mother's milk and fresh animal or artificial milk, or be fed first at both breasts, then given a ration of supplemental milk. The latter was generally preferred since the former method spaced maternal feedings too far apart, causing the milk to stay too long in the breasts.

In artificial feeding, nonhuman milk was given exclusively from the first days. However, it was reserved for grave cases, for it was not known to give perfect results even if all rules were scrupulously followed. Artificial feeding was known to disturb the nutrition and markedly increase the risk of disease and death, with indelible, lifelong effects. Moreover, if scrupulous cleanliness were not maintained, the child could easily develop oral thrush spreading over the entire alimentary canal (which was also said to happen in badly conducted maternal breast-feeding).

Modern science and experience were said to favor cow or donkey milk, in contrast to the popular affection for goat milk. The literature discussed in detail the merits of bovine milk's various forms, including raw, condensed, sugared, oxygenated, pasteurized, and powdered. Fresh milk had to be sterilized and "corrected" through dilution and other means. It was preferable to "artificial" forms, as the latter were associated with higher mortality and lower growth rates. Milk could be administered by spoon, cup, or bottle, but the latter was considered less hygienic. These themes were addressed in ONMI courses for health professionals, who then taught parents.

The method for both mixed and artificial feeding coincided with that used for maternal breast-feeding with respect to the time schedule, rations of milk, proper positioning of the mother and child, and maintenance of order and regularity in nutrition and digestion. The fixed daily ration of animal milk was divided among no more than five meals separated by at least four hours in daytime and six to seven at night, as in the following orario for hospitals and families: 6:00, 10:00, 14:00, 18:00, and 23:00. This rule was said to best guarantee tolerance of animal milk and ensure a more regular growth. It prevented errors such as too-frequent or too-abundant meals, which caused dilatation and weakening of the stomach, indigestion, and constipation or diarrhea, possibly leading to rickets or fatal infantile cholera.

Once again, mothers were threatened with extreme consequences including infant disease and death for failure to conform to medical norms of behavior. Women's ignorance and naturalness were contrasted against physicians' expertise and instruments, and the blood-mediated symbiosis between mothers and infants was now understood quite differently. The relationship shifted from communication through the placenta to synergism between the "natural" periodicity of the functions of the maternal breast and infantile gastrointestinal system. Educating and disciplining mothers and children to the importance of adhering to strict schedules therefore assumed overwhelming importance. This effort was supported by the assertion that incorrect and not simply imprudent maternal behaviors caused grave health consequences.

A new conception of the value of the infant and child in social and political terms was related to the decoupling of the mother-infant relationship at birth. As infants came to be considered the future of the fascist nation-state, their treatment and upbringing were dissociated from the needs or inclinations of their mothers. Medical ideas were connected to national political demographic aspirations, justifying the intervention of experts in women's behavior in the home and opening the private sphere into the public domain. The periodicity of biological functions was the essential theoretical basis for norms regulating excess through the spacing and metering of infant meals. It was a quintessentially biopolitical concept in an industrial-technological society obsessed with the rationalization of time, production, and output.

CHAPTER 6

Moral Obligation, Natural Duty
Consolidation of State and
Medical Authority

The changes in ideas about maternity and breast-feeding that we have discussed were mirrored in transformations in the organization and practice of medicine. The severed link between mothers and infants was reflected in the specialization of medical disciplines and the standardization of care. The authority of medical experts was contrasted against the alleged ignorance and ill-preparation of mothers for their maternal duties. Ancestral sentiments of resignation and fatalism were rejected in favor of faith in the efficacy of medical intervention and the importance of direct, informed maternal care. This justified medical surveillance and intervention in areas that had previously been considered the domain of families and traditional moral and medical authorities.

Fascist medical and political texts and propaganda unceasingly stressed the notion that every woman had a "moral obligation" to breast-feed, for her infant's vitality depended upon it.[1] By suppressing the influence of tradition and breast-feeding according to a rational method, mothers were to demonstrate their competence, modernity, and adherence to national political aspirations. Yet, relatively strong differences in social and economic conditions impeded the immediate, uniform acceptance of medical norms for breast-feeding. In the rural areas, hygienic conditions remained very poor while medical care was insufficient, if not nonexistent. While new child-rearing norms were embraced by mothers who lived in cities and had frequent contact with health professionals and government institutions, these norms were often ignored or dismissed by rural and working-class urban families.

The centralizing institution of fascist biological politics was the Opera Nazionale per la Protezione della Maternità e dell'Infanzia (ONPMI, later ONMI). Its scope was nothing less than the salvation of the nation through programs to lower infant mortality rates, bring about higher fertility rates, and impose more rational child-rearing methods, including regimented breast-feeding. These programs affected millions of mothers and infants, and drew health professionals into the fold of state influence. ONMI institutes were hailed as "schools for mothers" where women were submitted to frequent observation and taught how to be mothers. The foundation was laid for the medicalization of maternity as the public was brought into a close relationship with medical and state authorities. ONMI would continue to tighten this knot for another three decades after the war, contributing to greater cultural and medical control of the individual body.

Organization of Medicine

Medical Authority and Maternal Ignorance

Medical authority was a dominant theme in fascist-era texts on infant care, for it was considered the antidote to women's fatal ignorance. Meanwhile, political writers inaugurated the fascist period as a new era of activism in the care of infants, in contrast to the complacency of previous governments. Popular fatalistic and "Darwinian" concepts that had explained high infant mortality rates on the basis of divine will or differential fitness were now to give way to the belief that specialized medical intervention could make a difference and actually improve the physical and moral development of the stirpe. The first order of business was to correct women's "foolish customs" and deficiency of knowledge regarding breast-feeding and the upbringing of children.

A physician in Turin declared that "one could say without exaggeration that many mothers, even though they would be capable of every sacrifice for the good of their babies, kill them out of ignorance, out of obedience to prejudices."[2] ONMI courses for professionals taught about the "relationships between ignorance and infant mortality."[3] Borrino attributed the majority of infant deaths from gastroenteritis to the "prolonged and repeated damage which the mother herself has caused her own child during its upbringing, with disorder in meals, hyperalimentation, insufficient cleanliness, administration of inopportune and dangerous foods, [and] blind faith in old prejudices or the advice of tradition or fashion" (1937:viii).

In particular, "errors in breast-feeding" were thought to be the cause of infant suffering from diseases, including those of nutrition and the digestive tract (particularly acute gastroenteritis)—the primary cause of infant and early childhood mortality. Likewise, infectious diseases were caused by "intestinal autointoxication" owing to dietary irregularities, while anomalies in physical or psychological development could also be traced to feeding errors. The Fascist Confederation of Industrial Workers exclaimed, "*quante mamme hanno ucciso i loro nati con gli eccessi o l'irregolarità dell'allattamento!*" (how many mothers have killed their own

infants with excesses or irregularity of breast-feeding!) (1940:315). The
envelope for medical charts at the ONMI pediatric clinic in Sassari said,
"Give milk and all foods at fixed meals: disorder in diet kills one hundred
thousand Italian children every year."[4]

State and medical surveillance of maternal behavior was thought to
account for the decline in infant mortality rates and the victory over infectious diseases. Fascist civilization was said to have brought great progress
through laws protecting maternity and infancy, networks of medical clinics, and diffusion of a hygienic consciousness in the area of infant care.
Work for ONMI was portrayed as a moral issue of conscience, since the
physician's promotion and control of breast-feeding helped to reduce
infant mortality rates and improve the health and robustness of the population. This work also took part in the integral reclamation of the nation,
for improvements in communications and transportation permitted more
diffuse and constant medical surveillance.

In this view, the infant's right to proper maternal care took precedence over the mother's right to make her own choices. DeNapoli said that
physicians frequently saw gravely ill or moribund patients whose disease
or death would have been avoided if the mother had chosen to breast-feed
them, and he lamented "the liberty which the mother has to raise her child
as she pleases" (1934b:424). There was far too much voluntary abstention
from breast-feeding by the "modern woman." The fact that mercenary
and artificial feeding still carried much higher infant mortality rates than
breast-feeding (63, 32, and 15 percent, respectively, as reported in
DeNapoli 1934b:418) was taken as justification for suppressing alternative
methods while focusing on teaching mothers how to breast-feed properly.
In the countryside, the problem was acute since artificial feeding was "anything but infrequent," and natural feeding was "practiced completely irra-
tionally."[5] The Italian woman was exhorted to cooperate with physicians
and nurses in the "always greater diffusion of the norms that must govern
maternal breast-feeding."[6]

Mothers were told that they needed to acquire new attitudes and abilities that were not infrequently the opposite of what their "feminine affection" or "instinct" would suggest, no matter how important the latter were
for assuring loving and vigilant dedication. Intelligence and technical
knowledge, manual dexterity, and an exact memory were needed for
unerringly remembering and applying medical prescriptions. It was the
mother's duty to take the child to the pediatrician each month—and not
just to ask for a gift of milk or infant cereal. She must also continuously
and vigilantly observe the child's health and development, and seek the
physician's intervention in case of any possible disturbance. If the child fell
ill and the mother did not "rigorously and scrupulously" follow the physician's directives, there would be no hope of recovery. Statements like these

were made "not to scare anyone" but to convince mothers to observe medical norms faithfully, even if they did not understand their significance. Women should never treat illness by themselves, but "listen to the physician and silence the chatters" and "deadly prejudices" of midwives and "reckless milksops."[7]

Of all the untrained neighbors, friends, or relatives prone to give women "absurd advice," their mothers and mothers-in-law were singled out as the most meddlesome. Mothers and husbands were said to be the worst birth assistants because of their gross ignorance and superstitions. Mothers-in-law wasted their time giving advice about maternity and infancy that was "always perfectly annoying, almost always useless."[8] Indeed, it was considered easier to regulate artificial feeding than breast-feeding, because women's schedules were set by their mothers-in-law who, particularly in the agricultural households, had "direct and jealous command over the young wives and over the upbringing of the children, and tranquilly hand down obsolete traditionalism of the most tenacious ignorance."[9]

In order not to promote mixed or artificial feeding or the spread of knowledge about artificial feeding methods, the medical community was required by law to refuse technical assistance except in urgent cases in which it was absolutely necessary. The 1930 legislation regulating midwifery obligated midwives to try to convince all women to breast-feed. If a mother resisted or wished to renounce it, the midwife was to ensure that she was submitted to the physician's judgment. In fact, the midwife was required to defer to the physician's authority in all matters concerning breast-feeding, including difficulties in initiating it or ailments of the mother's breast or the infant's mouth. In teaching mothers the norms for breast cleanliness, diet, the scheduling and dosing of feedings, and periodic measurements of body weight, the midwife was always to follow the instructions of the physician.[10]

Transformations in Medical Knowledge and Practice

The interwar period overturned the old medical system and the ideas upon which it had been based. The autonomous medici condotti, levatrici, and liberi professionisti were channeled into an urban, laboratory- and clinic-based system in which research and cure came to replace comfort and care as the major mission of medicine. The relationship between health-care provider and patient changed as their interaction moved to the clinic, and diagnosis and treatment became standardized and dissociated from individual context. Physicians and midwives purposely changed their dress to express their sobriety, respectability, and authority.[11]

The old empiricism was devalued in favor of experimentation and clinical observation, setting the knowledge of experts apart from that of traditional authorities and the public. To further distance themselves, medical professionals attacked the credibility of local physicians, mid-wives, and folk healers of both sexes, but especially women. Physicians expanded their role in the care of maternity and infancy beyond that of assisting during complicated childbirth. The specializations proliferated along with the varieties of professional health-care workers, and this was accompanied by a rise in technological and instrumental interventions and treatments. The sophisticated specialist physician based in a clinic or laboratory was contrasted against the old, wandering, ignorant *medico condotto* or *medico dei poveri* (poor people's physician), who was considered an impediment to the proper practice of medicine. The practitioners of fascist political demography would be specialists, not generalists: hygienists, internists, pediatricians, gynecologists, obstetricians.

Given the widely proclaimed idea that it was the ignorance of mothers, grandmothers, and midwives that killed infants, one of the central aims of the new medicine was to supersede the traditional *levatrice* and female relatives in the care of pregnancy, childbirth, and infancy. Women were to submit themselves to the science of the hospital physician rather than empiricism of the trusted *levatrice* or medico condotto. Experts argued that midwives needed a more rational and thorough training. By teaching mothers about the midwives' dangerous limitations, physicians would convince mothers to trust physicians more and midwives less. Physicians questioned the need for midwives at all, saying that the tenacious Italian habit of calling them was backward and dangerous. Home birth was classified as unacceptable for "intelligent and modern" women, who should entrust the care of pregnancy and childbirth to the "physician-obstetrician-surgeon" only. Physicians argued that "many so-called *congenital* diseases, would be avoided if the pregnant woman made herself seen often by the physician (not by the midwives)."[12]

However, as in most things, contemporary thought regarding medical progress was ambivalent. One of the unwelcome consequences of progress was that the spotlight fell upon the negative health outcomes of urbanization and industrialization, rather than the equally acute problems of the rural areas. The fascist response to the poor living conditions of the countryside was a program of "rural health politics," involving the establishment of permanent or mobile health clinics to reach even the most isolated areas and the elevation of the status and capabilities of district physicians and midwives. While the medici condotti were more often criticized, it had to be acknowledged that, in spite of the "intolerable overbearing manner of certain authorities and the discomforts of life," they carried out the "highest and most humane, most worthy social function."[13] In practice, the effort to include district health workers meant drawing them into the state medical system through standardized and increasingly specialized training.

Medical Specialization

Until the early twentieth century, there had been few medical specializa- tions in Italy, and they had remained relatively generalized. While obstet- rics and pediatrics had been rudimentary specializations since Roman times, they mainly consisted of the inclusion of notions of maternal and infant care dispersed in ancient medical writings. In Italy, there had been few good treatises on obstetrics before the publication of Bumm's (1923) translated German text. The last edition of an obstetrics text by any pro- fessor at a university clinic had been published in 1887, and it was com- posed of his lectures compiled by another physician. The specialization truly began to grow only after the turn of the century; the first conference of the Italian Society of Obstetrics and Gynecology was held in 1912.

The specialization of the disciplines associated with maternity and infancy reflected both the splitting of the mother and child at birth and a new understanding of women and men, adults and children, as being essen- tially different rather than homologous. In the past, maternity and infancy had been treated as a single interrelated process from conception to wean- ing, and puericultura had been the main science devoted to them, in health and disease. The field was now bisected into puericultura prenatale and puericultura postnatale, while general puericultura was contrasted against puericultura infantile. Puericultura, as the science of upbringing, was sepa- rated from pediatrics, the science of childhood diseases.

The baby was no longer just a "little man," but a child with unique anatomical and physiological characteristics, giving rise to the new turn- of-the-century science of the nursling, nipiologia. Similarly, gynecology and obstetrics came to be based upon the idea that the female organism was not the same as the male, but had a different biology, physiopathol- ogy, and psychology. While midwifery dealt with normal reproductive processes, obstetrics focused upon pathology and was essentially con- cerned with obstetrical operations. The professionalization of maternal and infant care is evident in the shrinking of the categories of female birth assistants. In place of the trained *commari* (or *comari*), *riccoglitrici,* and *levatrici,* and lay *mammane* and *donnine,* there were now only the old-fash- ioned midwife or *levatrice* and the modern, university-educated *ostetrica.*

Within the specializations, there was a growing gender distinction. The treatment of disease (gynecology, obstetrics, pediatrics) was a heroic and esteemed "male" function consisting of wrenching lives from the grips of death and bringing new lives into existence. This work was supported by the "female" tasks of prevention, puericultura, midwifery, and social work.

There were also changes on the level of terminology, reflecting the separation and objectification of mother and infant. The mother's identity was effaced by terms such as *maternal organism* or simply *the organism,* and the *subject* or *terrain* on which one worked. Older, more general terms, such as *woman* and *child* or *creature,* were replaced by specific labels identifying discrete stages in the mother-infant relationship: women were *gestanti* or *gravide* in pregnancy, *partorienti* during childbirth, *puerpere* afterward, and *nutrici* while nursing. Children were *feti* during gestation, *nascituri* during childbirth, *nati* or *neonati* after childbirth, *lattanti* or *poppanti* while subsisting on milk or more generally for the first year, and *divezzi* during and after weaning. These words were not entirely new, but were now used more frequently, in the noun form, and independently of the simpler terms.

This parceling up and professionalization of the care of maternity and infancy was central to the standardization and medical control of breastfeeding.

Humoral to Mechanical Understandings of Childbirth

The shift away from thinking of mother-infant interactions in terms of continuous fluid interrelationships extended to the care of childbirth, especially in hospitals and clinics. It was accompanied by the exclusion of family members from the scene of childbirth, an interventionistic approach in medicine, and the physical separation of mothers and infants in maternity wards.

In medical texts and other writings, the wildly emotional and improperly prepared mother, father, and their relatives were contrasted against the calm, certain, authoritative physician. These and other "useless people" were only a distraction and had to be eliminated from the birthing room or maternity clinic. The physician represented women's salvation from harm or death due to their own ignorance and was referred to as a priest whose work was his "ministry." The mother was rendered silent and passive by the practice of referring to her as the *operanda,* the one being operated on, and the rising expectation that the physician would perform an operation (as in Vicarelli 1926a:3).

Contributing to the growing sense that childbirth implied an *intervento chirurgico* or surgical operation, medical texts enumerated many substances for reducing pain, including morphine, opium, or cocaine along with or as a preliminary to laudanum, ether, or chloroform. Medical texts also suggested epidural injections and an enema of olive oil and narcotic drugs. One physician, Gelli, advocated imitating other European countries and the United States by using general anesthetics universally, followed by the "almost habitual" use of the forceps. He maintained that this would make the mother suffer less and abbreviate labor and medical assistance, for anesthesia rendered "every kind of operation easier and more expeditious" (1931:530, 622).

One obvious consequence of this kind of thinking was a preference for the supine birth position. The obstetrical chair that had been around since Roman times was considered an obsolete, inappropriate, and dangerous instrument, all the more so because it was still used by some lay midwives and *levatrici*. Newly trained midwives placed women on their backs and supported their feet with chairs.

Prevention of infection was becoming an important part of hospital practice, for puerperal fever still accounted for three-quarters of all maternal deaths. Traditional understandings of the etiology of this disease had emphasized air currents, the shame of being examined by a male physician, or the lesser cleanliness of physicians' as opposed to midwives' hands. Now, it was said that puerperal fever was the result of bacteria entering the body through cuts and abrasions associated with childbirth.

While health professionals sought to keep themselves cleaner, the emphasis in medical texts was (and still is) on disinfecting the mother's body. The pregnant woman was to disinfect the genitals throughout pregnancy and was submitted to intrusive cleaning methods at childbirth. At childbirth, the woman—now an *operanda*—was treated the same as anyone about to undergo an operation on the abdomen or genitals. The decontamination of her abdominal-genital-anal area was accomplished through washing with soap and disinfectants; dietary restriction; preparation of the intestine with purgatives, disinfectants, and absorbents; disinfecting vaginal irrigation; and *tricotomia* (shaving of pubic hair). Governmental regulations specified that midwives were to use the tricotomia even for normal births, although some physicians argued against it due to the risk of abrasions.

The medical literature indicates a rise in enthusiasm for mechanical interventions in childbirth. This was supported by thorough research on and classification of varieties of *bacino ristretto* (narrow pelvis) (such as "total restricted pelvis, of elegant form," and "infantile" or "masculine" pelvis) or deformed pelvis (from rickets, scoliosis, or osteomalacia). Fascist-era texts are replete with photographs of skeletal remains, pictures of live subjects, and radiographs, often with the fetus present.[14] Birth through different kinds of narrow pelvis was a separate subject and was said to require frequent use of the forceps or craniotomy of a live fetus— that is, removal of the "cerebral substance" with scissors.

Operations were classified according to whether they were performed with instruments or hands, were *incruenti* (not bloody) or *cruenti* (bloody) for the fetus or mother, or both. The forceps, *rivolgimento* (version), and manual extraction were not bloody: all others were bloody. The latter

included craniotomy; embriotomy by decapitation or evisceration; caesarean section; and the cutting of limbs and other parts in the case of "double monsters." Texts described how the mother's hips could be enlarged
through symphysiotomy (cutting of the cartilage and ligaments of the
symphysis pubis with a scalpel) and pubiotomy (cutting of the pubic bone
with a saw), both of which were described as not just bloody but also
noisy.

Some of these operations had been around for a long time. Embriotomy was described by Sorano d'Efeso around A.D. 100 and Mercurii in
1601.[15] Symphysiotomy had been introduced in the late eighteenth century
but banished until almost one hundred years later because of high maternal and fetal mortality rates. Now, it was included among the well-accred-
ited operations, thanks to advances in antisepsis and operative techniques.

The operative acts may have been more captivating, but in reality the
various kinds of *rivolgimento,* together with the forceps, remained the primary methods of obstetrical assistance. Obstetrics textbooks continued to
devote many pages to them, and physicians and midwives recall using
them more than any other method. A district physician in Emilia-
Romagna named Gaspare Cenni, writing about the mid-1940s, described
his surprise at a "curious surgical-obstetrical coincidence" he did not think
common even in the great hospitals: "the execution of three caesarean sections in the brief space of one week!" (1965:120). Indeed, in both the countryside and the cities most births continued to take place in the home, in
the midst of family members, and without surgical intervention.

In the rural areas the midwife continued to be, in general, the only
health professional present, whereas in the cities it was becoming more
common to enlist the aid of a physician. It was not until well after the Second World War that the hospitalization of childbirth was complete. This
was a central factor in changes in the experience of childbirth and lactation, for hospitals were a major force in the propagation of norms for scientific mothering.

The Medicalization of the Maternal Condition

Medicalization in Italy did not mean a transition away from treating
maternity with indifference, for women and infants were subject to complex rules and treatments well before the rise of professional biomedicine.
Instead, it entailed a shift from the traditional authority of family members, midwives, clerics, and local physicians to the growing authority of
the professional medical community. The intrusion of the latter was
justified in the fascist period by the aims of political demography as well as
an understanding of maternity as a pathological state, in spite of its proclaimed naturalness. The perceived dangers of maternal behaviors and

constitutions and the damaging biological consequences of modern civilization made constant medical supervision necessary and the thwarting of disaster by preemptive intervention increasingly desirable. The cultural importance of the physician in managing gestation, childbirth, and breast-feeding consequently came to eclipse that of the mother.

The notion that even healthy people needed to present themselves for medical examination on a regular basis was entirely new. Experts such as Pende bewailed the public's reticence and perplexity in response to the idea that every working-class child should be sent to the ONMI clinics, even if "healthy and prosperous," and that all women should routinely procure prenatal medical care and give birth in ONMI maternity wards (1939:4). Beyond this, women were instructed to submit to a lifelong gynecologic "vigilance over the menstrual function" to control for irregular or defective periods indicating "scarce genital activity with consequent sterility."[16]

Maternity came to be perceived as a state of semisickness, in spite of the notion that gestation and lactation made women flower. This paradox was resolved through the principle that even minor, transitory disturbances commonly thought of as natural to pregnancy were to be included in the field of pathology, since they did not affect "normal" women. Pregnancy was said to induce true sufferings that could reach considerable intensity, especially in "subjects" who were feeble, sick, or congenitally weak.

In other words, although pregnancy was not a morbose state and the pregnant woman should not be considered diseased, the biological and mechanical phenomena of maternity did make her predisposed to get sick, and more sensitive to and defenseless against noxious influences. To obstetricians such as Bumm (1923a:131) or Vicarelli (1926a:5–6), these harmful forces included infection, exposure to toxins, modified circulation and digestion, anemia, and wounds caused by childbirth or obstetrical operations. Gelli believed that "pathological maternity" was the result of the progressive, heritable deterioration of the civilized races and their antinatural ways of life, which had created shoddy, gracile, sensitive races in which physiological maternity was unknown to women (1931:446–47).

If maternity was pathological, then the instrumental approaches of modern obstetrics were all the more important for bringing the child "to the light" unharmed. In a departure from a long tradition of making sustained efforts to save the mother's life while tossing the newborn to the side until the danger had passed—as seen in the birth stories recorded by Santandrea and Cenni—some experts began to express a willingness to risk the health and life of the mother for the sake of the child. Gelli explained that it would be morally correct to sacrifice the mother unless doing so would not be enough to save the child, for it was a sin against God and a crime before mankind not to "try with every means to conserve the life of the embryo or fetus, even with danger to the life of the mother" (1931:470).

In contrast, other physicians such as Bumm were against the "bad, active" obstetrics that always sought to operate and did not let natural childbirth proceed, making thousands of women pay with their lives (1923a:244). Vicarelli said that "operative obstetrics, in its highest ideals, proposes to bring to life a live, healthy child without damaging the mother," but because of the hazards of childbirth the obstetrician may have to risk the life of one to save the other (1926a:1). However, the physician's art must never be used without consent, particularly for an operation for the child's sake which the mother would oppose or refuse when conscious. Reacting against the tendency to intervene precociously or for the sake of convenience, he added that no inopportune intervention could be justified or legitimized by impatience, expedience, painlessness or near-painlessness of an operation, the safeguard of antisepsis, or the aid of anesthetics (1926a:5).

As maternal functions were displaced from the private to the public sphere, they came to be seen as the work of physicians, not mothers. This was evident in the notion that the physician's work in delivering a child was more difficult and heroic than that of the mother. As Gelli announced, he had to produce twice the physical force of the mother's contractions to extract the fetus manually or with forceps (1931:602). This shift in emphasis from the woman and her family to the physician and "his" instruments has been a central feature of twentieth-century changes in the care and experience of maternity.

Infant Feeding Patterns

Social and Economic Factors

The departure from empirical observation put increasing distance between medical and popular belief, and between specialized biomedicine and general medicine. Popular compliance with new medical norms was higher among the literate, urban populations in closest contact with university-trained health professionals. Well-off and urban women were much more likely than the "common women" to seek medical care during pregnancy, childbirth, and the puerperium, although they amounted to only a fraction of all mothers. These conditions changed little, as the growth of the middle class was slow in Italy and delayed until after the Second World War. Nevertheless, the nascent middle class did see an improvement in living conditions that prefigured the vast changes of the postwar period. Especially in the northern and central regions, new appliances such as radios, telephones, and cars appeared in increasing numbers. Most children went to school, and girls attended high school and college in modest but much larger numbers than ever before.

Overall, economic conditions did not improve over the interwar period, and there are many indications that they worsened in the 1930s. Wages in agriculture and industry declined, offsetting the highly touted fall in the cost of living (which rose again in the mid-1930s). The fascist government was unable to eliminate the problem of scarce and unfit housing, in spite of new regulations for builders and real estate owners and a substantial increase in new housing units. Showy efforts to support smallholding and clear new land for agriculture were not matched by any significant change in the level of peasant landownership. This was because fascism did not in fact provide much assistance to the rural economy and instead actually privileged industrial development.[17]

The goal of becoming self-sufficient in grain was met, but at a cost to the nation since cheaper grains were available on the international market. The outlawing of emigration kept workers in the country, but did nothing to improve wages or high and persistent unemployment rates. Provisions allowing city mayors to keep newcomers out did not stop urbanization, and living conditions in the crowded cities and outlying areas were still very poor. The Fascist Party itself published data revealing that 1.75 million families received public assistance in money and food and that 35 million rations of food were distributed over the winter of 1933–34 alone. Food sales had declined along with food consumption overall, especially in categories such as meat. Pawnshop pledges were rising along with the number of homeless people.[18] On the other hand, massive public works programs absorbed some unemployment, while the development of war-related industries eventually facilitated postwar industrialization.

In spite of fascist propaganda and efforts to extend medical care to all mothers and infants, there was virtually no prenatal care in the countryside until after the Second World War. This was blamed upon the "ignorant public's" resistance to prenatal medical visits, but there was also a real shortage of medical care. As one midwife recalls, "in those times women never had themselves checked, so that we midwives went to assist the patients [in childbirth] without ever having examined them."[19] Only 0.01 percent of all pregnant women were assisted by ONMI in 1926, a proportion that only grew to 11.8 percent in 1934.[20] Medical interventions in general were out of the reach of most people: in the 1930s top doctors charged more than ten times the average worker's annual salary for a single surgical operation.[21]

The distance between urban academic medicine and rural practice was extreme. Elite specialized physicians wished to do away with midwives and generalist physicians, and move childbirth completely out of the home. They were frustrated by the public's diffidence concerning hospital birth and argued that any medical care in a clinic was better than the incomplete, defective, and dangerous assistance provided in the home of even the wealthiest families. By contrast, the writings of health professionals who actually worked in the countryside indicate that physicians very often showed deep respect of and deference toward midwives. Likewise, far from being an annoyance, the untrained birth assistants who often substituted for the physician or midwife were "courageous, intelligent, generous and also often effective for their acquired experience."[22]

Childbirth still took place in the home for most people of every social or economic class and was assisted by the physician only in cases of necessity. Husbands and other relatives continued to be present. While many women remember sitting or squatting, the favored birth position began to conform to the supine standard, especially if an ostetrica or physician were present. Childbirth was still feared because of continued high rates of maternal hemorrhages, infections, and deaths. Women waited until the last minute to call the midwife, taking care of their work and families first. As a result, farm women sometimes gave birth in the fields.

Some families still preferred the lay midwife or were compelled to call her if the ostetrica could not arrive in time. This was not uncommon, for poor weather and a lack of roads and bridges impeded the travel of messengers as well as midwives and physicians. The latter had to do their best with limited supplies, and under hygienic conditions that were completely contrary to those enjoyed and expected by urban physicians. Postnatal care depended upon the availability of the midwife, who would make a visit to the house every seven or eight days for the first couple of months. These conditions persisted into the 1960s in places like Santa Lucia, in spite of the institution of new maternity clinics after the Second World War.

The social distance between families is evident in the contrast between the "common" women's on-demand feeding and the elite practice of having wet nurses express their milk and give it to the child by bottle, so that it could be measured and sterilized. The nurse also had to sterilize her nipples and all of the implements of artificial feeding. One Santa Lucia woman remembers doing these things for a baby she wet nursed in the early 1940s.

Well-to-do simple families also readily embraced the notion that infants should not sleep in the same bed or room as their parents. By contrast, ONMI social and health workers found it difficult to persuade large farm families whose housing arrangements and family traditions were contrary to the practice of isolated infant sleep. The goal was to reduce transmission of tuberculosis, but the practice also fit well with the new medical belief that cosleeping was damaging to infant health and development. Further, it converged with cultural beliefs about the child's place as external to the conjugal relationship, or rather the father's right to undisturbed sleep and access to the mother.

Continuity and Change

The infant feeding practices and beliefs of the interwar period reflected both an ongoing exchange and a rising conflict between medical and popular knowledge and practice. Areas of close concurrence between popular memory and medical textbooks and practitioners included the need to fast for several days after childbirth and the belief that a new pregnancy in the mother or wet nurse required hasty termination of breast-feeding. They also included the moderate but never excessive ingestion of wine during pregnancy and lactation, and the avoidance of many common foods thought to taint the milk during lactation. Parsley, in particular, was ingested in large quantities at weaning time, for it was (and is) considered a "poison" (and abortifacient, besides).

For the most part, medical and popular knowledge agreed that weaning should be avoided in summertime. This was based on the empirical observation that summer increased childhood gastrointestinal disease and the likelihood of food contamination. The novelist Natalia Ginzburg describes this with reference to Abruzzo in the 1930s: "The long sunny days on the low and stark hills, the yellow dust of the road and the dysentery of the children, end, and the winter begins" (1964 [1944]:1). The association with disease and death contributed to a cultural preoccupation with weaning that persists to the present day.

There was less agreement about when weaning should be initiated. We have seen that weaning was to be completed by one year and initiated at six months or earlier. While "modern" women complied and even went farther by starting weaning at two or three months, the "common" women obstinately continued to breast-feed more or less exclusively for a year plus another six, twelve, or more months thereafter. Experts attributed this to women's "unreasonable" and doomed aspiration to obtain healthy and well-developed children this way and to an instinctive, primordial, but futile and misguided attempt to prevent pregnancy. That women were still breast-feeding intensively and not running out of milk is evident in the fact that experts found it necessary to teach mothers how to get rid of the milk in their "painful, turgid breasts" at weaning time. Women were told to disregard the milksops' warnings that the methods of compression, dieting, diuretics, and saline purgatives compromised future lactation, indicating that mothers were reluctant to use these means for driving away the milk before its time.

The weaning foods suggested by physicians corresponded closely to traditional preferences, but were now supposed to be used under medical direction. Infant formula and supplementary foods were sold only in pharmacies. These products were considered both appealing because they were modern and expensive, and undesirable because they were not prepared at home.

While the specifics varied, the experts' recommendations tended to deny infants any flavorful or complex food until a relatively late age, reflecting the belief that such foods were harmful for children's development and gastrointestinal function. There was a further tendency to discredit commercial products, often on the basis of their preservatives and antiseptic substances. This was an expression of the traditionalist, antimodernist, anti-internationalist side of scientific mothering. That is, meals were to be made by a devoted and well-instructed mother (or cook) in the home, using precise methods, recipes, and schedules provided by physicians.

The first foods, beginning at three to six months, were predominantly the traditional cereal-based paps. Meat and vegetable broths with semolina, pasta, and vegetable puree were introduced after the ninth or tenth month, as well as bread, often grated into a pap. Water was to be given after meals; but diluted and sweetened milk during, never between, them. Throughout the first year, the child was prohibited common soups; sweets and biscuits prepared with sugar or honey; butter, margarine, and pig fat; sweet fruits such as bananas, pineapples, or dates; and fermented beverages, wine, tea, and coffee. Some experts allowed meat toward the end of the first year, but others did not permit it until the second or third year. Beginning at one year, slightly cooked eggs could be given. Egg yolk beaten with sugar and dissolved in tepid water or milk was described as a late afternoon infant meal. Legumes were to be given in the form of puree until the child was four and would be permitted to eat the family's meals.

These standards matched the actual practices of the interwar period and are still the basis of infant feeding today. Paps made with vegetable or meat broth, or milk and sugar, are generally offered at three or four months. People with farm animals commonly offer children freshly laid raw eggs whipped with sugar. Milk is used exclusively as a main or sole breakfast food, often in the form of *caffelatte* (with a little coffee or toasted barley). Children are given specially prepared soups and purees until the age of three or four, at which point they may share family meals.

Breast-Feeding and Alternative Infant Feeding Methods

Maternal breast-feeding continued to be the most popular method of infant feeding through the first half of this century, though mixed feeding was on the rise. A minority of mothers used artificial feeding, and there was still a residue of wet nursing. While women's "failure" to breast-feed was often blamed upon work outside the home, it was also attributed to whims and desires unrelated to any need to work.[23]

Since the middle of the nineteenth century, institutional and individual wet nursing had been more common in areas where manufacturing and industry employed many women, leading to geographical differences in breast-feeding patterns. In a discussion of ONMI inspections of 128 foundling homes in 1931 (almost two-thirds of which were found to be mediocre or very bad), Fabbri reported that, while the brefotrofio of the northern regions was better equipped and organized, breast-feeding was "almost an exceptional thing," whereas in the south it was "spontaneous," a "natural corrective" to the lack of well-organized institutions (though infant mortality rates still reached 60 percent of all births in some places) (1933a:140–42).[24] In a study of the conditions of infancy in Lombardy, Garzanti Ravasi pointed out that although the brefotrofi were relatively good in the north, pediatric clinics were rare or absent in many provinces and comuni. She observed that breast-feeding rooms in factories were so few that "you could say they do not exist," and where they did they were not used. Small business owners preferred to give women time off, but instead of breast-feeding, the mothers happily entrusted their babies to family members (1931a:89).

Mercenary breast-feeding was falling out of use due to increasing controls on the wet-nursing industry, the fashion for bourgeois women to raise their own children, and the relative economic well-being of the rural classes that had previously supplied nurses to the brefotrofi. Public health authorities and ONMI clinics reported fewer examinations of wet nurses and more maternal breast-feeding of illegitimate infants. Of the 670 to 780 infants given smallpox vaccine in their first six months in Faenza (population 47,200, including town and outlying areas) each year from 1932 to 1936, only 2 to 4 percent were fed by wet nurses. Artificial feeding was used in 5 to 8 percent of all cases, mixed feeding in 3 to 5 percent, and breast-feeding in 84 to 87 percent.[25]

A relatively long period of postpartum amenorrhea indicates that most women breast-fed for many months or years through the first decades of this century. Breast-feeding was said to "almost always" preserve women from pregnancy for at least ten months after childbirth, although half of mothers resumed menstruation in the sixth or seventh month.[26] These averages were reported by physicians, whose experience was limited largely to urban elite women. While these mothers breast-fed for six to twelve months, older farm women recall that mothers in the countryside did so for one, two, or more years, and remained infertile longer.

In the 1930s, urban women and elite women in the countryside began to supplement and wean their babies earlier. Among the women who attended Borrino's clinic, few breast-fed exclusively beyond the third or fourth month, and weaning was complete almost always before one year, usually at nine to ten months (1937:656). Formula was promoted heavily, in spite of political and moral opposition. By the early 1930s, there were several brands of formula on the market—most of which were from countries to the north—and Nestlé proudly advertised that its product Nestogen was used by ONMI in its free distribution program.[27] Although there were supposed to be tight controls on artificial milk, many people remember ONMI clinics mostly for the powdered milk, infant care booklets, and clothing they received there.

A wealthy landowning woman in Santa Lucia who had twelve children says that she never had milk for more than a month or so, until her penultimate child was born during the Second World War. There was nothing else to give the baby, and she found that she had plenty of milk. She concludes that "God takes care of us in times like that."

In addition to cultural trends, hospital birth favored reduced breast-feeding. A woman who moved to a city soon after marriage around 1930 breast-fed her three children for 13, 12, and 11 months, respectively, whereas her own mother had breast-fed her for three years. For the third child's birth in 1937, she went to the hospital, since there was a new law making it free of charge. She also attended the ONMI maternal refectory and medical clinic, and followed the feeding schedule closely. These phenomena were linked, for hospital birth and increased contact with ONMI institutes contributed to rising compliance with medicalized breast-feeding.

Compliance with Medical Norms

The insistence of medical experts on the importance of giving milk at long, equal intervals indicates that the common practice was to do the opposite. The common women were derided for tenaciously persisting in giving their infants too much milk, too frequently, under the mistaken idea that they would make them big and beautiful. Borrino complained that the importance of following parenting norms "except those of the oldest tradition is not at all penetrated in the popular consciousness" (1937:144). Consequently, the benefit of higher rates and longer duration of breast-feeding in Italy compared to other countries was canceled by unfavorable conditions for infants, especially the "innumerable prejudices" still governing mothers' minds. "Sure, there is the advantage among us of natural feeding, but *natural feeding* does not signify *rational feeding*" (1937:657).

Worst of all was the public's recalcitrance and skepticism about the rule of putting a regular distance between meals. Borrino observed that this necessity was the "least understood in practice by mothers and all superficial persons, who give the infant milk at any cry, repeating the usual

phrase, 'one needs to follow nature and in nature breast-feeding has neither meals nor rules'" (1937:141). These people needed to learn that the
feeding response was instinctive only initially, when the cry provoked
immediate aid and, according to certain "sensitive" mothers, a sense of
swelling in the breasts. With time, she maintained, the "necessities of life"
distanced these bonds, while the mother acquired improved understanding
of the infant's cries.

The owners of domestic animals put them on fixed schedules, while
wild animals respected the periodicity of function, spacing the feeding of
the young: "pauses and limits that we see completely lacking in the disordered breast-feeding of a great number of *donne del popolo*" (Borrino
1937:142). The most ignorant women and those dedicated only to housework were the most difficult to convince, for they knew neither discipline
nor orario, that "index of order." The illiterate *popolane* of the south and
islands exhibited the extreme of disorder, indolence, and obtuseness. For
example, the women of Sassari, who lacked work and observed the minimum of cleanliness and order in their one-room houses, had no need for
orari or punctuality. Borrino thought that at the least, the fundamental
rhythm of day and night should exclude nocturnal breast-feeding, "that
which instead we do not see happen at all" (1937:142). The long pause at
night, which brought such immediate tangible advantages as the family's
rest, "seems to clash so much with tradition, that it arouses surprise linked
to diffidence in those who hear of it for the first time" (1937:144).

Borrino added that even physicians were guilty, for some of them had
been repeating their advice about regular meals for many years without
intimate conviction. Midwives did so only because they had heard it or
read a box of infant food. Both were only bowing to fashion, for to them
the advice was somehow strange or foreign. She felt that Italy needed to
follow the example of Germany and the Scandinavian countries, where
artificial feeding was more common and as a result the norm of fixed meals
for breast-feeding was also better diffused among pediatricians and mothers. By contrast, in Italy, France, and England, the prescription of 8 to 10
meals per day in the first weeks with a slow reduction to 6 by the sixth
month was still popular. Some American pediatricians even suggested "ten
meals for weeks and months!" (1937:145–46).

Regarding the doppia pesata, contemporary medical literature
expressed physicians' frustration over the common mothers' resistance to
it, as well as both satisfaction in elite parents' acceptance of it and exasperation at their "over-zealousness" and "ill-preparedness" in using it.
Gelli, who enjoined parents to use the method and never deviate from it
unless authorized by a physician, rejoiced in the observation that the custom of "methodically weighing the infant is so diffuse today that all the
well-off persons for the most part acquire one of these instruments of con-

trol; the others go to the public and private clinics or to physicians and midwives themselves, some of whom possess portable balances or scales for the use of their clients" (1931:773).

By contrast, Borrino, who preferred greater medical direction as to whether the doppia pesata should be used in the first place, argued that, by obsessively weighing their infants, mothers "uselessly complicate things and upset themselves and err" (1937:147). In all cases, parents, as well as nurses and midwives, were told that they were unable, and should not even try, to interpret the results. Parents should not compare their measurements against averages or ranges printed as reference tools in popular infant care books, for "on the real value of variations above or below only the physician can be the competent judge" (Gelli 1931:773).

Among health professionals, adherence to new medical norms was not uniform or immediate. Borrino criticized the obstinate physicians who continued to depend upon traditional empirical means rather than regular weighings to monitor infant growth and health. She argued that the abuse of the scale in double weighings was "an error as grave as the other extreme case of not concerning oneself with the infant's weight at all" (1937:147).

The midwife Giuliana immediately promoted the orario among the women she treated in the interwar period. In response to their habit of giving milk whenever the baby cried, she taught that "if you don't wait at least three hours the milk is just water," and that it is better to give an infant with stomachache an enema than allow it to take more milk. On the other hand, she reserved the doppia pesata for special cases such as a nervous temperament, prescribing it more regularly in the postwar period. In fact, very few women say that they did the doppia pesata in the 1920s and 1930s, although many remember following a feeding schedule. Most did not weigh their infants at home, but some did so at the medical clinic. In contrast to the regimented breast-feeding practices followed by some mothers, breast-feeding without regard to time schedules and quantities persisted among many women in the countryside and smaller towns, while balie either with or without milk were still hired by some city and elite women.

Many women talk about having had the quality of their milk tested in a hospital or laboratory. As Rosa, a woman whose children were born in the 1930s, explains, if a baby cried and everything possible had been done, it was concluded that the mother's milk was defective. If it was "light" she gave the baby some "substance" (sugar or barley dissolved in water) after it had breast-fed. If the milk was "heavy" she gave the substance beforehand. The physician may also have had the milk analyzed and told the mother that it was not good, after which she used formula or animal milk.

Cow's milk was most common, in contrast to a generation earlier, when Rosa's aunt had fed her twins with goat's milk.

Rosa says that she fed her children when they were hungry, according to the expression she knew from her childhood, "babies must eat little and often." However, one of her children vomited often, so she gave him water before feedings to keep him from taking too much milk, indicating that she was probably spacing feedings at some distance. She eventually switched to barley-water because her physician told her that the child could not digest "any kind of milk." While she obeyed her physician and bought the new infant cereals, prepared fruit preserves, and other products at the pharmacy like other *signore,* she opposed universal norms for infant feeding, saying that "each mother has to understand her own child and his needs."

One of Natalia Ginzburg's novels described a young, urban mother's experience of the doppia pesata and orario. This woman felt that she had little milk and forced herself to eat, but the child remained thin. When she took her out in the carriage she was ashamed that her child was not as large and strong as her age-mates. She weighed the child at every poppata, and on every Saturday before her bath, and kept a special notebook for recording the weight before and after the poppate in green ink and the weekly body weight in red ink. On Saturdays, she woke with a great throbbing in her heart, always hoping that the child had grown . . . but was crestfallen when she found that the child had grown very little, and desperate when not at all. Her husband grew impatient and ridiculed her about the notebook and the way her hands trembled as she changed the baby's clothes, overturned the talcum powder, and worriedly bustled about the screaming child (1947:48–49).

This mother's trepidation indicates the power of rising cultural expectations of scientific mothering to put women's capabilities in doubt. It contrasts sharply against the parental detachment formerly common in the same sector of the population that was the first to embrace devoted, rationalized child rearing. Well-off mothers who complied with medical norms and directly participated in their children's upbringing with relatively little help were not at all prepared by their own childhood for this kind of domestic life. Their peers who did not make the same choice continued the old ways of hiring many servants to take care of the children and housework. Meanwhile, working and rural women fed their infants in various ways, using supplementary foods and animal sources as needed. Those who were in greater contact with medical professionals and urban life began to follow the feeding schedule and to check the infant's body weight more often. Others did what women before them had done, or what relatives advised.

Protecting Maternity and Infancy: ONMI

Combating Resignation and Fatalism

Changes in government laws and regulations affecting mothers and infants mirrored the overall shift in the character of fascism between the 1920s and 1930s toward greater state centralization and control. In the 1920s, there were legislative efforts to protect women's jobs and provide financial compensation during mandatory maternity leave. Women's work had been a critical issue for all of the political parties before the First World War, and there had been provisions for needy and abandoned mothers and women working in dangerous industries well before the inter-war period. The early fascist provisions were motivated by an awareness of the need to reduce infant and maternal mortality rates, an issue that had relatively little partisan content. ONMI was created in the middle of the 1920s as a parastate institution with high-level central-government representation, but an orientation toward the provincial and communal levels.

In the 1930s, the central government took a deeper interest in pronatalist and maternal and infant health programs, including those of ONMI. The expansion of ONMI took part in a larger strategy of mass involvement in state programs unified by the ideal of the fascist family. The voluntary character of the organization diminished as more paid personnel were hired. ONMI provided standardized courses and norms diffused from the center to health professionals, social workers, and mothers. Some ONMI functionaries began to complain that the organization was crippled by excessive centralization and overly detailed legislation and was unable to carry out its specified functions. As we will see, these problems were never resolved.

ONMI was one of the first fascist institutions. It was founded in December 1925. Related legislation in 1926 and 1934 built upon the 1890 law and sought to reconcile the existing lay and religious institutions for abandoned and needy infants with the national level organization. These laws reflected the new concept of public assistance as a duty of the state. They aimed to correct the demo-liberal "errors" of leaving the charitable institutions to their own devices and assuming that private initiatives with little state intervention were sufficient to provide effective aid.

ONMI was charged with unifying and "rationally" coordinating the existing 6,000 provincial brefotrofi, which were described as the legacy of a medieval system concerned above all with concealing the mother's guilt, rather than seeing to the children's moral salvation or the establishment of the family. There had also remained a few hospices for unmarried women awaiting childbirth, and around 100 institutions that granted subsidies. ONMI argued that these institutions needed an orientation toward education and hygiene, particularly regarding pregnancy and breast-feeding (1962:7–27). Since infants were most exposed to disease and death in the period from birth to three years, ONMI would see to it that they received a "rational upbringing" under the care of a pediatrician throughout this time, including rational breast-feeding and careful weaning.[28]

Those who wrote about ONMI frequently described it as the central institution of the regime: more important than the after-work organization, the Corporations, or the youth organizations. ONMI embodied legislative dispositions representing "in their spirit and essential lines a profoundly revolutionary act, exquisitely fascist."[29] It was the defender and guardian of the race, the "central and summarizing" institution of political demography, and the very essence and expression of fascist ideology and action: "not just the institution and character of a regime, but the solid stronghold and character of an entire civilization."[30]

The most important innovation of ONMI was to keep mothers and infants together for at least the first three years, with the explicit goal of ensuring maternal breast-feeding. As a former employee of the organization explained, in the past, unwed mothers had been permanently separated from their infants and forced to feed several others instead. Now, they could breast-feed their own infants either within an institution or with public assistance at home. Social workers assisted unwed mothers to remain within their natal families, become married, or achieve paternal recognition of their child. ONMI employees helped working mothers by monitoring and ensuring compliance with the legislation regarding maternity leave, subsidies, breaks for breast-feeding, and the creation of day-care centers. There were even provisions for incarcerated women to breast-feed their infants and have them cared for in special nurseries.

Breast-feeding was a requirement for public assistance from the very beginning. According to the 1926 law, "only those women who directly raise their own children can be admitted for assistance: except when it is a matter of a woman recognized as physically incapable of breast-feeding, or where reasons of hygienic-sanitary kind or special environmental conditions or reasons of moral order require the separation of the child from the mother."[31]

Another of ONMI's innovations was to provide prenatal medical care, which beforehand had been practically unknown. Previously, the only provision regarding maternity had been that hospitals were obligated to admit women in childbirth. ONMI created obstetrical services together with the dermo-venereal service that arose out of an overriding concern for venereal disease. A third innovation was the institution of preventive pediatric assistance, requiring comuni that did not already have an institution for infants to create one. Finally, ONMI provided training to physicians, midwives, health workers, and social workers and sent them out to

houses and businesses to inspect hygienic conditions and teach people how
to prevent disease. The latter emphasized the importance of breast-feeding, notions of breast and general cleanliness (including the acceptability
of bathing during the first forty days after childbirth), and the eradication
of the popular practice of sleeping in lofts in one-room houses.

ONMI's activities took four main forms. The first of these was the
provision of medical, material, and moral assistance to needy or abandoned children and pregnant and nursing mothers. The second was the
diffusion of "scientific norms and methods of prenatal and infant hygiene"
through medical clinics, theoretical-practical schools of puericultura, and
popular courses on maternal and infant hygiene. The third ONMI activity
was the prevention of or "battle" against tuberculosis and other infantile
diseases. The fourth was surveillance over the legal aspects of the protection of maternity and infancy and promotion of further legislative reform
in the interest of "physical and moral improvement of children and adolescents."

Initially, ONMI targeted only needy women and children, but soon
eligibility was extended to all pregnant and nursing women, as well as all
unweaned infants. Needy mothers included widows and unmarried
women who lacked sufficient resources or had been abandoned, as well as
married women whose husbands had abandoned them or were away in
prison, hospital, or charitable institutions, or otherwise unable to provide
for their families. Eligible children were those up to 3 years of age whose
families could not provide them with "all of the necessary attentions for a
rational upbringing"; children up to 18 years who were psychologically or
physically "abnormal" but capable of reform, needy, or materially or
morally abandoned; and children whose parents or guardians were in an
institution or had lost their financial position, or were abnormal, mischie-
vous, beggars, prostitutes, or criminals condemned to prison.

ONMI institutes included medical offices in cities and towns, as well
as mobile obstetric and pediatric clinics or "chairs" (like teaching posts)
serving remote areas on a periodic basis. There were demo-venereal clinics, and some medical-psychological-pedagogic clinics that provided prematrimonial counseling and psychophysical preparation for childbirth.
There were also social service offices, maternal refectories for pregnant
and nursing mothers, and day-care centers for infants.

Assistance to mothers and small children varied from medical care in
the clinics to snacks and meals in the refectories. Moral and material assistance in the home took the form of food, children's clothing and blankets,
subsidies, and training in hygiene and infant care. In the case of abandonment or need, children could also receive day care, placement with wet
nurses or foster parents, and admission into institutes for the prevention of

tuberculosis or the treatment of physical or psychological disorders. Older children and adolescents continued to receive similar assistance appropriate to their age, including admission into educational or vocational institutions.

ONMI's activities required cooperation with other institutions, including communal and provincial administrations, schools, the Federazione Nazionale per la lotta contro la tuberculosi (National Federation for the Battle against Tuberculosis), and the Istituzione Biotipologica Ortogenica (Orthogenetic Biotypologic Institute) for abnormal children. The social security institute (INPS) provided medical examinations and childbirth assistance to millions of women and children; the Associazione Educatrice Italiana (Italian Educational Association) created propaganda for day-care centers and the schooling of children in hospitals; and the associations of the party sent children to ONMI health camps. This collaboration helped to widen ONMI's influence on Italian life.

Structure of ONMI

The organizational structure of ONMI consisted of a central governing committee at the national level, a *federazione provinciale* (provincial federation) in the capital of each of the 94 provinces, and a *comitato di patronato* (patronage committee) in each of the 7,300 comuni. Although the lower organs were to have a high degree of autonomy, in general, organizational objectives and direction came from the top, while reporting on services and the needs of the population and institutions came from below. The central office in Rome published the monthly journal, *Maternità e Infanzia,* which reported on ONMI activities and funding as well as international news and studies related to maternal and infant health.

The central executive committee included top-level government officials such as the president of Italy, the vice president, and two others nominated by the minister of the interior. There was an advisory board of 13 members, including the ministers of the interior ministry, civil administration, and, later, the Fascist Union of Large Families. The ministers of finance, education, corporations, and the party each chose a representative, while the minister of the interior chose five representatives among midwives, pediatricians, biologists, hygienists, social physicians, psychiatrists, social service experts, and sociologists.

The provincial federations included a top-level provincial administrator, physician, public assistance and beneficence administrator, judge, and organizer of the fasci femminili. Six other members were chosen by nomination, including specialists in obstetrics and pediatrics as well as representatives of public and private institutions for maternity and infancy. The central office chose a *socio* (member) in ONMI who was an expert in assistance to maternity and infancy and resided in the province. The communal patronage committees were chaired by the prefect and composed of the secretaries of the fascio femminile and fascio di combattimento, a magistrate or justice designated by the president of the court, the local sanitary official, the president of the congregazione di carità, the director of education or a teacher, and a priest designated by the prefect. Other members of the committee (male *patroni* and female *patronesse*) were chosen by nomination.

While ONMI's administrative costs were kept low by the use of provincial and communal employees and volunteers, there was a paid staff of central office workers and technical personnel, mainly physicians specializing in pediatrics and obstetrics, ostetriche, and *assistenti sanitarie* (health workers, generally female, with the same two-year training as nurses, plus a third year of specialization). There were also physicians who specialized in dermosyphilography and psychiatry, puericulturists, child psychologists, and specialized *assisenti sociali* (social workers). Volunteer *visitatrici* or *visitatrici d'infanzia* (matrons or matrons of infancy) and *assistenti visitatrici d'igiene materna ed infantile* (visiting health workers of maternal and infant hygiene) carried out most of the work of visiting women at home. These volunteers were considered the connection between social services and the families, their function the basis of ONMI prophylaxis against infant mortality.

The professional assistenti sanitarie also made home visits, in addition to working with physicians and midwives in the clinics. Their duties included monitoring breast-feeding and the environmental conditions of mothers and children; teaching mothers to follow the physician's orders; giving the first medical assistance to children in the case of illness; and offering hygienic and dietary suggestions. They also worked in factories, monitoring hygienic conditions, finding ways to reduce injuries, observing the personal and family life of the workers, and acting as mediators between labor and management.

This activity was considered the continuation of a centuries-old tradition of Christian and lay charity work carried out by women. Although medical and social assistance became professionalized in the interwar period, nuns continued to staff hospitals, hospices, nurseries, and preschools in large numbers. In contrast to ONMI's mostly male administrative structure, the technical side of the organization was predominantly female, except for the male physicians and some male nurses, social workers, and health workers. The three levels of ONMI's organizational structure show us that there were high-level officials as well as medical, political, religious, judiciary, and social service workers involved in an organization with equally diverse activities and aims.

ONMI Programs and Services

Keeping Mothers and Children Together to Ensure
Maternal Breast-Feeding

One of the unifying symbols of fascist political demography was a mother with a child at her breast. Breast-feeding represented the conquest of infant mortality and solidification of family morality and relationships. This idealized morality was that of the Roman patriarchal family, glorified as the primary unit of the nation-state. The "regularization" of unwed mothers' family situation was therefore considered a double necessity, both in moral terms and because illegitimate infants were more likely to fall ill and die than legitimate infants. These priorities found expression in the requirement that women accepting public assistance breast-feed their own infants and that institutions do everything possible to secure maternal breast-feeding.

The effort to assist unwed mothers was based upon a contradictory interpretation of illegitimate birth, rooted in the cultural contradiction between the sacredness and impurity of maternity. On the one hand, women were to be assisted in performing their noble duty as mothers, even if they had reached motherhood in an ignoble way. On the other hand, they—not fathers—were considered responsible for their "guilty," "painful" motherhood. The unwed mother was told that she could redeem herself to some degree by giving attentive care to the child, "to love him all the more, for that which she has suffered for him and for that which he, later, will have to suffer" in having to associate her image with impurity, sensuality, and vice.[32]

ONMI proposed to "create motherhood" for these women, thereby keeping them from being pushed into crime. Minors deserved special attention, for they were considered the most pitiful and relatively innocent of all, and also the most likely to kill their infants and end up in jail. There was also the problem of parents abandoning their babies only to reclaim them from institutions or foster parents when they needed them as workers or farmers. Reformers sought to eliminate this practice and deny custody altogether to mothers who did not give their infants their milk and maternal care.

Beginning in 1926, a series of new laws changed the institutional care of illegitimate infants, regulated wet nursing, and imposed mandatory maternal breast-feeding in return for public assistance. The *ruota* (revolving door) for receiving abandoned infants was abolished by law in 1923. Foundling homes were required to make inquiries into the identity of mothers, to determine their health conditions, procure maternal breast-feeding for the foundling, and induce the mother to legally recognize the child (it was not until 1942 that the civil code expanded the number of circumstances in which paternal identity could be sought). In 1927, assistance to illegitimate children became an obligation of the state and province, provided their mothers recognized and breast-fed them. The 1934 law established that ONMI could found institutions of maternal assistance, maternity insurance funds, and auxiliary offices of the brefotrofi for the guardianship of "needy and abandoned women who breast-feed their own children."

These provisions required the brefotrofi to eliminate artificial feeding and entrust the children of unmarried or widowed women to their mothers for breast-feeding. Mothers who breast-fed at home received a trousseau, monthly subsidy, and medicines and food as needed. Those who breast-fed their babies in the brefotrofio also worked as wet nurses and fed a second infant, in contrast to the former institutional practice of forcing mothers to pay for childbirth assistance by breast-feeding two or three infants other than their own (who was immediately consigned to a different nurse or to foster parents). The staffs of ONMI "maternal shelters" for unwed pregnant women tried to persuade them to recognize and breast-feed their children, but if all else failed the child could be entrusted to a foundling home.

If the mother was judged incapable of breast-feeding and the infant was deemed immune to contagious diseases, the latter could be wet nursed at ONMI's expense or mixed-fed if wet nurses were lacking. No public institution could give infant formula to a woman unless she had a medical certificate stating that she was unable to breast-feed and competent in the "art" of artificial feeding. Artificial feeding was limited to babies infected (or suspected to be infected) with syphilis or another contagious disease, who could not be fed by their mothers or an infected wet nurse. Mercenary breast-feeding was against the law in this case, since the wet nurse could become infected.

The 1927 reform was considered one of ONMI's most important achievements, as services for foundlings had been functioning in a "way contrary to every hygienic-sanitary prescription" such that mortality of assisted children reached 50 percent and even 70 percent in many provinces.[33] This led to the idea that mandatory breast-feeding "should be prescribed for any kind of aid or subsidy."[34]

By the early 1930s, there had been an explosive rise in maternal recognition of children (the number of recognized children assisted annually by ONMI rose from 12,000 in 1928 to more than half a million in 1932). This was interpreted as the result of the breast-feeding requirement.[35] On the other hand, the initiatives to increase paternal recognition were recognized as being rather ineffective. This was lamented not only because paternal recognition brought a food allowance to the child, but also because the

solidity of the family was thought to depend upon the "blood tie" of paternity.[36] That is, women's moral salvation could be achieved through recognition and breast-feeding of their illegitimate children, but their relationship with them would not be complete in a social or biological sense
without paternal recognition.

Prenatal Care, Assistance in Childbirth, and Postnatal Care

ONMI was particularly concerned with the care of children during gestation and early infancy. Prenatal medical care promised to yield, "through
the treatments given to the mother, healthy and robust children."[37] The
care of the child after birth centered around breast-feeding, which was to
be promoted and managed through the maternal refectories, medical clinics, mobile pediatric and obstetrical services, home visits by the assistenti
sanitarie and visitatrici d'infanzia, day-care centers, assistance to working
mothers, and courses on infant care for health professionals and mothers.
These services had the central objective of diffusing "scientific" norms and
methods for breast-feeding and infant care to families and institutions.
ONMI staff thought of themselves as fighting a "battle" against ignorance, the root of errors in infant care and therefore the cause of elevated
infant mortality and morbidity. A modern outlook would emerge as physicians imparted new notions of maternal, infantile, and general hygiene,
"with particular regard to the practice of breast-feeding and dietary
hygiene in general."[38]

   The maternal-gynecological clinic was, in theory, staffed by an obstetrician or at least the medico condotto, with the assistance of an ostetrica
or *assistente sanitaria specializzata* (specialized health worker). The clinic
provided medical care and "hygienic surveillance" throughout pregnancy
and the puerperium, and prevention of sterility for all women from
puberty to menopause. If the physician deemed home care sufficient, the
visitatrici brought women leaflets with detailed norms for pregnancy,
childbirth, and infant care. The latter stressed breast-feeding and the
duties of maternity and included instructions for hygiene, vaccination,
dentition, and prevention of infectious disease. The visitatrici also checked
to be sure the instructions were followed by the mother and midwife, and
offered all other moral and material support outlined in the regulations.

   According to the legislation regulating ONMI, pediatric clinics were
to be instituted by the patronage committees in every municipality and
even every neighborhood, accepting all local children up to the age of six
or seven for free care regardless of social or economic status. The clinics
were to be staffed by a physician specialized in pediatrics or nipiologia, or
the medico condotto, with the assistance of a health worker. ONMI also

founded mobile clinics staffed by two physicians, one learned in "prenatal hygiene" and the other in "postnatal hygiene," each accompanied by an assistant trained in maternal and infant hygiene. They traveled to two or three communities each day, including remote and mountainous locations. The pediatric clinics provided medical care and surveillance, "hygienic education" of mothers, propaganda in favor of maternal breast-feeding, and instruction in and supplies for mixed, mercenary, or artificial feeding. Infants were charted for somatic and functional data, conditions of pregnancy and birth, personal and family characteristics, the method and duration of feeding, variations in weight in the first year, and notes from each weekly or monthly visit.[39]

ONMI maternal refectories built on a tradition begun in the 1870s and 1880s of providing food to needy and working mothers, but introduced a new function of medical-moral surveillance and instruction.[40] As a former ONMI employee explained, they ensured an adequate diet while also allowing physicians to look after women's health and behavior. This was considered an "exquisitely fascist action" favoring the next generation of citizens and soldiers, for women who attended the maternal refectories and obstetrical clinics gave birth to babies who "always" surpassed the average birth weight. The refectories offered a morning caffellatte and noon lunch to pregnant and nursing women who had obtained a physician's certification that their ordinary diet was qualitatively or quantitatively insufficient.

In the ONMI *asilo infantile* (day-care center, also called *asilo nido*), "maternal breast-feeding, exclusive or mixed, is practiced for all unweaned babies." Artificial feeding or nursing "at the breast of another woman" was permissible only if the mother were recognized as "physically incapable" or there were prohibitive "reasons of hygienic-sanitary nature concerning the mother or the child, or grave motives of moral order."[41] The same rules applied to permanent institutions or preventive sanatoriums, at which the mother was assumed as a wet nurse and constrained to breast-feed another child if physically capable. In some locations, the asilo was united with a pediatric-obstetric clinic and called the *Casa della Madre e del Bambino* (House of the mother and child).

The asilo admitted nursing and weaned infants up to three years of age, whose mothers were "regularly occupied outside the house" or housewives in poor financial condition overburdened with numerous children. There were also seasonal day-care centers for women working in activities such as the olive harvest or the winnowing of rice. The day-care centers were said to be extremely modern, providing "rational" assistance in nutrition, hygiene, psychological development, and education. In fact, many children enjoyed a better diet and hygienic environment than they did at home, and a large proportion of operating expenses in many asili was devoted to food. ONMI also helped unemployed mothers find work, and oversaw employer compliance with the labor legislation.

Schools for Mothers

The preparation of women for maternal duties involved both direct education of girls and women and professional training of health and social workers, experts in maternal and/or infant hygiene, school health workers, and midwives and physicians. Popular courses and public conferences were offered to teachers and women in general, while training materials were distributed in elementary, middle, and high schools, and vocational and teacher-training colleges. The organization of *massaie rurali* (rural housewives) was instituted in 1934 to involve farm families in the modernization of housekeeping and hygiene, extending the teachings of fascist visitatrici from working-class to farm families. In 1937, the Ministry of the Interior effected a provision in the 1926 law requiring ONMI to institute courses on puericultura for girls in the middle schools. This was the complement of the training for boys in "military culture," both of which were suppressed after the Second World War.

Courses on prenatal and postnatal puericultura were offered through the brefotrofi and medical clinics to physicians, surgeons, and midwives, while medici condotti received a similar but abbreviated training. Midwives and physicians who took these courses were treated preferentially in hiring decisions. Visiting health workers, scholastic health workers, and nannies or nursery school teachers received training through "theoretical-practical schools" in local health or social welfare institutions.

ONMI institutes were considered above all "schools for mothers" or "schools for breast-feeding," where physicians and their assistants provided assiduous, competent medical persuasion and direction, oversaw breast-feeding, and ensured that women visited and followed the norms of the medical clinics. In the maternity wards, women were obligated to breast-feed and learned fundamental principles such as the necessity of regulating feedings at the prescribed hours. The Casa della Madre e del Bambino taught mothers who were "still slaves of prejudice or unprepared for the rational and hygienic upbringing of the child."[42] Mothers in rural areas were trained in puericultura through mobile teaching units and medical "chairs." This effort was considered particularly important, since the rural areas had inherited so many ignorant traditions and "inveterate prejudices" and were lacking in "educational-hygienic propaganda."

The ONMI medical clinics were considered by fascist leaders to be of highest importance, for it was here that the "precious advice" of the physician corrected and prevented errors in breast-feeding. As Pende said, the often-catastrophic enteritis in newborns is the "consequence of errors in breast-feeding, which the physician of the consultation room can take away in time, suggesting opportune provisions." ONMI clinics conquered prejudices and "erroneous beliefs" coming from old grandmothers and neighbors, creating in mothers a "new mentality," a "new culture, more positive and more modern and above all more suitable for making their little one grow strong and healthy" (1939:14).

Disease Prevention and Treatment

ONMI's activities in disease prevention and treatment contributed to fascist national political demographic goals by improving women's health and fecundity and children's health and development. The opposition between gracility and robustness was central to this program. It was thought that individual physical robustness would be bolstered through "medical-hygienic guardianship," leading to a progressive improvement of the "physical integrity" of the entire race. This centered around Hippocratic and Roman ideas about the importance of light and air, physical exercise, and thermal springs.

One area targeted for natural cures was sterility and other reproductive disorders. The "battle against sterility" was aimed mostly at women, who were much more likely to be treated than men. Women were blamed for two-thirds of marital sterility (which was estimated to affect 10 percent of all couples) and were thought to suffer more from it. Women's purportedly higher morbidity overall and in the genital sphere was due to the "sometimes debilitating outcomes of maternity and lactation," the "more grave consequences of sexual contagions," and the "greater wear and tear of work in relation to their more delicate constitutions, to their more labile temperaments, to their scarcer powers of resistance."[43] Treatments included corrective *opoterapia* or replacement therapy for "constitutional weakness" of the genital tract.

While ONMI programs for women focused on maternal functions, those for infants focused on rendering gracile children robust, since gracility was considered a predisposing cause of tuberculosis and poor general health.[44] The new seasonal and year-round *colonie* (camps) located in the mountains or near water were said to be more modern and effective than those run by religious groups, for nuns and teachers were good moral elements but "absolutely insufficient from the technical point of view."[45] Solar cures were also promoted in the brefotrofi, day-care centers, and schools, where there was an increase in outdoor schooling and work in the fields and orchards—which favored the attitudes and abilities necessary for ruralization, besides. Children learned about hygiene and order, and followed a strict orario that ended with a fascist salute to the flag.

Millions of children attended the colonie and received medical examinations for prevention and treatment of disease. Beginning in the late 1920s, ONMI turned its colonie and most of the battle against tuberculosis over to the Opera Nazionale Balilla, the Italian Red Cross, and the provincial antituberculosis organizations. ONMI health services continued to include immunization and disease prevention through the obstetric and pediatric clinics, as well as efforts to improve and standardize nutrition in homes, schools, and camps. These activities contributed to change in medical and popular care of mothers and infants, including greater contact with health experts and rising acceptance of medical interventions.

Numbers Assisted

By all accounts, ONMI served a significant number of women and children during the interwar period, even without counting the families assisted by related organizations with medical care, subsidies, entitlements, tax exemptions, and prizes.[46] The annual participation of mothers in ONMI increased from under 400 in 1926 to over 245,000 in 1930, peaking at around 570,000 in 1937 and 1938. Thereafter, it fell into the 300,000s or lower until 1960. The number of infants assisted annually also increased rapidly, from around 1,700 in 1926 to 985,000 in 1930, peaking at over 2 million in 1937 but falling thereafter to 1.6 to 1.7 million until 1960. By 1960, ONMI had assisted 11.6 million women and 41.5 million children.

These numbers indicate that many more children were assisted than women. More nursing mothers were assisted than pregnant women. For example, in 1936, ONMI assisted 1,224,000 children, 183,000 pregnant women, and 251,000 nursing mothers. In addition, the numbers indicate that ONMI's activity was already rather extensive in the first years. Between 1927 and 1933, more than 200,000 pregnant women and 4 million infants were served by 301 mobile clinics, 558 obstetric clinics, and 8,193 pediatric clinics funded or organized by ONMI. Between 1926 and 1931, more than 128,000 children and adolescents received food allowances from ONMI, and more than 38,000 were placed in day-care centers where they received a "healthy daily meal."

In 1927 alone, ONMI paid for 180,000 children to attend mountain or seaside colonie. In 1928, the assistenti visitatrici visited 100,000 people in their homes. By 1934, ONMI had installed maternal refectories in the majority of provinces (serving some 148,000 people between 1926 and 1931) and instituted 59 mobile chairs of puericultura. The mobile units were later eliminated by regulations instituting permanent clinics and public assistance centers almost everywhere.

More than 6,000 needy pregnant women and mothers were assisted in finding employment between 1928 and 1931. Over the same period, ONMI helped more than 7,100 women obtain legal recognition of their children,

3,440 to legalize an illegitimate union, and more than 1,000 to obtain a declaration of paternity or food allowance from the father. This kept some 43,000 children from abandonment, presumably assuring them mother's milk as well. ONMI made marriage possible for thousands of "illegitimate" mothers through prizes for matrimony and the provision of goods for the establishment of a house and family. It assisted women living abroad to return to Italy for childbirth (1,210 in 1933), and the fascist Befana distributed gifts to children on the day of the Epiphany (1,668,802 in 1933).

By 1935, ONMI had created 9,000 institutes. This number did not grow much thereafter, reaching 10,555 in 1962. More than half of the ONMI institutes were pediatric clinics, and about one-fourth were obstetric clinics. The remainder were maternal refectories, permanent and seasonal day-care centers, "houses of the mother and child," and other medical and social-service institutes. These numbers understate the extent of ONMI's influence, for they do not count the thousands of institutes taken over or supervised by ONMI but created by other public bodies or religious or lay organizations. They included orphanages, day-care centers, medical clinics, maternal refectories, and milk dispensaries.

ONMI's administrative costs were only about 4 percent of overall expenditures, compared to 20 to 25 percent for other public institutions, since the only paid administrative personnel were in the central office in Rome. The majority of ONMI's "army" was made up of volunteers, whose numbers were many times greater than the number of paid technical personnel. There were 90,000 volunteers in the 1930s, including physicians, social and health workers, visitatrici, and volunteers on the local committees and subcommittees.

Effectiveness of ONMI

Contemporaries considered ONMI pathbreaking and innovative, a great advance in the history of the world and the civilized nations.[47] Fascist laws were a "truly imposing" legislative achievement putting the state, after the family, in charge of ensuring needed assistance and education to all children. ONMI was described as autonomous, rationally decentralized, free of "bureaucratic formalism," and blessed with complete freedom of initiative and action. By encouraging mothers to breast-feed and by providing effective "sanitary guardianship" and "moral defense" of children, ONMI created and maintained the necessary biological conditions for conserving and developing the national stock. ONMI "demonstrated itself one of the fascist state's best devised and most efficacious instruments of power and might."[48]

On the other hand, critics found ONMI's detailed legislation a serious obstacle to the realization of its stated duties. The 1926 law had 238 articles, and there were thousands of others affecting public services for maternity and infancy. ONMI's soon-to-be director, Sileno Fabbri, complained about imbalances in the administrative structure and the fact that ONMI had neither the means nor the organization it needed (1928:20–21). Informants confirm that ONMI institutes were not available in significant number or in smaller towns or cities until the postwar period and sometimes had to be housed in private homes for a decade or more before there was an appropriate building. In the postwar period, ONMI's fundamental defects (such as excessive centralization and overly detailed legislation) were not corrected. Much of ONMI's work was entrusted to the voluntary *visitatrici fasciste*, who were supposedly trained in hygiene and diet, but whose deficient knowledge was a cause for complaint among ONMI officials and physicians from the outset.

As a result, ONMI was not able to pursue its functions to the intended depth and extent, leaving a large gap between the grandeur of its conceptual aims and the reality of its activities. Even at the beginning, it was forced to face only the most urgent problems, which an ONMI history blames on the paucity of means (1962:13–14). By the 1950s, all that remained was the care of infancy in the hygienic and health fields. ONMI was dismantled in 1975, its functions and equipment absorbed by the regional administrations.

Critics have argued that Italy's efforts in public assistance were made just to catch up to other European countries. They note that social services only reached 1 percent of public expenditures in 1920 and rose no further until 1938, and that many of the provisions that were legislated in the fascist period had antecedents in earlier laws and either never came to fruition or were paid for by private donations. This does not mean that public services did not increase in character and scope over the interwar period. We have seen that volunteers and lower-level public administrators contributed most of ONMI's labor without adding to its expenses, and that ONMI represented an unprecedented attempt to coordinate and provide public assistance. The current seemingly indisputable conception of public assistance as a social duty and right of citizenship was a novelty then, as was the idea of extending obstetric and pediatric care into areas that had previously lacked or nearly lacked any form of social services.

Even the often-cited relentless fall in fertility rates does not rule out a role for fascist initiatives in influencing demographic trends, although it cannot be denied that birthrates were lowest in the very places—the large cities—where fascist action was most pronounced. Overall, Italy's birthrates remained high relative to other Western countries, thanks largely to broad socioeconomic and cultural trends, and perhaps to some degree to government policies. Birthrates fell from 27.5 to 23.4 per 1,000 inhabitants between 1927 and 1934, but this was roughly the same rate of decline as the previous decade. It therefore represents stabilization compared to the rapid drop immediately after the First World War. Indeed, there was a transient increase in natality rates in the late 1930s.

The fact that ONMI assisted only a minority of pregnant women, or that maternal mortality rates did not begin to decline significantly until after the Second World War, need not be taken as evidence of its failure. Many more mothers than pregnant women were served, and many times more children than women. ONMI's main achievements were in the areas of infant mortality and morbidity, rather than stillbirths or maternal mortality.

Although infant mortality rates had begun to fall a generation earlier, ONMI contributed to their continued decline, in a phase of epidemiologic transition in which, in principle, it is more difficult to achieve successive increments of change. Average life expectancy increased by five years from 1926 through 1937 alone, due almost entirely to a reduction in infant and early childhood mortality. Contemporaries enthusiastically reported that ONMI had conquered infant mortality and documented many local successes in reducing disease rates.

As a former employee from Emilia-Romagna said, "*l'abbiamo vinta*" (we defeated it). However, she noted, as did Fabbri (1933a:126), that infant mortality rates differed significantly among the regions and provinces, and that the care of maternity and infancy was not uniform given wide geographical differences in wealth and social services. In the early 1920s there was one asilo for every 2,846 inhabitants in Lombardy, but only one for every 24,450 in Sicily.[49] The central-northern regions were better able to increase the availability of ostetriche, physicians, and other health service workers in their territory; improve housing and hygiene; control the conditions of mercenary breast-feeding and the hygienic use of animal milk; and carry out the regulations designed to keep mothers and infants together so that all babies could be breast-fed. The same regions also experienced a more rapid decline in illiteracy rates, which itself may have contributed to the diffusion of norms for impeding transmission of infectious diseases, as well as other principles of disease prevention and treatment.

Through its thousands of new institutions and the millions of children and adults it reached, ONMI had a strong practical and cultural impact. It influenced behavior and affected women's and children's health. Together with other new organizations, ONMI represented a level of state and medical intervention into private and family life that previously had not existed. ONMI's emphasis on breast-feeding affirmed its political and moral value to the fascist nation. The standardized, orderly method specified by contemporary medicine fit well in a rapidly modernizing society infatuated with scientific-industrial concepts and implements. The principle of regularity in infant care also conformed to fascist political ideas presupposing identity between the individual and collective, such that dissent and rebellion were intolerable and regarded with disdain.

By extending its reach into previously inaccessible areas, ONMI diffused the precepts of scientific mothering and the expectation of frequent contact with the medical system. Particularly in the large urban centers, physicians assumed a predominant role as advisers to mothers and protectors of children. Rising cultural standards of order, rationality, and cleanliness applied as much to the care of infants as to housekeeping. However, because the state and its medical system had not yet succeeded in reaching into every social and geographical area, many families remained untouched by the new norms for infant care until the postwar period.

ONMI's enduring effect upon infant care shows that fascism did not, in fact, fail to influence private behavior. Some aspects of fascist ideology as well as many institutions outlived the regime itself. Regimented breastfeeding resolved the contradiction between the traditional, rural emphasis of fascism and its effort to modernize motherhood and housekeeping. By contrast, fascist "family values" and pronatalist programs rooted in the idealized rural family and economy were counteracted by the simultaneous favoring of education, urban-industrial development, and the aestheticization rather than repudiation of the body. The battle against falling birthrates was doomed not just by structural changes but also by internal contradictions in fascism. The same contradictions eventually brought enthusiastic compliance with the scientized model of breast-feeding developed by fascist-era medicine.

CHAPTER 7

Bad and Good Breasts
Medical and Popular Beliefs
in the Postwar Period

The conceptual divorce of maternity from infancy rooted in the interwar period allows for breast-feeding to be considered a distinct phase in the mother-infant relationship. ONMI fostered this division through the organization of its services and the method of breast-feeding it promoted, as well as its political mandate of producing healthy children for the fatherland. Mothers were intermediaries between the state and its future.

As industrialization has progressed, the language and analogies of mechanics and industry have come to describe all kinds of bodily functions, including lactation. Breast-feeding is metered and timed through a method that also accords with current health concepts and the belief in the centrality of methodical nutrition and digestion to health and well-being. Scientific and folk notions agree upon the importance of regularity in bodily functions, which are considered to be interlinked in such a way that imbalance in one brings disorder in another. Mothers' bodies are held to be particularly fragile and irregular, increasing the need for order. This must be imposed from without, for women are considered especially vulnerable to destabilizing influences, even if they are also seen as agents capable of directly affecting their secretions.

Breast-feeding is increasingly thought of as exhausting, debilitating, and disappointing for the mother since she so often fails at it. The current method and the concepts supporting it ignore her needs and capacities, failing to produce conditions favorable to breast-feeding. They help to harden fascist-era ideas about infant stomach capacity and digestion time which make frequent, unregulated breast-feeding unthinkable. In the past, since maternal behavior was thought capable of directly harming or killing the fetus or child, any failure to comply with precautionary norms was said to reflect either ignorance or malice. Today, enduring ideas about the negative influence of maternal behavior also ensure compliance with medical norms and add to the difficulty of lactation.

The continued tendency for the literature to elaborate upon impediments to breast-feeding before discussing breast-feeding itself contributes to the belief that it is inadvisable or impossible for many women. The establishment of universal standards assumes that women have uniform time schedules and sufficient economic resources to buy or rent a scale. Whatever the other demands upon them, mothers are expected to never fail to feed their babies at the appointed time and with the proper dose of food. The onerousness of breast-feeding is exacerbated by the competitive atmosphere created by scientific mothering, in which breast-feeding becomes a performance to be judged against abstract cultural standards as well as other women. It is ironic, in light of fascist intentions, that this competition may actually contribute to women's reluctance to have many children, or any at all.

Understandings of Maternity and Infancy

Good and Bad Breasts

Earlier this century, the ancient belief in the transmission of the mother's essence to the child through breast-feeding gave way to an emphasis on the production of a nutritious and digestible substance adapted to the latter's developmental needs. More recently, the focus has shifted to the psychological importance of breast-feeding for both the individual child and society. According to advice books for parents, breast-feeding is still valuable for the first few months because it provides an optimal food for healthy and harmonious growth, but its advisability depends upon the quality and quantity of the milk and the mother's health, personality, and willingness. What matters is that the child is transmitted "calm, serenity, availability."[1] This may be better accomplished with the bottle, so long as the mother does it herself (at least at the outset), for breast-feeding is beneficial only if she wants it profoundly: "one could conclude that women's milk becomes bad when the desire to give it is lacking."[2] It can even disappear.

The postwar literature frequently describes an overtired, discouraged, anxious mother who breast-feeds as being much inferior to a contented mother who bottle-feeds lovingly and devotedly. The former inadvertently mistreats her baby in her exasperation, preoccupation, tiredness, and pain, and she reacts poorly to its cries. This seems to be expected, for lactation is described as debilitating, causing weakness and exhaustion. Women who are tired from life in the big cities or hard labor are thought to have no milk.

An extremely popular and long-lived book by Miraglia, Orlandini, and Micheletti claims that mothers who breast-feed unlovingly or distractedly are the cause of character disorders in children, indeed "all the troubles of modern society"—from class conflict to drug abuse, greed and corruption to sexual deviance (1984:62–64, 69, 166, 331–32). The authors explain that in the first, two-year oral phase of psychological development, the breast-fed infant "makes love" with his mother, as manifested in the male's erection and the mother's experience of pleasure in proportion to the "authenticity" of her "affective gift." Based upon this experience, the infant forms phantasmagoric representations of the "good breast" and "bad breast," drawn in the text as a fairy and witch. The latter is said to cause irreparable psychological deficiencies, leading to isolation, autism, and sucking or gnawing of the fingers or other objects; nervous hunger leading to obesity; alcoholism; and masturbation. This is nature's "vendetta" against mothers who commit errors on the affective plane: all responsibility falls upon their shoulders. In reality, teachers and parents do attribute many psychological problems in children to a bad relationship with the mother, including constipation and anorexia nervosa.

The "good" breast requires attentive preparation, care, and sterilization, for the baby's sake. This is a subject that no medical or advice book fails to address. The nipples are described as such delicate organs that they need little abuse to be rendered unsuitable for breast-feeding. Insufficient preparation and "incorrect conduct" in breast-feeding lead to painful cracks and inflammations that make breast-feeding impossible and open the way to mastitis. Accordingly, the breasts must be prepared during pregnancy with daily massage, cleansing, and oiling. After birth, they are cleaned daily with soap and water, the nipples washed before and after each feeding to avoid putting germs into the baby's mouth. Some experts advise expressing a few drops of the "polluted" old milk left in the breasts before each poppata. Afterward, the breasts are cleaned and dried lest contact with the residual milk should make the skin rot or inflame. Mothers must never touch their own nipples with unwashed hands.

Before today's sterilized water and prepackaged cotton discs soaked in disinfectant solution, women washed their breasts with boric acid solution before feedings and alcohol afterward. Between feedings, they put sterile gauze over the breasts, but today women use another packaged disc, possibly dampened with a lotion or medication, after wiping with disinfectant. These products are sold in pharmacies, and women are expected to buy them unless they have asked for professional advice in using homemade products.

In addition to cleanliness, women are encouraged to take care of the attractiveness of their breasts, for it is assumed that breast-feeding constitutes a sacrifice of their looks. Only after weaning will the mother return to her usual appearance, and then only if she has followed the rules for breast hygiene, diet, and maintenance of tissue elasticity with lotions and "medical exercise." The belief that breast-feeding makes the breasts sag is not only left unquestioned, but sustained by suggestions that they can remain firm and attractive if the woman wears a suitable brassiere or does special exercises often illustrated in advice books.

Breast-feeding is also discouraged by the practice of introducing it in popular and medical texts by first discussing artificial feeding. These books state that newborns will be given supplements of formula unless the mother manages to "succeed" in breast-feeding right away. They recommend that if the mother wishes not to breast-feed she should tell the hospital staff immediately to procure the appropriate medicines.

It should not surprise medical experts that breast-feeding can make mothers feel nervous or irritable, considering the expectations of failure and the behavioral restrictions and time-consuming, anxiety-producing obligations of the doppia pesata and orario. The norms for breast cleanliness imply that milk is a source of uncleanliness and infection, contributing to the unidirectional understanding of lactation as secretion of a product made for the child which the mother is likely to sabotage. Women are told not to breast-feed if they lack sufficient willingness and availability, but the impact of regimented methods on their sense of calm is never explored, and neither are the reasons why fathers are not expected to have any appreciable domestic responsibilities. While claiming that what matters is the mother's devotion and love, experts argue that there is a wrong way to breast-feed, and they penalize women for being tired or unavailable. The switch to bottle-feeding is construed as a liberation that also allows mothers to regain their strength and figure.

Utility and Interrelation of Physiological Functions

A century ago, it was believed that all people needed to regularly exercise every physiological function in order to maintain fluid balance and therefore health. For women, reduced or forsaken reproduction and breast-feeding led to ailments and diseases such as breast cancer. Over the first half of this century, this understanding was replaced by a focus on the introduction, through the sexual act, of male elements into the woman's body. By the 1950s, the importance of this transfer for female physical and psychical well-being was said to be beyond doubt. As the focus shifted to the impact of men on women, so it shifted to the effects of women on their infants, and soon the path of return influence was forgotten.

For many years after the Second World War, experts continued to describe the beneficial effects of conception and spermatic impregnation on the female organism. Male elements were assimilated by the woman and finished in her organs and blood circulation, stimulating metabolic and secretory processes, helping to resolve intestinal stasis and chronic mastitis, and making the woman "reflower" and appear younger after matrimony. Their absence brought physical and psychical troubles, as shown in the successful treatment of women's skin disorders and sexual and nervous-psychical disturbances with semen-replacement therapy. This treatment was also effective for hormonal and nervous disequilibrium due to "voluntary" spermatic deficit caused by birth control practices. Sex and reproduction benefited women above all through the delivery of male elements.[3]

Meanwhile, the growing trend toward thinking of breast-feeding as a one-way transfer of milk to the child further reduced awareness of the impacts of maternal functions on women. Protective effects with respect to breast cancer have been completely forgotten. A spirited rejection of traditional knowledge about contraceptive mechanisms of lactation has accompanied an actual decrease in its efficacy due to rising acceptance of regimented breast-feeding methods. Breast-feeding is not thought to affect women's reproductive cycles in any predictable or useful way. Those cases in which women do not get pregnant during lactation are attributed to certain women's "natural parenthesis" of sterility, or a "hormonal antagonism" between the mammary glands and ovaries that is terminated at random.

In the early postwar period, it was said that menstruation would resume within two months if the woman did not breast-feed, but three to six months if she did, and that there was a good probability of becoming pregnant again in either case, whether or not the menstrual cycle had resumed. Today, experts and the public agree that the first ovulation takes place at 40 days, and menstruation returns at that time or within a couple of weeks if the woman does not breast-feed. If she does breast-feed, amenorrhea lasts two to six months.[4] Experts flatly refute any protective effect against pregnancy, calling it a "simple superstition" which it would be an error to take seriously. "Absolutely do not believe the rumor that breast-feeding functions as a contraceptive method." "It is absolutely not true."[5]

The principal maternal benefits of breast-feeding mentioned in the literature are economy and efficiency. Rarely, someone will go against the grain and suggest that it helps the mother return to her previous body weight. Psychological benefits deriving from its greater "naturalness" are also mentioned, but usually overshadowed by reference to the child. In short, the main reason women should breast-feed is that the benefits to the child are numerous and evident.

Yet, although the utility of breast-feeding to women's health and fertility has been denied, some humoral notions have been retained. The menstrual cycle is still believed to harm or threaten the child, during both gestation and lactation. Sex in pregnancy is considered dangerous during the missed menstrual periods, when the uterus is said to be more sensitive and the mother's general equilibrium less stable. Women are advised not to take baths, go swimming, or travel during those times. If their abdomen feels hard and contracted for a day or two, their obstetrician may tell them that this probably coincides with the days they would have had their menstrual period. After childbirth, baths are prohibited for as long as locha-tion persists, and routine hospital practice allows no showers or baths for the entire postpartum stay (recently reduced from a week or more to three to five days).

At the capoparto at 40 days, whether or not there is a menstrual period and for all successive cycles, breast-fed infants are said to experi-ence uneasiness, dyspepsia, modifications in the appearance and number of bowel movements, and refusal of the milk. This is attributed to feminine hormones and histamine-like substances passing in the milk, or simply a change to "less good" or less abundant milk. Experts try to reassure moth-ers by telling them that they need not suspend breast-feeding during the actual or missed menstrual period. Yet, by enumerating the alterations in the milk, they instead fuel popular fears. Similarly, they describe how pregnancy produces a decrease in milk secretion, but argue that there are no ill effects for the infant so long as the mother ceases to breast-feed after the first trimester and so avoids straining her organism too much.

These examples show how medical thought juxtaposes denial of the interrelations that cause lactational amenorrhea against affirmation of those that produce noxious effects on the infant. This minimizes awareness of the utility of breast-feeding to women, while maximizing attention to the myriad ways in which their bodies and behavior can make it fail.

General Health Beliefs

Today's health beliefs are largely the same in popular and medical thought, though some experts complain that the public observes protec-tive behavior to an excessive degree. Infants and mothers are regulated very closely since imbalance is thought to cause discomfort, illness, and disorders in milk production. One area of particular care is body tempera-ture, which is thought to have a homeostatic or equilibrium state that may easily be upset. Temperature is kept within a proper range by covering the body and avoiding exposure to cold, dampness, and heat. This becomes complicated at hot temperatures because deep fears about sweating and exposure of the skin preclude actions that favor the body's attempts to cool off. In short, taking cold or getting wet is tantamount to getting sick. Getting hot also implies getting sick because afterward one must necessar-ily cool down.

The midwife Giuliana says that when she first began working in the 1920s, infants who died in winter died of bronchitis and bronchopneumo-nia: "they were struck by a draft, they began to cough." Infants who died some time after birth were victims of gastrointestinal disease provoked by their mothers' hard labor. She explains that work gave women a *bella sudata* (great sweat) that inflamed their milk glands. When they fed their babies from their *gran piene mammelle* (great full breasts), it caused inflammation of the little intestines, illness, and death. Others who are less precise simply say that the sweating spoiled the milk and killed the infant. A sure way to evoke an immediate reaction of horror and harsh criticism is to breast-feed in a sweat on a hot day. The mother is expected to wait or take a cold shower to cool down the "hot," "boiling" milk.

Even if it is summertime, sweating or being exposed to wind (or especially both) is sufficient to cause the most varied kinds of illnesses and discomforts. These include fever, cough, sore throat, loss of the voice, respiratory diseases, backaches and neckaches, gastrointestinal disorders, and cysts or other problems in the eyes and ears. There are terms for different forms of sweatiness, such as "lightly sweaty," "soaking-wet sweaty," and "dirty-sweaty." Baths and showers are taken with the windows closed to keep out drafts, no matter how hot it is outside, and sleeping with the windows open is to be avoided because it brings backaches. Failing to dry one's hair, even while at the beach or at the height of summer, is said to automatically cause neckache and backache, and it brings the automatic reproof that sooner or later the practice will lead to *artrosi cervicale* (arthrosis in the neck). When a cyclist on a military team sprayed a teammate with his water bottle during a July ride, the latter exclaimed, "don't do that, I'll get sick!"

Illness can also result from changes in general atmospheric conditions such as the different air and water encountered on a trip or move. It is considered harmful to the kidneys and digestive process to drink abundant water or to take it during meals. Athletes used to restrict their water intake during competitions and training, and older ones still do. The shock of a refrigerated beverage is blamed for painful abdominal "congestions," vomiting, and general malaise as much as a day later. Prevention entails adding a warm liquid to the drink (water, fruit juice, beer) and is never transgressed in the case of infants and children.

In addition to muscular and nervous disorders, infectious, contagious illnesses can be caused independently by an uncovered abdomen or a sweat followed by exposure to wind or cold. As a result, fans and air-conditioning units are rare, women going through menopause wear winter clothing in summertime because of hot flashes (which they fear even more if it is windy), and until recently there was practically no market for antiperspirants because people avoided sweating. A 1994 television advertisement for Neutro Roberts deodorant showed a man in a white lab coat saying the unfamiliar: "*diciamo la verità: sudare fa bene*" (let's speak the truth: sweating is good for you).

Children are covered heavily and clothed in shoes and cotton or wool undershirts year-round from the moment of birth. Infants are never permitted to remain in a place where the wind is blowing, regardless of the season, and may be encased in a clear plastic cover snapped on to their strollers if they must be taken out on a windy day. The abdominal area in people of all ages is unfailingly kept covered. Shirts and undershirts are tucked deep into pants or skirts pulled high over the belly to protect what is considered a particularly vulnerable part of the body. Children are scolded for running on summer evenings when they might sweat, or playing barefoot in the damp grass. One father told his infant son to stop crying because it would make him sweat. Another told his preschooler on a hot August evening that if he didn't put his slippers on, he'd get a cough (although some nursery school teachers have begun to encourage the children to play barefoot in summertime). In winter, parents and grandparents keep children from playing outside by promptly putting away bicycles and outdoor toys at the first sign of fall. This is widely thought to fall definitively on the holiday marking the end of summer, *ferragosto* (August 15), whether or not the heat continues for many weeks thereafter.

A local pediatrician describes the fear of children taking cold as a "wall around people's thinking that I can't get through." Even if parents can be convinced to cover their children a little less, they still worry about drafts and sweating. One mother told her five-year-old son, who had had a slight fever the day before, to get out of the doorway on a scalding hot day because of the drafts. As a mother of a sick four-year-old said, "I was told to keep her cool by not overdressing her, but what about all of the air currents?"

The retired midwife Marina believes that in the old days infant death was caused by the excessive covering and protecting of infants in both summer and winter. In summer, they became overheated and died of gastroenteritis. In winter they died of bronchopneumonia because at night they were moved from their place near the hot kitchen fire to freezing cold rooms with uncovered windows, open roofs, and cracks in the walls. She observes that older people are especially concerned about keeping children warm, for they remember the cold and cover infants even when they know the heat is on.

In addition to atmospheric insults, germs circulating in the environment are thought to constantly threaten to enter the body, especially if the equilibrium is upset. Riding on a moped can be blamed for a viral illness caught from the outside air. Carpets evoke disgust and aversion because they can never be perfectly clean. Tile floors are washed and "disinfected" every day. At most swimming pools one is obliged to walk through a basin of disinfectant solution, because warts are said to be rampant there, but at the same time pools are considered sterile compared to natural bodies of water. There are products for disinfecting food, the household, the air, the body's surface, and children's clothing, linens, and toys on a regular, daily basis. Boiling water is used for sterilizing these things as well as cleaning dishes and clothes. Athletes soak their water bottles in bleach. Parents of young children invariably keep a store of chemical products for cleaning bottles, pacifiers, and human or artificial nipples. A main reason they try to avoid sending their child to day care is that they fear they will catch diseases.

On the other hand, some treatments recognize the valuable presence of internal microorganisms, while others use naturalistic elements. Diarrhea is treated with *fermenti lattici,* huge doses of lactobacillus. The food of the queen bee (*pappa reale*) is considered a wondrous nutritional supplement for athletics, pregnancy, or illness. The dark sticky substance bees use to repair their nests (*propoli*) is used as an antiseptic, anesthetic, and antibiotic; its uses include treatment of bronchitis and prevention of maladies associated with the change of seasons. Thermal springs are used to treat everything from gastrointestinal and cardiovascular disorders to lymphatic and skeletal diseases.[6]

Whatever its origin, illness is commonly treated with antimicrobial drugs. Most children have taken several rounds of antibiotics before their first birthday. Once, an infant's ear produced an unusual smell in springtime (due in the end to pollen). The physician attributed it to a gust of wind and prescribed antibiotic drops. Another physician interpreted an insect bite to a woman's eye as a "nice case of conjunctivitis," caused probably by a gust of wind, and prescribed antibiotic drops and boric acid. The latter is a traditional treatment that older people remember using for irritation from having dust blown into their eyes.

Fever is greeted with particular alarm. A grandmother in her eighties, restraining her feverish grandson, looked out from an upper-story window in a raging wind, waved her arms about, and said that the fever was "out there." A local pediatrician complains that she makes more than a dozen house calls per day in wintertime because of parents' "terror" of their children taking cold and getting a fever. Parents aggressively treat fever, even of viral origin, with antibiotics and antipyretics (often in the form of suppositories), but are fearful of removing the child's clothes or blankets.

While treatment stresses germs, prevention stresses environmental factors. Children are not discouraged from kissing, sharing dishes or food, or exposing other children to infection through contact with their hands or mucus. Instead, they learn not to expose themselves to wind, water, or immoderate temperature. A six-year-old did not want to swim or get wet one summer day because she had a cough, which she and her mother both attributed to a previous day at the swimming pool. When questioned further, she said that sickness is always around, just like fever, and comes in when you sweat. Similarly, one father said that his year-old infant fell ill because he took him out on a bicycle ride. He added that the child either got sweaty or was struck by a gust of wind, and the virus that had infected his brother a few days before entered through his skin.

Some people disapprove of the overprotection of children, saying that it renders them immunologically unable to overcome illness without antibiotics. One such woman attributed her friend's six-month-old child's frequent febrile illnesses to the way she and her husband kept him from being exposed to any germs. Their desire to protect him was so extreme that to avoid having to put him on the floor when visiting a second-story apartment, the mother and her friend—who had her arm in a sling—carried him inside his carriage, unstrapped, up two flights of stairs.

Many infants never touch the ground. This stems from both a rejection of what is thought of as a dark, miserable past—when newborns and infants were left upon the dirty floor or ground—and what the midwife Marina describes as a "mania for cleanliness." She believes that this excessive care makes children weak, for "babies need to form antibodies and be exposed to what's around. . . . If not when they do get infected it's even worse. . . . Babies need some freedom, they need to crawl, it's good for them." The pediatrician mentioned earlier in this section urges parents to let their babies crawl, but finds that they simply refuse to do it. Instead, infants remain night and day in their carriages or cribs for six or eight months, then are moved directly into a playpen or onto a spotless mat.

The concern for environmental and microbial threats leads to a relative lack of regard for other health risks such as accidents and injuries, as in the case of the baby carriage on the stairs. One mother who becomes very concerned if a child does not wear an undershirt allowed her three-year-old daughter to sit in the bed of a tractor while several people threw wood into it. Infants' bedrooms give the impression of a hospital room, with a bare tile floor and a shelf for the digital scale and sterilization equipment. Yet, there are dangers everywhere in the house, including hard floors, furniture with sharp corners, and unscreened windows in the upper stories. Children very rarely wear helmets as they ride their bicycles along with the cars and motorcycles, and often do not use seatbelts or car seats. Construction workers do little if anything to protect themselves or the people who walk through their work sites. People drive long distances at breakneck speed to collect water from favorite springs, admiring the beneficial effects of the water on the liver while ignoring the dangers of driving and its contribution to environmental pollution.

The overwhelming concern for equilibrium that justifies such seemingly incongruous behaviors also forms the foundation for beliefs about the centrality of regular digestion and nutrition to health and happiness.

Digestion and Nutrition in Maternity and Infancy

The intestine has a special place among the organs. It is the very center of well-being, and its management is essential to proper breast-feeding. To regulate intestinal function is to maintain health, while to empty the intestine is to cure many disorders, such as headaches. When one woman's mother called the dentist because of a childhood toothache, he asked if she had emptied the child's intestine. A cyclist who was sluggish one day was mailed a laxative pill from his friend, with instructions to take it the night before the next ride. Many older people recall being given hot enemas made with camomile, boiled herbs, salt, or olive oil and believe that their current digestive problems, including intestinal tumors, stem from being burned by these concoctions. A nursery-school teacher is so tired of answering parents' daily questions about their children's bathroom habits that she has started to write a *c* on the hand of every child who produces a *caca* at school. She says that parents give their children an enema if one or two days go by without one; the children are terrorized to the point of sitting on the toilet after lunch until they are red in the face.

There are innumerable products available in standard pharmacies, herbal medicine shops, and general stores for improving digestion and intestinal function, including laxatives, enemas, herbal teas, yeast-based "vitaminic integrators," elixirs, and herbal bitters. Most of them promise extra benefits such as healthier hair and skin, greater vitality, or improved immune response. One advertisement for an overnight laxative shows a woman in lacy underwear standing before a mirror. It asks the reader if perhaps she finds herself not quite in form, her figure not as slim as it should be, her skin less luminous and her gaze not as limpid as she would like. "Listen to the mirror: it is warning you that, probably, something in your organism is not regulated. . . . Maybe the intestine."[7]

The emphasis on what goes in and out of the body is so overwhelming that the way in which food is utilized is almost completely neglected. Physical activity is considered a distant second in the determination of health, body weight, and appearance. Foods such as red wine, horse meat, and concentrated sugars are taken to treat low blood pressure, which is considered as serious a health problem as high blood pressure. Products claiming to improve well-being, prevent disease, and reduce body fat without any need for physical activity include garlic concentrate, fish oil, ginseng, *pappa reale,* and a dazzling array of lotions, drugs, and machines to combat cellulite. One newspaper article about getting rid of the postpartum belly says that the "only solution" for subcutaneous fat is diet. Further, it states that this layer, which increases during pregnancy, can also expand afterward, "especially if the woman breast-feeds."[8]

Although men and women demonstrate equal concern over intestinal function, women are considered more constipated "by nature," as one pharmacist put it. Pharmacists say that older women wait only a day before coming to ask for an enema or laxative. One pharmacist recalled an advertising campaign for a laxative called "pearl," which declared that to make a woman happy you should give her a pearl.

An advertisement for baked goods entitled "Fiber: Equilibrium to the female" brings together a number of pertinent themes about women's health and behavior. It presents women's reproductive processes as pernicious transformative events, and their participation in an active "male" life as unnatural and disequilibrating. It affirms women's need to take care of themselves in order to be attractive and avoid becoming overweight, and it directly blames them for the lifelong health problems of children.

The advertisement is illustrated with a photograph of a male physician-dietician from the University of Milan, who explains that women have special nutritional characteristics because of the hormonal changes of puberty, procreation, and menopause. Because modern women, "immersed in the whirling of an active life (like a man's)," do not always succeed in conducting their lives properly, they must pay special attention to fiber. Fiber prevents overweight and lower-limb venous and lymphatic disturbances affecting even young women. If taken in insufficient amounts, the ensuing constipation and intestinal dysfunction increase abdominal tension and aggravate circulatory disturbances, harming the legs' appearance and inviting the "much-feared cellulite." Pregnancy exacerbates these disturbances, especially now that modern women postpone the age at first conception, causing the "rise in congenital malformations and above all the birth of overweight (macrosomic) babies which increases the phenomenon of obesity in our population."[9]

Advice books on pregnancy and the puerperium affirm that in recent years "a correct diet has become one of the fundamental pivots of our society."[10] Of all the rules for pregnancy, the most important is the avoidance of any imbalance through maintenance of a healthy, "rational and correct" diet: this is the "fundamental pivot" on which the fetus counts. For the mother, a proper diet is "literally the secret" for combating constipation, cellulite, nausea, insomnia, and other disturbances of pregnancy. Its transgression can bring more difficult labor, greater probability of premature birth, and difficulties in breast-feeding. On the other hand, specific measures such as increasing the intake of tryptophan in the last two weeks are said to make childbirth easier. Traditional knowledge holds that consumption of beer should begin during pregnancy in order to have the effect of improving the milk supply.

Books for mothers contain extremely precise schedules for daily nutritional and caloric intake, including meal plans and even meal times, depending on the stage of pregnancy. They advise weekly monitoring of increases in weight, in grams, for the sake of the fetus and to control those "overeaters in excess" whose weight gain with each pregnancy will remain "forever." This threat works against breast-feeding, for medical and advice books confirm the popular belief that a four-kilogram reserve of fat is necessary for good breast-feeding, and that weight loss after childbirth coincides with the termination of lactation. Indeed, slim women with scarce fat reserves are said to have "no little difficulty in producing the milk necessary for the nutrition of the child."[11] In general conversation, a thin body constitution is described as *secca* (dry).

Women are admonished to "scrupulously" regulate the intestine during pregnancy and afterward, when it is said to be "habitually lazy." This requires eating the proper foods, living a hygienic life, and taking common laxatives and purgatives as needed. In addition to the obligatory enema just before childbirth, the woman is routinely given a purgative or medicated enema on the second day and her food intake is restricted for several days. The "unplugging" of the stomach and intestine is done before the initial engorgement of the breasts, to release the "residual material of digestion" before it can cause local infections and the absorption of toxins. Mothers who choose not to breast-feed are given a saline purgative to increase loss of water and thereby diminish the milk secretion. Some experts say that the purging of the new mother is not necessary, but family members and friends take great interest in her bowel functions and ask openly about them, even helping with enemas.

Some women take tablets that are said to empty both the intestine and the breast, highlighting the presumed connection between regularity of intestinal function and regularity of milk production. A parallel connection is seen in the practice of clearing the infant's digestive pathways before it takes any milk. In the past, when it was believed that infants did not enjoy colostrum and that it caused vomiting and gastrointestinal problems, this was done with lemon juice, barley tea, sugar water, or mashed apple. As the purgative properties of colostrum were better appreciated, it was given after a wait of a day or two, to allow the mother to overcome her exhaustion and clear her intestine. Even now that mothers are encouraged to begin breast-feeding within 24 hours, "very early" attachment means several hours after birth.

Experts discuss constipation in infants at length, dividing it into subtypes and defining the normal frequency for emptying the bowels, even while complaining that mothers and their relatives and friends obsess on the subject. It is little wonder they do, given that methodical intestinal function is said to be linked to proper growth and development and to the avoidance of gastrointestinal disorders. This brings regimentation of diet, daily sittings on the toilet after a meal at exactly the same time, and the use of enemas, suppositories, and oral purgatives whenever there is not a daily bowel movement. Otherwise, the matter is said to transform itself into an intestinal block and cause the absorption of toxins. In breast-feeding infants, constipation is thought to be caused by an insufficient diet due to frequent vomiting or scarce production of mother's milk, illustrating the convergence between regularity of maternal secretory and infant digestive function.[12]

Ideas about Maternity and Infancy

Threats to Pregnancy and Childbirth

Today's ideas about the protection of mothers and infants from grave health consequences are solidly rooted in past conceptions of the dangers of exertion, stimulation, imbalance, and humoral stagnation. They also continue to promote medical authority against women's presumed fragility and tendency to commit immoderate or imprudent acts. Traditional health beliefs intersect with political and gender ideologies in beliefs such as the inadvisability of women's exerting themselves in sports or work. The ancient fear of sweating blends with the more recent belief that athletics are incompatible with maternity, or femininity itself.

In the cultural memory, the hard agricultural labor of the past is equated with stillbirth and miscarriage. Those with a more romantic vision tend to think that women were hardier back then and had no trouble giving birth, and they believe that stillbirth rates were lower (they were not). According to the midwife Giuliana, by the 1920s most infant deaths were stillbirths, and they were beginning to decline because there was *meno fatica* (less exhausting physical effort) for farm women thanks to mechanization and shifts to other kinds of work.

During pregnancy, Italian women today are expected to exercise moderation in sleep, dress (including wearing moderately high heels), exposure to the elements, emotions (which must never be strong), and physical activity. Physical strain and trauma, as well as certain kinds of work, are said to directly harm the fetus or lead to problems in childbirth by causing deviations of the mother's skeleton or pelvic organs. This means that pregnant women must not carry heavy shopping bags or children, or work in agriculture or jobs requiring hard labor, a prolonged standing position, an overly long period of wakefulness, or the use of pedal-driven sewing machines. During the last three months, they are advised to take extra rest, climb stairs slowly and rest at each landing, stop doing chores requiring raised arms, and abstain from moving to a new house, painting the baby's room, making useless trips out, or going on vacation or away for the weekend.

Expectant mothers must also avoid temperature changes and the "congestions" and circulatory disturbances they cause, given their especial lability in thermoregulation and their vulnerability to taking cold. Their susceptibility to "local circulatory stasis" is considered the root of common disturbances such as dental caries and gingivitis. Wool undershirts are recommended because they keep the body temperature constant and prevent "cutaneous vasoconstrictions." Cold baths or showers are said to provoke congestions and dizziness, while hot permanent waves cause circulatory disturbances leading to congestions and disturbances of the cerebral circulation. The elevated temperatures experienced under the hair dryer have the same effect and must be avoided.

Travel is also considered disequilibrating, especially if it involves mechanized transportation. Miraglia, Orlandini, and Micheletti advise pregnant women not take trips, or even travel by motorized transportation for daily life, and never for frivolous motives: "the physician must decide if and when you can travel and with what means" (1984:205). Women should travel only after gynecological examination, after which they will be given a sedative based on progesterone and antispastics. If going by car, they should insert an antispastic suppository and sit on a pillow, even for short trips. Forleo and Forleo's contrary advice that trips by motorized vehicle are not dangerous, as long as they are not long or tiring, indicates the severity of the more general view: "It is not true that [such trips] cause abortion and premature birth: the child is not like a pear hanging from a tree which falls with any jolt!" (1989:130).

The assumption that women and their unborn children are extremely fragile and vulnerable is especially clear in discussions of physical activity during pregnancy and lactation. Exercise is considered beneficial, so long as it is moderate, controlled, and supervised. Activity is said to favor psychological independence and physiological functions, facilitating digestion and regulating the intestine, keeping the proper muscle tone for childbirth, and preventing stretch marks, hemorrhoids, varicose veins, excessive weight gain, back pain, and other "typical" disturbances of pregnancy. Just as the woman who practices excessive or competitive sports must abstain from them, so the woman who lives an idle life must conquer her laziness by doing "sweet," rhythmic, noncompetitive stretching exercise or "bedroom *ginnastica*" of the type proposed by Pende and others in the fascist period. Sports are said to harden the muscles and render them unable to relax, in contrast to the enhanced elasticity achieved through *ginnastica medica* that is needed for a happy childbirth.

Any activity, including housework, must be stopped before the pregnant woman feels any sense of tiredness. In fact, tiring or isolated exercise and fast or violent movements are "always harmful" because pregnancy reduces tolerance of physical effort and increases recovery time. In addition, muscular activity increases energetic needs and cardiovascular labor, harming the fetus through the production of lactic acid. Miraglia, Orlandini, and Micheletti second a popular apprehension that athletic women are not suited for maternity by stating that the "woman [who is] athletic by instinct, often has a musculo-skeletal structure of masculine stamp (it is the result of a certain hormonal situation)" which makes her not "well equilibrated in the attributes of femininity" and therefore subject to gynecological problems, including sterility (1984:203).

All exercise must be "dosed" and monitored by the physician, who decides whether the woman may exercise in the first place. In addition to up to a half hour of light exercise of the muscles used in childbirth, women are encouraged to walk or swim (excluding the crawl, diving, and water skiing). Bicycling is sometimes advocated, but other times discouraged because, like equitation, it causes pelvic congestions. It has become less common for experts to exclude dancing, but after the first few months it is still discouraged. With the physician's approval, after normal childbirth the woman may begin gentle exercises in bed for a few minutes during her hospital stay.

It is consistent with general health beliefs that physical activity for pregnant and puerperal mothers is nearly always described as secondary to diet, even though it is said to promote health (if done in moderation). Discussions of exercise typically begin with a statement that a healthy *diet* is the foundation of well-being. Similarly, prenatal exercise is considered far less important than learning the "correct way" to give birth using psychological methods against pain. Indeed, the exercises and respiratory relaxation of "psychoprophylactic" preparation for childbirth are said to provide all of the benefits of aerobic exercise, such as avoidance of accumulated toxins, without any excessive exertion—which, incidentally, would require sweating. Self-reinforcing beliefs such as these conspire to circumscribe women's behavior in everyday activities such as exercise, travel, or work, throughout pregnancy and lactation.

Imbalance and Debilitation during Lactation

Women's supposed delicacy and fragility reach an extreme immediately after childbirth, when they are considered to be exhausted to the point of anorexia. However, by the 1950s the belief that women should remain immobile in bed began to give way to the idea that they should be treated just like other patients after surgery (even though very few actually underwent surgery!). By moving around in bed and getting up after the acute period is over, women could prevent vascular complications, favor the involution of the uterus, stimulate intestinal motility, and prompt spontaneous urination.

In the 1950s, this meant allowing women to rise for bodily needs and sit in a chair for a few hours a day during the two weeks after a first birth, or one week after a subsequent birth. A generation later, women could get out of bed for a few minutes on the first day under the supervision of medical professionals, who would "dose" their movements and the time allowed. If healthy, the woman could "already" walk alone on the third day. Her diet would be nearly completely liquid until then, including meat or vegetable broth and cooked fruit. Thereafter, the caloric content and quantity of solid foods would gradually increase to reach normal levels within a week or two.

Today, it is still thought that women thoroughly lack strength and appetite for at least a week after childbirth, but that they need to replace lost fluids through a liquid diet. After the intestine has been cleared, the woman may gradually return to a normal diet, but must avoid foods such as cold beverages or ice cream that could cause dangerous forms of diarrhea due to the lability of the intestine. Women are told that "even if on the first day one is always very weak," they should get up for a few steps. Somewhere between the third and fifth day, after having built up strength by doing exercises in bed and laying on the stomach for brief periods, they may get up and walk the hallway, even alone. But they must not exaggerate: "to walk is still very tiring and the energies are few."[13]

The state of weakness induced by childbirth is thought to produce uniform, predictable nervous and psychological consequences. This makes it necessary to have the woman sleep in tranquillity at the right temperature and light, with limited visits from relatives and friends, and to give her sedatives, sleeping pills, nutritional supplements, and medicines for regulating the nerves, heart, and intestine. For the first couple of months, the fragility of her nervous system does not permit her to face too many things at once. If she breast-feeds, her weariness will be extreme. When a mother in her forties observed my trouble in threading a needle in a dark room, she attributed it to the "exhaustion of nursing" and said that she was so fatigued when she was breast-feeding that she could not read.

As in the past, women continue to exercise extreme care and extra precautions with regard to destabilizing influences during the first 40 days. For the first week or longer, they do not bathe or wash their hair, exert themselves, or sweat. The baby is taken outside only after a ritual eight days or longer and is completely covered and protected from the elements. A young mother explained that the shock she experienced upon the death of an aged uncle was enough to deprive her of milk at 40 days.

By having instituted a period of inactivity associated with maternity, legislative initiatives elaborated during the fascist period buttress the assumption that women (and infants) are in an extremely compromised physical and emotional state after childbirth. At each period during the past century, women have been considered physically or psychologically incapable of working during an interval of time that happened to match the one set by the law. Today, it is a minimum of two months before and three months after childbirth, but very often comprises the entire pregnancy and many months thereafter. Even the most benign kinds of work are considered advisable only for the first six or seven months of pregnancy. Although it may be admitted that "under a certain point of view it is even true that the woman is not to be treated as a sick person,"[14] this concession itself embodies the deep presumption that the mother and infant are extremely delicate beings on the verge of ill health, if not already diseased.

Protection of the Nursling

The ideas we encountered from the fascist period about the importance of the breast-feeding mother's conduct for her child's health and development continue to circulate today. The nursing mother must continue the hygienic, methodical regime of life begun in pregnancy, under the direction of the physician. She must pass her days in constant serenity, getting sufficient sleep, fresh air, and light exercise, while avoiding disease and any other morbid influence such as physical exertion; strong emotions; environmental insults; closed, crowded, or impure environments; and substances containing toxins such as smoke, liquor, or too much coffee.

The "training" of the breast for lactation begins in the first months of pregnancy, when women must wash and rub their nipples twice a day, first with hard crinoline and later with a nylon brush. After the ninth month, the already robust tissue may be softened with an emollient cream massaged into the breast. The *irrobustimento* of the skin covering the nipple may be favored by applying alcohol and glycerine or lemon juice and eau de cologne.

To avoid damaging her milk or digestive system, the nursing mother must eat a well-regulated diet in terms of quality, quantity, and the scheduling of meals. This means abstention from cooked fats, fatty sauces, gassy drinks, and all very spicy or salted foods. Medical and popular texts offer special meal plans, with tables of caloric and nutritional values and the amount of beer, wine, and coffee allowed. They explain that, by learning to use "autoregulation" and avoiding excesses, the nursing mother keeps herself efficient and useful to her child.

The child also must follow an orario for all activities, including dressing, outings, baths, rest, and meals. Cleanliness, orderly bowel activity, and "rational" clothing and bedding are part of the infant's regime of life. This is part of the "healthy, ordered, serene, and welcoming environment" and "loving, wise, rational assistance" that favor the infant's physical health and nervous and somatic development.[15] Through the 1970s, mothers were urged to visit pediatricians at the ONMI clinics and listen to the assistenti sanitarie in order to learn to raise their children correctly. Today, they no longer need to be coaxed.

One point on which the impulse to regulate behavior intensifies is the exact orario of feedings. The mother is told never to deviate, regardless of her social life or the child's sleep, unless the physician makes an exception. The mother must resist the temptation to offer the breast between feeding times, for the baby must digest the last feeding before any more milk is introduced. There have always been experts who will permit mothers not to wake their children for a feeding, but this indulgence is usually accompanied by a limit (say, half an hour past the feeding time) and the requirement of rescheduling all subsequent meals accordingly.[16] This is because "one could almost say that every delay in feeding is a delay in growth."[17]

At night, the "good little mother, who knows how to arrange her time" places the child in its crib definitively after the last feeding and sleeps eight hours before waking him for the first morning meal.[18] In the early weeks, she may possibly give one or at most two more feedings during the night. The child must learn the difference between night and day, to avoid disrupting the family's rhythms and exhausting the mother. By the fifth week the baby is expected to sleep seven hours in a row, provided it weighs at least five kilograms and has overcome any problems with digestion. Infants are said to sleep even longer by the end of the second month, and within a few weeks after that the last feeding is eliminated.

Medical norms also control infant access to the breast by specifying how long suckling should last at each feeding. In the first few days, the newborn is allowed 15 to 20 minutes at each breast, but thereafter only 5 to 10 at each breast or for both breasts together. This is considered sufficient to stimulate and empty the breasts, and allow the child to obtain the rich hind milk after first satisfying the thirst. Significantly, while many experts discuss the infant's need to suck and consider the merits and drawbacks of the thumb or pacifier, nobody connects this to the limitation of the duration and frequency of meals.

Just as in the interwar period, infants are expected to conform to rigid time limits, quickly learn to keep their place in the family, and adjust to restricted access to the breast and milk. This requires an effort on the part of the mother, who must resist her desire to feed her baby more often or at night. Together with the difficulty of meeting standardized time and production schedules, the need to discipline one's own behavior and bodily functions makes breast-feeding vulnerable to failure.

Norms for Breast-Feeding

Qualities of Mother's Milk

As in the fascist period, mother's milk is considered at once integral and ideal, *and* incomplete and deficient. Equivocation about the quality and quantity of mother's milk reflects a lingering suspicion that it is fundamentally insufficient and defective. Most medical and popular texts introduce the topic of breast-feeding by enumerating impediments to it. They repeat the contradictory message that, as long as there are no contraindications, mother's milk is the optimal food for the infant. Some mention a recent reduction in cases in which breast-feeding is discouraged, before proceeding to discourage it. This ambivalence is at the root of the common practice of "integrating" or "completing" mother's milk with formula beginning in the early months, if not in the hospital.

Whether implicitly or explicitly, experts conclude that mother's milk is not complete after all, even while presenting all of its wonderful qualities and the reasons why mothers must fulfill their natural duty. In contrast to "artificial" or "unnatural" feeding, breast-feeding is described as a "natural" maternal function that delivers a "natural" nutriment to the child. It is a "logical" form of feeding that provides an unmatchable quantity of elements necessary for "rational" and "complete" nutrition in the first few months. The milk is uniquely suited to the human infant, perfectly digestible, and blessed with the proper content and balance of mineral salts such as phosphorus and calcium. The milk may even be compared to blood, for it too is created by the organism and reflects its characteristics: it is a unique, very special food, a "biological," almost "live" liquid. Yet, it does not measure up to the umbilical cord in delivering everything the child needs.

Beyond nourishment, breast-feeding provides the child many other benefits. It enriches both the mother's and child's personality, significantly contributing to the latter's psychointellectual development. The milk and colostrum contain antibodies, function as a tranquilizer, and are sterile, always ready, and of the right temperature and composition. They come in a transportable container, which allows the child to regulate its nutrition. Of 14 reasons for the uniqueness and superiority of mother's milk listed in Maglietta's medical textbook, all refer to qualities that serve the infant, except for the last: "breast-feeding favors the mother-child dyad"——and even this refers mainly to the benefits the infant receives if the dyad is a healthy one (1985:308).

While the benefits refer to the child, the ways in which the product can be easily damaged and therefore rejected point predominantly to the mother. It is not uncommon for discussions of the advantages of breast-feeding to begin with a statement that, for many maternal or neonatal conditions, artificial feeding is undoubtedly the obligatory and also most convenient solution. Readers may be told that it is not always possible to carry out breast-feeding without drawbacks. Alternatively, women are criticized for so often thinking their milk is indigestible or too heavy or light, but experts then affirm that in fact the milk can be a bit too fatty or watery and has an inconstant composition that varies from one person to another, one pregnancy to another, and one hour to the next. The milk changes with the seasons, the infant's size and manner of sucking, and the woman's way of life, diet, health, and use of medicines.

At bottom, the milk is understood as only an *almost* complete food: insufficient to nourish a growing organism by itself, especially after the first months; often deficient in nutrients; and always low and declining in minerals and vitamins. Accordingly, to supplement with a dose of formula is to *integrare* (complete) the mother's milk, and is considered necessary from the very beginning. The routine hospital practice of "integrating" with formula is considered justifiable by the delayed arrival of the milk and the newborn's weight loss in the first few days. If a woman wants to breast-feed, she is not advised to refuse other foods for her child, but told to limit them and ask for sugar-water instead of formula.

In a clear industrial analogy, one text says that, like other "highly esteemed" products, mother's milk maintains its characteristics intact only when the "productive structures" are in perfect function and the inputs are ideal. "If a factory lacks supplies of primary materials, production will not be able to maintain itself at a reasonable level."[19] The expectation that milk quality is compromised by imperfect health, behavior, or nutrition practically presumes failure and is implicit in the testing of mother's milk. Laboratory testing was common into the early 1980s and continues to be recommended in cases such as suspected allergy in the nursling. A less exact method is to swirl expressed milk in a glass to see if it leaves a veil (indicating good quality), which physicians used to recommend and many people still mention.

The mother's diet is considered capable of making the milk simply unpleasant, or causing more serious disturbances in the nursling including allergies (from foods such as strawberries or mollusks) and digestive disorders. If the child does not seem to enjoy the milk or has intestinal problems, the mother is told to reconstruct her diet over the past day to determine whether it included something disagreeable. Experts confirm popular fears by saying that "it is true" that foods such as onions and those containing B vitamins alter the taste of the milk. All sorts of vegetables including broccoli and asparagus are thought to taint the milk, together with game, smoked meats, marinated and fried foods, most spices and herbs, spirits, and chocolate and cream-based sweets. Mothers are warned, "the little one—let us keep in mind—has tastes a bit different from ours!"[20] If an infant "sucking avidly what he expects to be the usual sweet milk, feels arriving in his mouth an atrocious and pestilential spurt of garlic," he will energetically express disapproval by letting out "inhuman screams" and "categorically refusing to attach to the breast" next time.[21]

While suggesting that it is extremely easy to damage the milk, medical experts declare that it is difficult or impossible to improve its quality or quantity—though they are quick to point out that modern hormonal preparations are highly effective in *inhibiting* milk secretion in mothers who do not plan to breast-feed. Mothers are reminded that the efficacy of milk-enhancing substances is uncertain aside from a possible placebo effect, but they nevertheless methodically ingest milk, beer, and foods high in protein, vitamins, and minerals held in high popular and medical regard. They put fennel drops in their water and take concentrates of herbs, special herb teas, homeopathic drugs said to stimulate prolactin release, hormones, vitamins, and organ extracts.

The food and behavioral restrictions to minimize the mother's negative impact on the milk are not mentioned among the inconveniences of breast-feeding, but are certainly inconvenient. They subtract many basic foods from the diet—including the nearly universal seasonings of garlic, onions, and parsley—forcing the mother to eat completely different dishes from the rest of the family. The belief that her diet can spoil the milk to the point of it being refused by the child remains firm, reflecting the depth of cultural doubt over the quality of breastmilk.

Characteristics of Milk Production

The traditional knowledge that milk production depends upon both nipple stimulation and the emptying of the gland has been verified by postwar science, which nevertheless upholds certain practices that can disrupt lactation, rather than supporting baby-led feeding. The perceived necessity of spacing meals at least three hours apart is based upon the ideas that the gland must be completely emptied in order to be free to produce new milk and that the infant's digestive system must be allowed to rest for at least half an hour after the two and a half hours of digestion time. While it is considered common sense that the mother's emotional state can gravely affect mammary function, it does not seem to occur to anyone that this regimentation might disturb the mother psychologically.

The classical idea that stagnant secretions are harmful finds expression in the belief that milk left to pool in the breasts causes rhagades, mastitis, and blocked milk secretion, especially if the breasts are very engorged. To prevent this, women are advised to completely empty the breast at each feeding, finishing the infant's work manually or with a pump if necessary. The child must not be allowed to suck for too long, for this is thought to damage the breast if it is empty. If the breasts are very hard and distended, the mother should express some milk before the feeding, so that the child is able to attach and suck effectively. She may also apply ice to the breasts or take a sublingual compress of oxytocin or other drug suggested by her physician. Some experts advise that even during pregnancy and after childbirth, colostrum must be expressed many times a day to keep the glandular tubes clear.

Ironically, the problem of engorgement, requiring interventions such as pumping the milk before or after feedings, is exacerbated or in fact created by the regulation of feedings by the clock and scale. Similarly, the method of alternating breasts between feedings compromises lactation in two ways, by reducing nipple stimulation and introducing supplementation. This system has been recommended in the literature for decades and is still preferred by some experts and mothers.[22] The supposed advantages are that the infant is able to take the richer hind milk because it spends more time at one breast and that the breast is allowed at least six hours to refill between feedings. If production is low, mothers are advised to offer the other breast or give a supplement of formula.

Breast-feeding mothers are said to have an "internal clock" for feeding, while infants are said to be able to "autoregulate" their nutrition. At the same time, infants are believed to "naturally" put themselves on a feeding schedule, given that they all feel the stimuli of appetite according to a "certain periodicity." The optimal functioning of their gastrointestinal system is said to depend upon respect for this rhythm. Like hunting dogs that run home at a fixed hour to feed their puppies and then run back to their work with the same haste, mothers of normal, unspoiled infants put them in their cribs after each meal, in a continuous alternation between eating and sleeping. These infants do not ask for food between feedings, while their mothers do not interpret their cries as hunger and never answer them with milk.[23] It is widely agreed that, on average, the interval between meals initially should be two to three hours, becoming fixed in the first weeks. Thereafter, it increases to four or more hours, with a longer interval at night.

Just as the feeding schedule is not thought to conflict with infant autoregulation of nutrition, so the doppia pesata is not considered antithetical to the idea that a certain amount of flexibility in breast-feeding is tolerable because it prevents the baby from taking overly high or low "doses," as is more likely with artificial feeding. Even if one does not weigh the baby at each meal, the scale cannot be abandoned. It is said to be often necessary to measure whether the child is being fed the correct amount, and always important to weigh the infant every day in the early times and then once a week thereafter.

During the first few days of "familiarization" after birth, feeding times and amounts are relatively free, but thereafter parents are expected to search for a reason if their baby eats more often than every three or four hours. That is, the child is given a few weeks or up to a month to learn to "regulate himself alone." This is what is meant by "autoregulation" and conveniently matches the mother's presumed need for nipple stimulation and emptying of the gland at uniform intervals of time.

Contraindications and Impediments to Breast-Feeding

As in the interwar period, mothers today receive the contradictory message that although all of them should breast-feed, many must not. Popular and medical texts continue to introduce the topic of breast-feeding by outlining impediments or contraindications to it, or stating that errors in infant nutrition can cause permanent harm to the child. There is the added condition that the pregnant woman must have her breasts examined by her obstetrician, who will judge their anatomical suitability for breast-feeding and assess possible contraindications. The physician's judgment must not be disputed, for to insist on breast-feeding against it constitutes an "extremely risky" or "gross" imprudence that could seriously harm the child.

Usually the reason for advising against breast-feeding is a condition or disease in the mother, but there are also a few infant causes. The latter include prematurity, low birth weight, harelip, inability to suckle, and milk intolerance or "allergy" in the infant (attributed to the passage through the milk of allergens such as protein in cow's milk, ovalbumin, and medicines). Maternal contraindications constituting a "very grave danger" to the infant include tuberculosis, diseases of the heart or kidneys, tumors, hyperthyroidism, serious chronic diseases, and certain contagious diseases. However, medical experts point out that some conditions commonly thought to contraindicate breast-feeding are not true impediments, such as maternal syphilis, Rh or ABO autoimmunization, return of menstruation, and new pregnancy.

Other contraindications include malformations of the breasts or nipples that make them unsuitable for breast-feeding. Mastitis and rhagades or lacerations that appear during breast-feeding may be considered sufficient reason to discontinue breast-feeding, or more as useless suffering than an absolute impediment. They are attributed to the mother's failure to observe the norms of breast preparation beginning early in pregnancy (although washing with soap in fact increases susceptibility to them!). Until the 1980s, mothers with anemia or eye diseases or vision problems including myopia were categorically excluded from breast-feeding. Today, they are sent to specialists for a determination of their eligibility.

The physician may also advise against breast-feeding on the basis of psychological obstacles, the woman's personality, or indefinable negative conditions of her organism. The causes of depression, exhaustion, anxiety, and fear rather than pleasure in breast-feeding are said to elude even the woman herself. Some women are said to simply lack the "vocation" of breast-feeding, or the desire to practice it as an act of love.

One contraindication dwarfs all others: milk insufficiency (*ipogalattia mammaria*). This condition is considered a common biological phenomenon that often thwarts even the most willing mothers' attempts to breast-feed. Recent medical texts are more precise about the causes, but for many years postwar authors affirmed the notion that the "aptitude of the female organism for the function of breast-feeding is progressively declining."[24] Today, milk insufficiency is attributed to individual causes such as mammary hypoplasia, defective nutritional states, disease, psychological causes, or bad attitudes toward breast-feeding.

Advice books endorse popular fears by asserting that breast size, shape, and richness or otherwise of glandular tissue determine the sufficiency of milk production, while the type of nipple determines the effectiveness of nipple stimulation. Further, they claim that milk insufficiency affects women randomly and unpredictably: it does not depend upon the dimensions of the breast, for tiny breasts can provide adequate milk while "prosperous" breasts can reveal themselves to be completely arid. Alternatively, the milk secretion may never begin because of hormonal disequilibrium resulting in insufficient production of prolactin.

While the ability to produce milk is thought to depend upon a number of intrinsic and uncontrollable factors as well as willingness to breast-feed in a loving and self-sacrificing way, lactation is equated with exhaustion, discouragement, mechanical difficulty, and insufficiency of quality and quantity. This makes bottle-feeding appear a much happier solution. Indeed, it becomes unavoidable since conditions such as milk insufficiency or the child "not growing as it should" are treated with supplements, not more frequent feedings—with the predictable result that milk production ceases completely.

Technique of Breast-Feeding, Supplementation, and Weaning

The Feeding Schedule, Double Weighings, and Regularity of Infant Growth

Although behavior and constitution are still considered to impact upon lactation, method takes precedence over maternal conditions. This method centers around the orario, which is grounded in the idea that the infant's gastrointestinal system and the mother's mammary glands need time to rest between active phases. Over the past decades, this notion has hardened into an indisputable fact, while the schedule has maximized the inviolable rest period. This has come about even as experts observe that on-demand feeding has been increasing in popularity—particularly in America—and reflects both the infant's desires and the mother-infant relationship. Many tell mothers that they should not be too rigid in applying the feeding schedule, but very few are those who abstain from providing one in the first place.

The most common schedule over the past decades, which is found in both medical and popular texts and is essentially the same as in the interwar period, is six or seven meals during the first week at 6:00, 9:00, 12:00, 15:00, 18:00, 21:00, and 24:00, which is then reduced to five or six meals at 3½-hour intervals between 6:00 and 20:00 or 23:30. The last meal is skipped if the lesser number is chosen, and it is permissible to shift the schedule by an hour. After a few weeks or at most a couple of months, the number of meals is reduced to five and redistributed at four-hour intervals: 6:00, 10:00, 14:00, 18:00, and 22:00 (or each an hour later). From some time between the second and sixth month on, the meals are reduced to four, given at 8:00, 12:00, 16:00, and 18:00. Notably, no nighttime feeding is specified in the schedules. This is because even demand-fed infants are said to stop taking a nighttime meal within ten to twelve weeks after birth. As in the past, it is considered always better to give one fewer meal than one more: nothing will happen if a meal is skipped, but damage will readily happen if an extra meal is taken, especially if the error is repeated or becomes habitual. The stomach does not get enough rest and sooner or later ends up sick.

The even spacing of poppate, together with the ingestion of a fixed amount of milk at each meal, is thought to ensure that the child's overall weight gain will be regular. Growth in stature is also expected to be regular, but it is considered less susceptible to illnesses, disorders, and hygienic or dietary errors and is monitored only twice a year for the first year and once a year thereafter. Body weight, by contrast, cannot be measured frequently enough.

After the first seven to ten days, infants are expected to progressively increase in weight without interruption. While experts usually mention that individuals can vary considerably from the averages and should not all be expected to follow the same rhythm, they nevertheless present standards for growth. In the 1950s, these standards referred to *monthly* growth. Infants were said to grow 600 grams per month in the first six months, 500 in the second six months, and 250 in the second year. A generation later, although experts observed that many parents weighed their children every day, most standards were for average *weekly* weight gain, such as 170 to 210 grams per week for the first three months, 200 in the second quarter, 100 to 140 in the third, and 70 to 100 in the last quarter of the year. Today, the averages are narrowed down to *daily* weight gain through the first year: 25 to 30 grams per day in the first three months, 20 to 25 in the second, 15 to 20 in the third, and 10 to 15 in the fourth.

It is hardly surprising that parents and relatives become anxious if a child's weight gain is lower than expected, even for one day. Many call their pediatrician immediately, which some physicians and writers describe as annoying and erroneous. Medical experts may suggest weighings only once a month during the first year, but in practice most parents weigh their infants every day or week. The standard regimen, outlined in ONMI charts from the 1970s and used in pediatric offices today, is to record the child's weight once a week for the first six months, then biweekly and eventually monthly by the end of the year. The same scale must be used to weigh the child undressed, on the same day and at the same time every week, at least three hours after a meal.

Weight gain is also monitored at each feeding. Rather than rely on "subjective" observations of infant nutritional status, parents and health professionals adopt the doppia pesata to obtain a mathematical and therefore "exact" measure. The doppia pesata is praised as useful not only for the physician but also the mother, who, "especially in the early times . . . can feel the necessity to verify if the milk administered corresponds to the child's need; that can give her a sense of security and help her investigate other causes of possible disturbances."[25] The child is weighed before and after every poppata either naked or in the same clothes. The results may be averaged over the day (since consumption tends to decrease in the afternoon and evening meals) to allow for "judgment of the sufficiency or less of the mammary secretion."[26] That is, milk production is almost expected to fail—an assumption encountered often above.

If the child receives insufficient milk, it is said to suffer hyponutrition, with arrested growth and weight loss. Symptoms include scarce, rare, brown or olive-colored "feces of hunger," and restlessness and crying, especially after meals, which then turns to apathy and sleepiness during and after meals. Overconsumption arouses equal or more alarm, and immediately calls for limitation of the duration of meals. Excessive milk intake is said to cause hypernutrition and excessive weight gain, with long-term damage. It is also blamed for gastric expansion and dyspepsia leading to perturbations of the entire digestive apparatus, with weight loss and other consequences. Symptoms include agitation, acidic vomit just after a meal or within the hour, abdominal pain, strong perianal erythema, and acidic, greenish diarrhea rich in lactose, lactic acid, and fatty acids.

Medical and popular books, forms distributed at hospitals, and packages of infant formula indicate the allotted amount per poppata according to age or weight, which is said to respect infant nutritional needs, metabolism, and normal growth patterns, as known through scientific studies. The rationing of meals begins even before the milk arrives, with colostrum: 10 to 30 grams per poppata on the first two days, 30 to 40 on the third day, and 30 to 50 on the fourth or fifth day. The amount rises to 60 to 70 in the second week, working up to 100 grams at one month.

Today, the ration is calculated in various ways. One of these is the formula presented in chapter 5 that specifies that the child needs 140 grams of milk per kilogram per day.[27] To simplify the calculation, one may use 150 grams of milk per kilogram: a 3-kilogram child needs 450 grams per day; a 6-kg child 900 grams. This quantity is then divided by the number of meals per day. This means six (exceptionally seven) in the first three weeks, five until the end of the first month, and four thereafter, so that the child takes 70 to 90 grams per feeding in the third week; 100 to 110 in the fourth; 130 to 150 in the second month; and 160 to 180 in the third month.

Another rule is to take the child's age in days minus one and multiply by ten to calculate the rations in the first week: a three-day-old child will take 20 grams of milk per meal. After the first week, if the child takes seven meals a day, then the ration is two times the first two digits in the child's body weight: for a 5,000 gram child, the meal is 100 grams. A third method is to give the child as many grams as one-hundredth of its body weight in the first week: an infant weighing 3,200 grams at birth will take 32 grams per meal. For the rest of the first month, the ration increases by 30 grams each week. From the second through the ninth month, the month is inserted between the 1 and 0 in the number 10: in the second month the infant takes 120 grams; in the fifth it takes 150. From the ninth month on, the ration is 220 grams.

Flexibility and Rigidity in the Rules for Breast-Feeding

The same experts who enthusiastically discuss the doppia pesata and include tables and formulas for determining exact levels of milk consumption and production also warn parents not to use it excessively or obsessively. They complain of parents' misinterpretations of infant nutrition and describe an all-consuming "complex of the scale" leading to incessant, insistent, and irritating questions about how much the baby should eat at each poppata. Some experts suggest that the chore or "tedious rite" of double weighing need not be considered indispensable, and that parents may simply ensure that the meal lasts no more than 20 to 30 minutes and observe whether the child seems satisfied or falls asleep soon after eating. Yet, parents continue to insist upon knowing how much the child eats, and they are not satisfied with signs such as the infant's appetite, behavior, or change in body weight.

Experts admit that medical writings fuel or confirm parents' fears that their children eat too little and feel hunger, or eat too much and suffer indigestion. Their assertion that normally these conditions are extremely rare does not go very far toward calming these fears, given the gravity of the health conditions associated with hyper- and hyponutrition. Even though some experts recommend against the doppia pesata in the home, no one questions its use in hospitals. It may be argued that the doppia pesata is only advisable when the infant does not seem satisfied, wakes too early, or gains little weight, but in practice this is taken to encompass all babies. Further, the unshakable, incontestable belief that regular weekly weight gain is the only definitive proof of infant health makes it unthinkable to do away entirely with the scale.

In contrast to the "rigid discipline" of past decades, today's experts consider themselves progressive and permissive in allowing a degree of flexibility in feeding times and amounts. Current medical texts may suggest double weighings only in special cases or during the first weeks, until it is certain that the child nourishes itself well, but continue to insist upon weekly weighings thereafter. A parenting magazine discusses how international authorities agree that it is best to breast-feed whenever the baby gives signs of hunger, but also states that by the middle of the first month the child "almost certainly" will have begun following "a precise schedule for meals."[28] Likewise, most advice books and medical texts express admiration for the infant's capacity for autoregulation and urge mothers to learn to respond correctly to their child's unique constitution and behavior rather than external norms. Yet, they also insist upon verifying that growth is normal and provide standards for infant feeding and weight gain.

The recommendations of an unusually strong advocate of baby-led feeding put prevailing views into relief, but not without equivocation. Albani refutes the idea that the babies should be fed on a precise orario, for "*it is not true that the nursling, left free to eat as much and whenever he wants, can eat too much, expand the stomach, develop indigestion*, become obese, etc., or, by contrast, eat too little and therefore not grow sufficiently" (1990:14–15). Parents should not wake their babies because "the hour has arrived" or let them cry desperately because it has not. The processes of digestion will *not* be altered if the baby eats after waiting as little as a half-hour since the last feeding. While many mothers worry whether their milk is "light" or "heavy" and ask if they need to have it analyzed, "mother's milk, even though it has variations in composition from one moment to another in the day, *can not ever be qualitatively inadequate* to the needs of the nursling" (1990:16). Finally, each child is an individual with normal fluctuations in growth and should not be expected to grow by the day or week with "perfect regularity, or according to certain theoretical predictions" (1990:26).

Yet, even in Albani's book there is the assumption that milk insufficiency is common, and that there is a precise relationship between the timing and duration of feedings and the adequacy of infant nutrition. If a baby wants to eat every hour or two and seems to be constantly hungry, Albani says that it is not succeeding in obtaining enough milk from the breast and the mother's milk will have to be "completed" with formula. A pair of drawings shows a woman breast-feeding under a clock that reads 9:10, then bottle-feeding at 9:25. The caption says: "If it happens that the maternal milk is not sufficient to satisfy the needs of the infant, after having attached him to the breast it is necessary to also give him the bottle" (1990:17). Thus, even those who seem to promote baby-led feeding sow the seed of doubt regarding innate autoregulation and impose quantitative standards for judging and regulating the mother's milk secretion.

In spite of the experts' warnings that their standards should be used with flexibility, from the infant's first moments they are imposed with rigor.

Supplementation and Weaning

The foregoing discussion indicates that few mothers breast-feed beyond the first few months and that experts consider this period normal and desirable. One text says that mothers should breast-feed for four to six months ("If you want to, you can also breast-feed afterward") so long as varied foods are also included in the baby's diet since the milk begins to be less nutritious.[29] That is, while experts suggest that weaning should *begin* some time before six months, they also assume that it will be *completed* by six months. This is evident in Maglietta's weaning diets, which allow four milk meals (maternal or artificial) in the fourth month, three milk meals ("if still mother's milk" or "if no longer mother's milk") in the fifth, and two meals of cow's milk only in the sixth and seventh (1985:340–42).

In the 1950s, medical authorities decried the common women's continued habit of breast-feeding intensively through the first year and beyond. Mothers did this "a little for weakness toward their own little one," but more often for "the fallacious illusion" that in so doing they could avoid an undesired pregnancy. They needed to learn that protracted breast-feeding not only did not protect against pregnancy, but almost always brought a visible deterioration of mother and child: she because of loss of humor and he because, "spoiled by the tepid sweet taste of that nectar" which was no longer of much nutritional value, limited or refused important foods for good nutrition and health.[30] Weaning should begin at 6 months and be completed by 12 months, avoiding the summer season and following month-by-month medical meal plans.

Over the following decades, the seasons lost much of their relevance to weaning, though older people still talk about avoiding the summer months. Meanwhile, the age at which weaning should begin declined together with the age at which mother's milk was said to become inadequate or "incomplete." In general, this has been four or five months—the time when mother's milk is said to no longer satisfy the infant's needs and the infant must learn to habituate itself to new flavors. In contrast to "monotonous" mother's milk, weaning brings a more differentiated, rich, complete diet. It represents "dietary *enrichment,*" a "leap forward," and an abandonment of infant ways in favor of exploration of the "terrain" of diet suitable for mature individuals. Weaning is compared to the explorations of a traveler or pioneer, solid food to an "adventure." Infants who are loath to embrace this challenge are compared unfavorably to "curious and robust eaters" who have no difficulty with weaning and with whom "life is certainly easier."[31]

In the 1960s, mothers' milk was still recommended through the first year, but other foods were to be introduced by the end of the fourth month. In the 1970s and early 1980s, breast-feeding was to be definitively abolished much earlier than one year. Experts argued that supplementation with small amounts of "integrating elements" from the moment of birth, or at least during the second month, gave better results in terms of growth and health than exclusive breast-feeding. If the child were not completely weaned by the time the teeth appeared, the mother would "inevitably" anticipate the poppata with apprehension and might tear the breast away, compromising the relationship. That is, dentition and breast-feeding were now considered incompatible, in contrast to the age-old practice of waiting for a full set of teeth because they were needed to chew food.

Early supplementation was further justified by the expectation that most women would run out of milk within a few months. Advice books from the 1970s warned mothers that they could be left inexplicably without milk at any time. The mother might have to return to work, and the child could fall ill and require suspension of breast-feeding. This meant that it was only prudent to supplement the milk from the outset. Some experts defended lactation, saying that women are endowed with the capacity to breast-feed, "let us suppose, for six or eight months"; it would be against nature to shorten this and it would bring about a disequilibrated, insecure character in the child. The more popular view was that mother's milk is imperfect even in the first months. To introduce other foods early on was to stimulate the digestive system to a more rapid and efficient functional development and to allow the child to grow up more entrepreneurial, independent, vital, and active. As in other areas of human endeavor, in infant nutrition "one must go against nature, in the sense of improving her with opportune dietetic interventions."[32]

Today, the initiation of weaning before the fourth month is discouraged because of the risk of excessive or untimely introduction through baby food of certain minerals and proteins as well as colorings, additives, and other unsuitable substances. However, because the child is thought to need extra dietary iron and copper from the fourth to sixth month on, iron- and protein-rich foods such as meat and eggs are introduced then, even if this is earlier than was thought to be proper in the past. This is said to represent a very "precise stage in the nutritional, psychological and sensory evolution of the nursling."[33] The tongue-thrust reflex has been extinguished, and the infant has acquired head control, is able to sit, and no longer pushes food out of the mouth. The mother must favor the progress of her relationship with the child by ensuring that it acquires new capacities for assuming different kinds of food. If she continues to give only milk, the child will utilize only the most elementary mechanisms for eating and become more resistant to taking other foods.

The focus is clearly upon the nursling, to the exclusion of the mother. Yet, it is she who must submit to medical direction and surveillance, and put significant time and effort into the preparation of foods for weaning. To illustrate, the written instructions given by a pediatrician to parents in Santa Lucia initially allow four or three meals of milk (maternal or powdered) of 180 or 220 to 250 grams each, depending on whether the infant takes five or four meals. The noontime milk meal is substituted with a 180 to 200 gram ration of vegetable broth made according to specifications regarding the length of cooking and the exact quantities of water, peeled potatoes, carrots, beet greens, rice or corn flour, tapioca, and corn or olive oil. Over the next few weeks, as more milk meals are replaced by broth, freeze-dried or homogenized meat is added, increasing in concentration along with the amount of cereal. Another set of instructions explains how to boil and dilute specific quantities of cow's milk from weaning through the second year—extending regimentation well beyond the breast-feeding period.

Weaning is presented as an adventure and a test of character and skill, whose renunciation implies retrogression or stalling of development. The mother must enthusiastically participate in the passage to an unquestionably beneficial independence from a now-incomplete food. Because it is begun early, this brings mixed or artificial feeding in the vast majority of cases.

Mixed and Artificial Feeding

The need to time and meter meals is proclaimed as forcefully for artificial feeding as breast-feeding, and there is an equal concern for giving the child a controlled amount to prevent overconsumption. While today formula is used exclusively in place of mother's milk, treated and diluted animal milk was common through the 1970s (mostly cow and goat). These substitutes were and are administered with the same regularity as breastmilk, if not an even stricter adherence to the orari of meals. Women are told to carefully follow the pediatrician's directions for the doses, with no approximation or improvisation, for disturbances will "inevitably" arise if they vary the concentration of the milk and thereby give too much or too little. Mothers must never use formula without the physician's authorization since they may use the wrong kind of milk or the wrong doses.

As with breast-feeding, the number of meals is reduced over the first months from six or seven, to five and then four, while the intervals between them increase from 3 or 3½ to 4 hours. The rule that it is always better to give one fewer than one more meal is imposed with even more severity than in breast-feeding, in which a transgression of this kind may even be pardoned since mother's milk is more easily digested and overworks the stomach relatively less. Mothers are told never to take such a risk with artificial milk, for it will be paid very dearly in disequilibrium of the intestinal functions.

In mixed feeding, the mother must first use the doppia pesata for breastmilk, then calculate and compensate for the missing caloric value of the meal with a ration of formula. This "complementary" feeding is generally preferred over alternating meals of breastmilk and formula, since it provides more frequent nipple stimulation. For similar reasons, the spoon may be recommended, to keep the child from preferring the bottle's easy flow. More often, the bottle is preferred for the pleasurable sensations it is supposed to give the child.

Mixed feeding is recommended most often for *ipogalattia* (low milk supply) and twins. In the former case, the infant is attached to the breast until both have been completely emptied; in the latter until the allowed amount has been taken. Some experts recommend not using the doppia pesata because it prolongs meals and shortens the interval between them, tiring the infant's stomach. They suggest allowing the infant to take breastmilk and formula for equal periods of 10 to 15 minutes, following the orari exactly and paying due attention to its intestinal function.

So long as it is well-regulated, artificial feeding has long been considered equal if not superior to breast-feeding. A celebrated pediatrician gave the following address to a national conference in 1964.

These investigations contribute to unmoor us from the old concept of the absolute perfection of the milk of woman, demonstrating that, thanks to the modern advances of technics, a well-conducted artificial feeding favors growth better than exclusive and prolonged maternal breast-feeding . . . And it is not impossible that the ever wider, nearly complete diffusion of artificial feeding has influenced the acceleration of growth.[34]

About a decade later, the same pediatrician repented and declared that artificial feeding was one of the worst disasters of the century, saying that only the most ignorant and ingenuous pediatricians could still recommend it.

Medical experts are reluctant to acknowledge their role in encouraging formula feeding, blaming it on factors such as women's work, advances in the production and preservation of infant formula, and advertising and publicity campaigns. They berate the public for thinking that artificial feeding is quick and convenient, prevents the falling of the breasts, is more nutritious, and makes children more beautiful. Yet, these ideas did not emerge spontaneously in the public consciousness, but were promoted by professional medicine itself—in much the same way as experts discouraged gracile urban women from breast-feeding a century ago by promoting wet nursing. A major difference is that today's experts are in contact with a much wider portion of a more receptive population and can have a much stronger impact than they did in the past.

The norms discussed in this chapter illustrate a high degree of complexity and precision in standards for infant feeding and growth, and continuity in belief and practice with the fascist period. Today's rules continue to appear alongside contradictory notions of women's instinctual or intuitive maternal knowledge and "common sense," as well as capacity for autoregulation shared with the child. Although most women are said to be capable of breast-feeding, frequent discussions of contraindications, ipogalattia, and the damaging effects of women's behavior and bodily functions presume that many women will not be able to breast-feed or will do so poorly. It is not surprising that most women give up breast-feeding rather soon after starting, given the complicated technique they are expected to follow and the pressure to breast-feed properly or the child will die (as claimed in the interwar period) or grow up to be psychologically and physically damaged or deviant (as asserted today). As compliance with medical management has increased, this outcome has been ensured given the conflict between regimented norms for breast-feeding and the psychobiology of lactation.

CHAPTER 8

Scientific Modernization of Parenting
Maternity and Infant Care
since the Second World War

The norms for breast-feeding and the general care of mothers and infants presented in the last chapter reflect a strong element of continuity with those of the fascist period. The cultural and political concerns of the fascist period themselves had fused with older health beliefs to yield new norms of behavior and treatment. These included mechanical-industrial analogies for the body and its functions, and the rationalization of time and production. The idea of national cultural necessity lent a sense of urgency to political and medical intervention in maternal behavior. Regimented breast-feeding was promoted through standardized norms and a specialized, expanding medical system developing its own professional culture and body of knowledge in opposition to the public's "ignorant traditions." Through an overwhelming attention to the infant, the impacts of maternity and maternal functions on the mother fell into the background.

As medical care has been enclosed within hospital and clinic walls, health professionals have stopped making home visits and personally knowing patients and their surroundings. Not coincidentally, they have increasingly imparted universalist notions about the care of maternity and infancy. This general trend of Western medicine was furthered by fascist-era studies and conclusions about the purportedly uniform nutritional needs and functions of infants.

Compliance with medicalized breast-feeding methods has risen steeply over the postwar period. This has brought a decline in breast-feeding, notwithstanding changes in its prevalence, since the methods interfere with milk production. The rise in compliance is rooted in increased cultural uniformity, greater contact between individuals and professional medicine, social and economic transformation, and changes in family structure, size, and relationships. These changes have continued to draw the private, family sphere into the public arena. There has been an enormous expansion of the welfare state, whose public health service has carried forward the aims and practices of fascist medicine. Even such private matters as sexuality and birth control continue to be affected by fascist-era ideas and legislation.

Today, Italy is on the other end of the transitions begun a century ago. Birth, death, and infant mortality rates have settled at very low levels, with the result that there are relatively few children and many older people. The economic structure has shifted from a predominance of agriculture to industry and administrative and service work in government and business, while the agricultural system itself has moved toward an industrial-capitalistic model. The state has grown in administrative capability and extension throughout the country, touching ever wider areas of public and private life.

The material conditions and professional and economic opportunities of various social classes have become relatively equalized, contributing to greater national cultural uniformity. Improvements in transportation, communications, and educational levels have led to reductions in local and regional cultural autonomy and in the isolation of farm families and communities. The dissolution of the multiple-family household system in favor of simple families has diminished the influence of family members and traditions. These changes have contributed to the effectiveness with which state and medical authority has reached into private life.

We will now connect the norms of the previous chapter to actual infant feeding patterns and analyze them in terms of changes in medical care and authority, family life, and the institutional care of maternity and infancy. The final chapter will take up the wider cultural context for today's high degree of compliance with medical norms for infant care.

Organization of Medicine

Medical Authority and Maternal Ignorance

By the present time, it has been widely accepted and internalized that maternal behavior is the main determinant of infant well-being and survival, or rather that "maternal errors" are responsible for infant suffering and distress. In the 1950s, maternal ignorance of hygienic principles was blamed for the relatively slow decline of Italy's infant mortality rates compared to other countries. Relatively high death rates from gastroenteritis were blamed upon the suspension of middle-school education in puericultura after the fall of fascism and the "chaotic and insufficient" functioning of ONMI.[1] Even today, dietary errors are said to reverberate dangerously on the child's development, with permanent effects, and inadequate or inappropriate nutrition is considered the direct cause of numerous infectious diseases. Of these, infantile gastroenteritis is said to be "for the most part indeed provoked by denutrition and dietary dysfunctions" and the cause of 2.4 million infant deaths in the first year of life in Italy between 1887 and 1964.[2]

Accordingly, experts maintain that women must be taught how to undergo pregnancy, childbirth, and breast-feeding for their children's sake, given that they are incompetent and uninformed even with respect to the main "natural" purpose of their lives. Medical pedagogues proudly announce that they will teach women what is going on inside them during pregnancy—as if they could have no idea otherwise—and how to give birth with less pain and in such as way as to minimize their effects on the child. After childbirth, the physician must manage the relationship with the infant in order for the mother to behave properly. The loving and sensible mother will find this a comfort, for she will be furnished "a technical base, so to speak, for her behavior."[3]

ONMI infant health charts from the early 1970s proclaim that the pediatric clinic provides "answers to all of the questions" and "all of the most appropriate advice" for maternal upbringing of the child to ensure growth and the development of the personality (ONMI 1970a:1). Ferrari and Bonelli advise mothers not to visit the pediatrician only when their child is sick, but to "ask him how to behave oneself in that infinity of occasions which fall within the daily life of the neonate." The physician's delicate work of intervening in the family's intimate personal affairs may even require his having to "interfere in the mother-infant relationship" (1989:217). These statements represent the apex of decades of increasing political and medical intervention in the private world of the family.

Remarkably, experts find it necessary to tell women of their dependent condition or "state of regression" during pregnancy and childbirth: "few women know it: during their pregnancy they relive the story of their early infancy."[4] Pregnancy is construed as an extraordinarily disruptive time in which the woman searches for safety by turning back into a little girl and seeking the protection her parents once provided. Her insecurity and anxiety render her incapable of taking care of the child initially. "The first time you take the baby in your arms and move it close to your breast, you probably will not feel very sure of yourself." "You will not know well what to do." Mothers must not take fear, but learn how to breast-feed under expert guidance in the hospital. "You'll see that within a few days you will become very expert 'nutrici' and that the baby will nestle in your arms with ever greater naturalness."[5]

The idea that it takes an outside expert to teach women how to be mothers is explicit in advice books and prenatal courses for parents. The premise is that, unless they are taught properly, women interfere with the natural birthing process and make it painful. The preference for psychological methods as opposed to other forms of pain relief was also evident in the interwar and early postwar periods, when "psychoprophylactic preparation for childbirth" was one of the responsibilities of physicians working in ONMI obstetrical clinics. Monsignor Prosperini, professor of religion and professional ethics at the School of Obstetrics of the University of Rome, wrote that severe pain was the result of certain women's "morbose excitability." Their agitation exaggerated the normal sufferings that were women's "title of honor and merit" and the price they paid for the joys of motherhood (1954:131–32). In 1956, Pope Pius XII advocated psychological methods in a speech on obstetrical anesthesia to an audience of Western European gynecologists.[6]

Nowadays, experts say that there is no natural reason for pain in childbirth, sometimes making reference to the work of the British physician Grantley Dick-Read. In their view, childbirth is a physiological act like any other—a basilar function like digestion or respiration. There is no anatomical "obstetrical dilemma" between a rigid pelvis due to upright posture and a capacious cranium to hold a large brain. Uterine pain is nothing but the realization of the woman's sensations. Whether because of ignorance or a cultural tradition holding that painful childbirth is woman's payment for the sins of all humanity, she is afraid. Her primordial fear leads to irrational behavior, complaints, inadvisable movements, and bad respiration. Neuromuscular tension in the uterus impedes the dilation of the orifice, and the result is real pain.[7] Modern medicine liberates woman from her "typical fatalism" and teaches her that her child's development depends upon her "having or not [having] suppressed atavistic fears and ignorance in material of behavior, hygiene and diet."[8]

We saw in the last chapter that the physician is the "only authority" in decisions regarding infant feeding. It is the physician, not the midwife or puericultrice or especially the mother herself, who interprets the results of the *doppia pesata* and determines whether a supplement will be needed. The physician must be consulted before giving any infant formula, whatever the motive, and for the choice and "dosing" of weaning foods. The mother must never "give in to the temptation" to make "personal variations" or "arbitrary modifications" in the diet, but scrupulously follow instructions so that the physician can properly evaluate the infant's growth and tolerance of milk.[9] Albani's somewhat unconventional text encourages parents to think of themselves as capable of raising their children on their own; however, it criticizes not medical experts but relatives and friends who incessantly interfere with bad, confusing suggestions (1990:46).

The predominant view is that women must be taught how to undergo maternity instead of submitting to ancient irrational fears and a tenacious ignorance about which experts have been writing for generations. Women are said to become children again during pregnancy and to need to sleep like babies for days after childbirth while not engaging in relationships with adults. They must ask for help with breast-feeding since they inevitably feel ill at ease and know not how to behave. Only through the intervention of science do they learn to use their instincts to the proper ends in correctly caring for themselves and their infants.

The Hospitalization of Childbirth

Most of the hospitalization of childbirth has taken place since the Second World War. Compared to the past, it has brought uniformity and anonymity in the care of maternity and infancy, which is split at childbirth. The structure of the state medical system does not permit the physicians and midwives who care for pregnant women in the preventive clinics to assist at childbirth in the hospitals. The hospital staff and procedures focus upon mechanical aspects of childbirth as opposed to humoral interactions between mothers and infants. Hospital practices ensure an immediate and prolonged physical separation for several days, interrupted for feedings at precise intervals through medically mediatêd interactions.

Until after the war, most towns had few or no facilities for childbirth and were served by a handful of midwives, physicians, and liberi professionisti. In Santa Lucia today, there is a midwife, gynecologist, obstetrician, and assistante sanitaria working at the public health service clinic, in addition to the liberi professionisti. Now that there is so little in-home care, the personal relationship between patient and health professional has been lost, as has an appreciation of the former's domestic, family, and professional circumstances. Medical care has become more uniform, while health professionals have, by necessity, become interchangeable in the minds of patients. This is especially difficult for older women, who no longer go to the clinic because it is run by a changing staff of outsiders they do not trust.

Through the 1950s and early 1960s, the midwife continued to be the principal health-care provider for women and children. According to medical texts and informants such as the midwife Marina, who came to Santa Lucia around 1960 and worked there for some 30 years, only those few women who were seen by a health professional in the ninth month and diagnosed with an abnormality of the fetus or hips gave birth in maternity wards.[10] In Santa Lucia, this ward was simply a few large rooms with normal beds, and no equipment. All other births took place at home, sometimes under such poor conditions that she had to ask the women to hold a candle since there was no other light. Women did not request prenatal care or take their children to the pediatric clinic unless they were quite ill. Marina worked alone, whether assisting in childbirth or in the town's pediatric clinic, in part because one of the physicians was a lung specialist and did not care much for obstetrics and gynecology.

The first childbirth experience of a woman named Paola was typical for the early 1950s. She was at home with a midwife and her husband, mother-in-law, and sister-in-law. The latter brought an image of Saint Anne, protector of pregnant women. Paola was laid flat on her back, her legs raised, the assistants pushing on her abdomen. Labor lasted a long time, so her husband went across the way to his mother's house to sleep, but the child died just after it was born. To spare him from seeing it, her sister-in-law went to tell him. Paola says that she was not well afterward because she did not have the pills women take today to get rid of their milk. She got up after three or four days, because her house was small and required little work, whereas her own mother had gotten up the next day.

When Marina first arrived in town, "every house was in mourning, whether for a mother or a child." Resolving to combat the public's diffidence about preventive medical care, she visited expectant mothers as soon as she heard of their pregnancy and sought to persuade families not to call for untrained assistants instead of midwives. The former often did not recognize complications until it was too late and used the traditional birthing chair instead of the more proper supine position. After the birth, Marina visited the mother and neonate every week for two months, weighing the child and giving it a bath herself in order to diagnose potential developmental abnormalities. After two months, the "infant defends itself alone."

During the 1960s, women began to give birth in a new maternity clinic in the next town or the new private hospital in the city. By 1970, Marina says, "people stopped having babies altogether." She accompanied those who did to the hospital, where she remained for five or six days. She deplores today's practice of releasing women from the hospital a week or sooner after childbirth, with little instruction in how to care for themselves or the child. However, the midwife Carolina says that she telephones mothers at home and visits them three or four times if needed, but that not all midwives make home visits.

Even though home birth was the norm until only a generation or two ago, and in spite of recent talk of its psychological and emotional benefits, it is now dismissed as too risky—for it is "always better" to give birth in a specialized hospital or clinic.[11] Women cannot be admitted too soon during labor, and the hospital stay can never be too long. In the early 1990s, it was still a week (ten days for caesarean section), but in recent years it has been reduced to as few as three or four days. During those days, constant surveillance and frequent bodily interventions pave the way for medical manipulation and control of breast-feeding.

Medical Interventions in Maternity

Over the past few decades, a standard regimen of visits and procedures has emerged in the care of pregnancy. Expectant mothers see the midwife or physician once a month through the eighth month, and two to four times during the ninth. Routine screening tests include ultrasound examination once each trimester. When labor begins, the woman must keep the intestines empty by not eating or drinking. She is submitted to an "abundant" enema in the hospital—described by one woman as an opaque, industrial-strength chemical "bomb"—purportedly to make her feel more at ease, prevent embarrassment, and give the baby more space. Routine pubic shaving is described as a hygienic norm in preparation for the almost inevitable episiotomy. Women and experts agree that if a woman is bothered by these procedures she should do them at home, but no one raises the possibility of refusing them altogether.

In addition, women are repeatedly subjected to pelvic examination and disinfection during labor, involving washing of the pubic zone with disinfectant solution every one to three hours and before every examination. This implies that it is the woman, rather than the hospital personnel or environment, who is the source of infection. Likewise, because the mother touches the infant and its food and other things, women are told to wash aggressively and scrupulously several times a day for six or eight weeks or until lochation stops, keeping the intimate parts and hands clean.

Within the hospital, childbirth is sharply divided into labor and delivery, which are handled in two different rooms shared by several women at once, as are the recovery rooms. While most delivery rooms look like operating rooms, there are some (most often private) hospitals that provide labor-delivery rooms that conceal the heavy equipment. The woman is usually assisted only by the midwife and may not see the physician at all. In general, she is attached to a fetal monitor during labor and kept in bed, giving birth laying on her back. There is little awareness of the inadvisability of laying flat on the back during pregnancy because of the pressure on the vena cava.

In recent years there has been more flexibility regarding birth position, movement during labor, and episiotomy, especially among newly trained or very old physicians and midwives. They may seek to avoid the latter by massaging the uterus or peritoneum and lubricating the infant's head. The Santa Lucia midwife Carolina says that it is permissible to use the monitor only once every half-hour for five minutes. She encourages women to walk in between or take a shower if they have a private room. When it is time to push, she has them sit on the toilet or squat on the bed. One woman used an old-fashioned birthing chair because her midwife was a relative.

While some health professionals maintain that an intravenous drip is not always used, most admit that it is given to all patients to keep them from getting thirsty, to induce labor, and in case of caesarean section. Several health professionals told me that about one-half of all deliveries are induced artificially after a few hours of labor. Italy now has the highest rate of caesarean birth in Europe, at 22.2 percent (up from 3 to 4 percent in the 1950s), a rate exceeded only by the United States, Canada, Brazil, and Australia.[12]

In light of the other interventions in pregnancy and childbirth, it may seem contradictory that pain relief is not routinely offered, and epidural injections are rarely used. While one woman who calls her labor pains *dolorini* (little pains) believes that she was given a sedative through the intravenous drip, most women do not think they received any chemical pain relief. One woman says that "maybe around here they're a little behind" with respect to epidurals, implying the persistence of ideas about the "naturalness" of childbirth and women's responsibility for pain. A midwife explains that her prenatal classes are oriented toward teaching women to relax and "control themselves" through breathing exercises.

After the birth, the child is taken to the nursery. In theory, breast-feeding is allowed in the delivery room, but conditions such as the intravenous drip or a stomachache are enough to postpone it until 6 to 24 hours after birth. Newborns are immediately bathed, clothed in a heavy wool garment, wrapped tightly into a blanket that is tucked into the mattress of the crib, and lined up before the nursery window. To the dismay of parents and relatives, the nurses will not bring them out except at scheduled feeding times. In spite of wide criticisms of these procedures, most hospitals are reluctant to undertake the organizational changes needed to allow rooming-in.

Common hospital practice therefore violates several of the fifteen recommendations of the World Health Organization regarding childbirth.[13] Both caesarean birth and induced labor are more frequent than the recommended limits of 10 to 15 percent and 10 percent, respectively; enema, pubic shaving, and electronic monitoring remain routine practices; and the supine position is used for labor and birth. On the surface, hospitals comply with some of the recommendations promoting breast-feeding, but end up contradicting them. There is little support of breast-feeding under the expectation that all women are able to breast-feed, for this concept has not been truly believed by Italian medicine or culture for many decades. The recommendation that healthy infants must stay with their mothers, given that no observational procedure justifies their separation, is openly disregarded.

The doppia pesata and orario are procedures that interfere directly in the mother-infant relationship. If the amount of colostrum or milk is deemed insufficient, the infant is promptly taken to the nursery for a supplement. As one father wrote in a letter in 1994, "during the poppata a midwife tears the baby from you and, among screams and shouts, weighs him under the astonished gaze of the mother . . . Our midwives are inhuman." Observing that triple weighing is now practiced for the first six months, he adds that "at bottom we are a people full of contradictions; we permit trains and airplanes to not even arrive on time, but one does not trifle with the poppata."

Another father concludes that it is more "natural," "simple," and less complicated to bottle-feed. He finds that after a medicalized pregnancy and childbirth some women prefer the autonomy of bottle-feeding. Contrariwise, to one woman it was all the more important to breast-feed after having had an "unnatural" caesarean birth, but she saw nothing "unnatural" about following the orario and doppia pesata with extreme precision.

Whatever the case, parents are put into close contact with the pharmacy, for they must rent a scale and buy formula and sterilization products for bottles or the mother's nipples. Infant formula and most infant foods are available only at pharmacies, reflecting the sense that these products are medicines. Pharmacies also sell pacifiers, strollers, toys, and shoes. They have become a visible expression of the medicalization of infant feeding methods and the displacement of expertise and ability away from parents and home.

Intersections between Medical and Popular Knowledge and Practice

The interventionist approach to maternity fits within a broader context of intrusive health practices in Italy. Enemas are standard hospital procedure for any surgical intervention, as one man explained with reference to his arthroscopic knee surgery. They are also used at home. Many drugs are given in the form of suppositories or injections. The latter are administered with materials purchased without a prescription, and most people are capable of giving them. Thermal cures are taken not only for illness but also to improve general well-being, prevent against conditions such as arthritis or osteoporosis, and treat the skin. There is a wide range of herbal products and natural antibiotics said to improve overall health and cure particular conditions, and many pharmacies promote themselves as herbalists at the same time. These treatments reflect an overwhelming emphasis on influencing the body through medicines and foods as opposed to physical activity, rest, or time.

Data gathered by the national statistics bureau in 1996 suggest a high level of pharmaceutical consumption in Italy. Although 93 percent of children under 15 were reported to be in good health, 17 percent of the nearly 8.5 million children had taken medicines in the two days before the survey (24.2 percent of 3- to 5-year-olds). Most were given drugs according to medical prescription (87 percent), but in a large proportion, 39 percent, the medicines were already in the house. With increasing age, the proportions of people reporting good health declined while the proportions who had taken medicine in the previous two days increased steadily to 33.2 percent of 45- to 54-year-olds, and 76.9 percent of people 75 and older (ISTAT 1997:82–84).

Newspapers devote long sections to news about health, a large proportion of which concerns maternity and infancy and advocates medical supervision and advice. For example, a single health section of the newspaper *Corriere della Sera* contained articles on the doubling of multiple births over the past decade; "those strange secretions" of the breast; a pregnancy diet for not gaining too much weight; the necessity of early, frequent professional examination of infants' eyes (six times in the first year and two in the second); and the American physician John Smith's opinion that only women should become gynecologists.[14]

By now, the gap between medical and popular knowledge has been largely closed. As professional medicine dissociated itself from its traditional, empirical base early this century, local differences came to be replaced by a relatively uniform body of biomedical knowledge. Now that literacy and national cultural uniformity have increased dramatically, so has the degree of acceptance of the authority of health experts—whether physicians, herbalists, pharmacists, or representatives of pharmaceutical or medical-equipment companies. This has been counterbalanced by a declining appreciation of mothers' knowledge and capabilities. In fact, very few women complain about the high degree of medical intervention in labor and childbirth, and some say that they would not benefit from one of the newer birthing rooms because the hospital atmosphere does not bother them at all.

The convergence of medical and popular belief is evident in shared ideas about the importance of digestion and nutrition in the determination of health and well-being. It is also apparent in the relative roles of atmospheric, behavioral, and microbial factors in causing disease, and in the presumed delicacy of the menstrual period and its effects on pregnancy and lactation. Identical food prohibitions in the medical literature and popular tradition forbid pregnant and lactating women from eating tasty, rich, or elaborate foods based on the belief that maternity requires moderate, sober behavior in all areas, but especially diet. The modern interpretation is that proscribed foods are not tolerated in pregnancy due to hormonal variations, while cravings represent nutritional deficits.[15]

Medical and popular ideas have settled upon the time to initiate weaning—the fourth or fifth month—whereas until a generation ago there was considerable variation in timing in spite of conformity in the choice of foods. Within a month or two, the infant passes to a diet of cereal-based paps made with vegetable or meat broth, complemented by pureed fruit.

With time, vegetables, small pasta, meat, and eggs are added to the diet, but broths seasoned with olive oil and parmesan cheese continue to be the primary food through the first year and beyond.

In the first decades after the war, paps were made at home from flour or grated bread mixed with milk and sugar or olive oil. People remember the rule of avoiding weaning in summer, but say that it was no longer applied, in agreement with contemporary medical advice. Meanwhile, there was a shift from the spoon to the bottle. Parents who had children in the 1950s and early 1960s say that they always fed paps and cow's milk with a spoon. As experts began to promote the bottle for administering liquids and pureed foods, it became more popular. The bottle is still used today for serving broths, fruit, and dissolved cookies.

The tradition of preparing broths at home continues, but the recipe most often comes from the pediatrician or a book, and the cereals are purchased at the pharmacy or in certain grocery stores. Some parents only use prepared infant foods, including fruit and vegetable purees and homogenized meat or fish. To pay high prices for these products, as for infant formula, has always had an element of conspicuous consumption and has been equated with participation in modernity and scientific progress.

Ideas about weaning foods illustrate the two-way exchange between popular and medical knowledge. The common weaning foods suggested by professional medicine reflect the country's culinary traditions, while cooked fruit is thought to be more healthful and digestible than raw fruit, especially for "delicate" people such as infants, small children, and the infirm. Medical advice, in turn, dictates the exact timing of the introduction of foods, and parents tend to follow the schedule very closely. In general, there is little difference between medical and popular belief. In the area of breast-feeding the public even goes beyond medical prescriptions with behaviors some health professionals find excessive.

Infant Feeding Patterns after the
Second World War

The Immediate Postwar Period

Three dominant trends in breast-feeding since the war include an increase in compliance with biomedical norms; a decrease in the duration of breast-feeding; and a fall then a rise in the prevalence of breast-feeding. The first trend has been related to the increased cultural uniformity, economic well-being, and access to and provision of medical care of the past 50 years. Because medical norms have either precluded or biologically obstructed breast-feeding, compliance has meant a reduction in its duration. Between the mid-1960s and mid-1980s, compliance meant using the doppia pesata and orario in breast-feeding, but more often abandoning it in favor of bottle-feeding. Since then, the medical community has promoted breast-feeding. Most women do so initially, but compliance with regimented methods has become so complete that few continue past the first few weeks or months.

Through the 1940s and 1950s, there were still many isolated farm families who remained outside the state medical system and emergent national culture. Many people born at that time say that their mothers breast-fed their babies for three or four years. The midwife Marina recalls that several families in Santa Lucia continued to earn a large part of their income by wet nursing foster children from the cities or nearby towns. Many people born before 1960 were wet nursed (or dry nursed) and fondly describe the affection they share with their milk mothers and milk sisters and brothers. Scholars lamented the disregard of laws regarding mercenary breast-feeding, indicating that it remained fairly common, and noted that mothers breast-fed intensively, and sometimes exclusively, through the first year and beyond.[16]

To be able to breast-feed was considered extremely important, for infant deaths were interpreted as the result of the mother's lack of milk. One woman whose neighbor's child died recalls that living conditions were very poor, and women had little to eat. They subsisted on pasta made without eggs and therefore of little substance: "If they did not have anything to eat they did not have milk." Many mothers also died, leaving this same woman to raise two nephews on cereal paps and cow's milk.

By the late 1950s and early 1960s, there was a growing tendency to renounce breast-feeding. Scholars were concerned because artificial feeding was senselessly being used even for neonates.[17] Compared to their mothers, women breast-fed for a short time and were also more likely to give birth with medical assistance. Marina found that most women she encountered in Santa Lucia and surrounding areas wanted to be "modern" and not breast-feed at all, though some did so for six or seven months. She says that she was caught between them and their mothers-in-law, whose traditional culture had long maintained that a good mother was a good nurse. Marina took the young women's side, giving them pills to get rid of the milk and telling the mothers-in-law that the breasts were dry.

Marina found that pediatricians fed the fire by telling women that it was better not to breast-feed because it ruined the figure and by prescribing an extremely precocious weaning. Women began to give rice pap in the first days, unless she convinced them to wait two or three months (but not longer). She advised against weaning in summer, especially if the child would be fed cow's milk rather than formula (provided the mother's milk had not already dried up by then). She explains that mothers tried to pass to cow's milk as quickly as possible since formula was expensive.

While some well-off couples hired wet nurses, they increasingly used formula-feeding, animal milk, and early weaning instead. As one Santa Lucia couple explained with reference to their three children born over a period of 31 months in the mid-1950s, parents had to go to pharmacies in Bologna or other cities to buy formula and prepared infant foods. Those who breast-fed increasingly kept scales in their homes for the doppia pesata. One woman in Forlì is proud to say that she was among the first to do so, but does not link this to her having to give the child "milk from the pharmacy" (formula) after a few months (which the child did not like, so she switched to cow's milk mixed with water). However, she notes that infants began to lose weight as the orario became popular, since she knew that they needed to eat "little and often" rather than at the long intervals demanded by the schedule.

Many women blame their having breast-fed a short time or not at all on fever, milk insufficiency, or the child's refusal or intolerance of the milk. This was a time in which more and more women were judged unsuitable for breast-feeding, and children incapable of drinking or digesting breastmilk. Laboratory testing was becoming a routine procedure, so it is little wonder that many women were told or believed that their milk was inadequate in quality or quantity.

The orario was a standard medical practice applied from the first moments of breast-feeding, for by then it was taken for granted that after childbirth the infant would be presented to its mother "from time to time."[18] Marina considers it more important for artificial feeding and says she allowed greater flexibility in natural feeding unless the infant ate "too much" or the milk was "heavy." She also insisted upon it in cases of mothers who were distracted, mentally deficient, or older or recovering from a caesarean section. She says that these mothers would have forgotten to breast-feed if their family had not been given the schedule.

Marina carried a scale in her medical bag, since she was required to record the weight of newborn children. She was and is very enthusiastic about the doppia pesata, for "with the weight one understands everything." She recommended it at each meal for the first two months, including waking the infant at night in some cases. Provided all went well, the mother could thereafter simply take a measurement of body weight once a week and, later, every 15 or 30 days.

After explaining this regimen, Marina noted that lately she had read that it is not necessary to do the doppia pesata every day, but only every second or third day. Significantly, she had never heard of women feeling their milk descend in response to thinking of their child or hearing its cry, and instead asserted that they feel it arrive every three and a half hours. However, she then said that psychological factors might indeed influence lactation, since nervous women do not have milk while relaxed women produce it in abundance: "the milk requires tranquillity and rest."

Marina's own case helps to illustrate the changes between her mother's generation and her own. When she was born in the 1920s, her mother suffered a hemorrhage and was told not to breast-feed, so Marina was fed goat's milk. Her husband was fed by a balia who also breast-fed her own daughter, whom he calls his "sister." The balia was the wife of one of his family's industrial workers and tenants in Forlì; she received a discount on the rent in return for the service. Marina's husband says that the balia fed him for at least six months before he was given cow's milk, but that by the 1950s wet nurses were not needed since most urban women used formula or cow's milk under safer hygienic conditions. When their child was born, Marina's milk disappeared after 20 days and did not return in spite of injections, teas, and other remedies.

The infant feeding practices of the time were even respected by Italians living abroad. One Santa Lucia woman had two children in a hospital in Somalia in the late 1950s, with the assistance of a female Italian physician in the first case and midwife in the second. She says that the medical care was the same during pregnancy and childbirth, and that all of the Italians used the doppia pesata—as they did back in Italy when she had her third child in the 1960s. She nursed each one for three months, stopping then because the milk was no longer nutritious. She knew her milk was "watery" because it was analyzed by the hospital, so she bought formula and other infant foods imported from England and Italy. She disdainfully explains that earlier generations, including her own mother, were like the Somali women who breast-fed "forever, for years." They allowed their babies to "always pull at the breast, so the milk kept coming"—intimating that prolonged, unregulated breast-feeding is barbaric and irrational.

"They Said That Babies Grew up More Beautiful
with Formula"

By the 1970s, the conditions were right for artificial feeding to be practiced on a large scale. At the same time, those women who breast-fed were much more likely to regulate feedings with the orario and doppia pesata. Women of all social classes, from farmers to college professors, participated in these trends. The postwar economic boom had produced the well-being necessary for the added expense of formula and a scale for weighing the baby, while medical advice tended to undermine or prohibit breast-feeding, especially baby-led feeding. The promotion of early supplementation and weaning with formula meant that all infants would be fed sooner or later with formula—the logical outcome of doing things with "good sense and due prudence."[19] In a reversal of past practice, no child was to be breast-fed until the moment it could eat table food.

Even when experts complained of modern woman's failure to breast-feed and sought to encourage it, they described breastmilk as an ideal but not irreplaceable food for the first few weeks or months. Boschetti et al. offered proof in the fact that in northern Italy 8 out of 10 infants were bottle-fed, but the frequency of intestinal diseases and defects of development was much lower than elsewhere (1975:86). This argument not only indicates how popular bottle-feeding was, but points to an ongoing assumption that infant health is exclusively shaped by diet, irrespective of the vast differences in economic and hygienic conditions between the north and the rest of the country.

Whatever the infant feeding method, parents increasingly adhered to medical advice and submitted to ONMI surveillance. The first of eight statements or rules on the opening page of the ONMI infant health booklet kept by parents in the 1970s reads: "Respect of the orario of meals from the first days of life constitutes an educative rule and a protection against disturbances of digestion and other diseases of the child" (ONMI 1970a:1). The booklet concentrates on the first year, beginning with details regarding feeding, whether maternal, mixed, artificial, or mercenary. There are charts for recording weight and stature every week for the first 26 weeks, every month for the next six months, and every six months for five more years. While there is a place for data on immunizations, illnesses and laboratory tests, and physical and psychomotor development, the frequent measurement of body weight is one of the things people remember most about the ONMI clinics, aside from the distribution of milk and formula.

As part of the modern approach to infant feeding, it became increasingly common for parents to put their infants in a separate room to sleep. Both the Church and bourgeois reformers of the late nineteenth and early twentieth centuries had equated cosleeping with ignorance, backwardness, and danger of suffocation. During the fascist period, it was opposed also on the basis of transmission of tuberculosis. In the postwar period, the infant's separate place found firm ground in the simple family and the commonsense equation of cosleeping with the miseria of the past. Lone infant sleep came to be considered unquestionably essential both for the psychological development of the infant and for the resumption of the parents' sexual relations. This has led to the curious circumstance that infants under one or two years of age are not permitted to sleep in the same room or bed with their parents, but children from three to eight often do so.

Over the 1960s, 1970s, and early 1980s, the idea arose that there is a fixed reservoir of milk, both in the individual woman and the population, and that its volume was much greater in the past. This is linked to the belief that the woman becomes "exhausted" by breast-feeding a second child, particularly if it is born soon after the first. Many women who had children at this time breast-fed their first child for six to nine months but their subsequent children for two or three. As they say, "there is less milk after the first child."

Surely the rising popularity of formula as well as medicalized breast-feeding methods played a large part in the diminishing duration of breast-feeding from one child to the next. Parents describe a "mania for formula," for "everyone" used it. A teacher remembers that 9 of the 13 women in the maternity ward with her started off by using formula. It is often observed that "they said that babies grew up more beautiful with artificial milk." Women were also told that breast-feeding ruins the breasts, debilitates the body, and delays postpartum weight loss. Many women were not allowed to breast-feed because they wore glasses, whether for nearsightedness or farsightedness.

Routine hospital practices often made it impossible for women to breast-feed, for infants needing special care were sent to hospitals far away from their mothers. One husband was prepared to drive pumped milk 70 kilometers to the hospital where his baby was being treated for a congenital disease, but his wife's hospital roommates ridiculed her, and her physician said it was inadvisable and gave her hormones to get rid of the milk. A friend's prematurely born infant was kept in a separate ward. The mother was not allowed to breast-feed, but she pumped her milk and gave it by bottle in spite of negative pressure from peers and hospital staff.

Parents who started their families at this time were at a crossroads between traditional and new knowledge, set in the context of the large-scale abandonment of farming and the rapid reduction in family size. Though they may have been born at home to families with anywhere from one to a dozen children, their few children were born in hospitals. They knew about their parents' ways, but they were exposed to new ones. For example, couples recall that many women ran out of milk and fed their children goat's or cow's milk, and remember the particulars of how it was done (using the same nonpregnant animal and starting early on). Sometimes, the milk was taken directly from the animal, though this was more common during their own childhood.

Mothers say that they listened more to their midwives and physicians, because many of the things they were supposed to do did not exist for their mothers. While their mothers weaned them when they had a full set of teeth, they were to wean their infants when they had few or none. Often, they say that they followed the midwife's and pediatrician's advice with respect to infant feeding, swaddling, and washing cloth diapers with a sterilizing powder. However, while many scrupulously respected the orario, some either fed their babies at night or failed to wake them for scheduled feedings. While some believe it is important to know how much the child takes at each meal, others did not use the doppia pesata.

One woman says that her first child was "bad" and cried a lot, making it more difficult to respect the feeding schedule. She believes that "good" infants enjoy weaning, which should be completed by six months, and openly disapproves of prolonging breast-feeding any further. She is unaware of any connection between breast-feeding and the prevention of pregnancy. Her college-educated daughters do not share their mother's beliefs: they know of lactation's contraceptive effects and favor prolonged, baby-led feeding.

Women who had little or no family support often depended more heavily upon medical guidance. A homemaker named Costanza, who has lived since childhood in a city she does not consider her own, did not breast-feed any of her three children. Her physician forbade it because she wore glasses. She unfailingly followed the orari and weighed her babies weekly on a rented scale. Her husband agrees that it is wrong to feed infants whenever they want, or even a half-hour before the scheduled time: "a baby has to cry to develop its stomach muscles." To Costanza, it is "right" for infants to sleep in a separate room, even if this means the hallway. Significantly, Costanza says she does not get along with her mother and has few relatives nearby, but keeps 20-year-old books about child rearing on her shelves.

Margherita's case is illustrative because of the age difference between her older children, born in the mid-1970s, and her youngest child, born around 1990. She explains that there was still enthusiasm for breast-feeding when her first child was born, but by the time the second one came four years later, everyone was using formula. Perhaps it was not a coincidence that she breast-fed the latter for only a couple of months, due to a liver problem. By the time her last child was born, breast-feeding was again in favor. Margherita says that she did not use the doppia pesata or orario, never had any problems producing milk, and was always more likely to follow the advice of her relatives than the instructions of hospitals and physicians. She lives in an extended family and helped to raise her two brothers, who are 8 and 13 years younger than she. Like other farm children, she brought them out to her mother in the fields for feedings, or kept them outside all day in order to stay closer. Consequently, she was not inclined to find the doppia pesata and orario useful or appealing.

Breast-Feeding Practices Today

Prevalence and Duration of Breast-Feeding

Since the 1980s, there has been a renewal of interest in and approval of maternal breast-feeding. Today, at least 85 percent of all mothers in Santa

Lucia and the region begin by breast-feeding, as measured through interviews, observation, discussions with health professionals, and questionnaires. A practicing gynecologist and midwife state that all mothers attempt breast-feeding, except those who have grave myopia or other vision problems, but that the proportion drops to 70 to 80 percent after a few days.

The average duration of breast-feeding for mothers reported in questionnaires compiled by parents of young children is roughly 3½ to 3¾ months in two cities and 4¼ months in the town. When those who answered that they did not breast-feed are excluded, these averages rise to between 4½ to 5 and 5⅓ months, respectively, but when the single highest value is excluded they drop to 3⅓ and slightly over 3¾, respectively. When compared with ethnographic analysis, these numbers suggest an average duration of 3 to 4 months. Miraglia, Orlandini, and Micheletti (1984:328) report that 70 percent of mothers stop breast-feeding by the routine medical visit at 40 days, and another 20 percent stop by three months.[20] According to local health professionals including the pediatrician Chiara and the midwife Carolina, the few women who continue beyond the three-month mark do so until the baby is six or seven months old. A few young mothers reach the one-year mark.

In most cases, the reason for terminating breast-feeding is that the milk has become scarce or has disappeared. Two-thirds of the mothers who responded to questionnaires attributed it to exhaustion of the milk supply, with the remainder divided among weaning, maternal illness or tiredness, resumption of work, nearsightedness, or maternal thinness with consequent effects on milk quality. As a woman who stopped after two months said, "I felt a sense of anguish that I would not have enough milk for the next feeding, and that it would not be very nutritious."

This fear is shared by many women, who find that their milk begins to disappear in the mornings or afternoons or from one breast or the other, which only increases their anxiety. In addition, they may believe that the doppia pesata must be done with the infant completely undressed, which makes it scream all the more when placed on the scale. Larger infants try to roll over or crawl away. As a result, although most women state that they believe babies should be breast-fed for at least six months, and medical texts and personnel agree, their milk rarely lasts that long.

Curiously, women's lack of milk is attributed not to regimented breast-feeding practices but rather to their supposedly insufficient will to breast-feed or to a natural tendency to run out of milk. Carolina believes that 10 percent of mothers are biologically incapable of producing milk. A gynecologist told me that women can breast-feed up to seven or eight months "if they have the milk," seeming to consider it normal that most do not. Mothers and health professionals know that infants usually lose weight in the first week, but do not see anything odd about using the doppia pesata at precisely that time.

Many people and books argue that young women simply do not want to breast-feed or are just waiting for an excuse to stop—such as the milk disappearing after a week or two, or their physician finding them very exhausted and making them stop. A grandmother describes how her daughter-in-law ran out of milk after 1½ months (after which, she points out, the baby immediately fell ill) and had no milk at all for her second and third children. Her physician scolded her: "*voi donne moderne dovete allattare!*" (you modern women must breast-feed!).

The duration of breast-feeding does not seem to be dictated by the required maternity leave of three months, since homemakers also begin to give supplements before then. Very few infants never receive formula, which on average is given beginning at two or three months. Respondents to the questionnaires report that their mothers breast-fed them for about twice as long as they breast-feed their own children, averaging over six or seven months. This is about the same as the average length of time working women remain at home after childbirth, as well as the duration of breast-feeding parents consider ideal.

The reason for the discrepancy between the actual and ideal duration of breast-feeding is the high rate of compliance with the doppia pesata and orario, including the rapid elimination of nighttime feeding. These methods are used by more than three-quarters of mothers. Even when the feeding schedule is not respected exactly, mothers tend to space feedings at intervals of at least three hours and eliminate them at night. "Not following the orari" often means that the parents find that the baby does fine on one fewer feeding so they eliminate it, or perhaps they are flexible during the day but refuse feedings at night. When nighttime feeding is allowed, it is limited to one or at most two feedings. Parents try to quickly work the child down from six to five to four feedings a day, introduce solid foods in the fourth month, and complete weaning at six months. Under these circumstances, it is not surprising that the duration of postpartum amenorrhea is lower than in the past, averaging 2½ to 3¼ months according to the questionnaires.

Popular and Medical Expectations of
Breast-Feeding Mothers

Although some women realize that the doppia pesata and orario make them anxious, they are unable to renounce them. It does not help that, once home from the hospital, mothers are incessantly asked by relatives, friends, and even acquaintances they run into on the street, "*gli dai il tuo latte?*" (are you giving him [the child] your milk?). Everyone wants to know about the quantity of milk produced and the number of feedings the mother gives each day. After visiting a new mother in the hospital, people always talk about how many grams of colostrum she gave the baby at its most recent feeding. This social reinforcement makes it inconceivable to breast-feed without following at least some regimen.

There is a strong belief that it is possible to overfeed an infant on breastmilk, not just formula, and that it is necessary to feed on schedule in order to achieve regular infant growth. This leads many parents to wake their baby for a scheduled feeding. Alternatively, they may make the baby wait for the next feeding, in spite of screams or discomfort, even for hours and during the night. It is not at all uncommon for parents to call or visit the pediatrician if the child does not gain weight for a day or two. The booklets mothers and fathers fill with data often contain not only the weekly and mealtime weights, but also the composition of the paps given to the child.

Together with the food restrictions and the idea that breast-feeding women must take extra care to avoid sweating or taking cold, these beliefs about scheduling and rationing mother's milk lead to the conclusion that bottle-feeding is less complicated and requires less work than breast-feeding—helping to ease the transition when the mother runs out of milk. According to numerous women and the pediatrician Chiara, when this happens early on the mother feels rather guilty, but if she makes it until three or four months she is satisfied. The midwife Carolina says that she was one of those mothers who have little milk at the outset and have to "integrate" right away. Within ten days she had stopped breast-feeding, which she felt was a "liberation" from a "*gran male*" (great ill-being). She says that the mother is sorry because she fears not having as direct a relationship with the infant, but then finds that she can if she always gives the bottle herself.

Bottle-feeding is like breast-feeding in many ways, for parents are expected to keep a scale in their homes and closely observe medical norms for infant feeding and care. One mother named Maura who never breast-fed explains that in the hospital it was determined that she was not producing enough milk, so the child was started on formula. She was not upset by this, for she observed how much trouble the other women in her recovery room were having with breast-feeding. She was extremely conscientious about following the pediatrician's directions regarding formula-feeding and the measurement of weekly weight gain, and has kept the schedules she followed for introducing diluted fresh milk and solid foods.

Maura took her son to the clinic once a week for several months, once a month through the first year, and every other month through the second. At this point, she faltered by not taking him to each of the biannual visits that are expected until the age of six. Interestingly, for the first two years, she and her husband insisted that he sleep in his own room, but for the past three he has slept in their bed. This timing indicates a transition out of a period of close medical surveillance and high compliance with medical norms in the child's early infancy.

Some health professionals complain that patients are overly obsessive about the doppia pesata and orario. At the same time, the latter may believe that physicians (more than midwives) promote the methods for their own convenience. Chiara finds that in cities such as Bologna, physicians are less rigid about the orario than in outlying regions, except, justifiably, in the case of formula-feeding. She tells parents to use the doppia pesata only once a week if the child is growing well. If it seems that they may need to supplement, they should do it for two days and take an average. However, she says that giving this advice is useless, because women are "fixated on the scale" and want to scrutinize milk production at each and every poppata. She describes mothers in towns and cities as being equally "abandoned and insecure."

Yet, Chiara also assumes that every woman has a scale in her house, indicating that she is not prepared to do away with it, either. This is a fair assumption. In an episode of a popular television show in which a police officer and his friend have to take care of an infant, two women waiting in line with them at the pharmacy want to be sure the men have acquired a scale. A scientist from Florence who had lived in the United States for ten years before expecting his first child astonished his American wife by presenting her a digital scale just after the birth.

Carolina confirms that everyone buys or rents a scale. She advises not using the doppia pesata at all, since it "becomes a nightmare," and tells parents to weigh their infants undressed only once a week. She is frustrated by the town's "old way of thinking," and "forms of anxiousness" especially with respect to the first child and finds that mothers cannot accept freedom in the timing of the poppate. They reject her advice not to stand around with a watch ready to make their infants eat according to the schedule they received at the hospital. She finds it senseless and cruel that they get up from their own sleep and wake their child for the 23:30 feeding, but leave it to cry until the next one at 6:00 even if it wakes at 4:30.

While medical textbooks seem to promote baby-led feeding by arguing that it is popular and successful in other countries, they nevertheless continue to stress feeding schedules and the calculation of rations. These methods are taught in medical schools and used in hospitals all over the country. Health professionals give lip service to the benefits of baby-led feeding, but contradict themselves with other recommendations. For example, physicians and midwives invariably advise parents to have their children sleep in a crib, which should be in a separate room, within a few weeks from birth, if not from the very beginning. This reinforces the tendency to reduce and eliminate nighttime feedings, taking away an important stimulus to milk production.

Health experts know that once mothers start supplementing with formula their own milk disappears, but their advice does not counteract this process. One of the pediatrician Chiara's patients was getting only 40 grams of breastmilk at the first feeding, and she predicted that soon the mother would have to stop breast-feeding altogether since she already was unable to produce milk during the rest of the day. She explained that in such a situation her advice is to be sure to attach the infant at each of the usual number of feedings for its age and give the supplement after each feeding rather than alternate between meals of formula and breastmilk. These are considered the best ways to stimulate milk production.

To increase the number of feedings never seems to come to anyone's mind. Chiara confirms that women are never told to go beyond the standard number of feedings. They may be allowed to feed the child a few minutes before or after the scheduled time, but that is the extent of the flexibility they are permitted. This seems inconsistent with the assertion made by many physicians and parents that infants know how to autoregulate themselves, and that women's milk production depends upon nipple stimulation.

Clara, a teacher and the mother of two children born in 1989 and 1992, did triple weighings at every feeding and abolished nighttime feeding after the first few days. Within a month of the second child's birth, she began to have days when she had no milk in one or both breasts and had to give him formula. One day when Clara's infant cried, she explained that he probably had a stomachache from drinking 150 grams of breastmilk and 20 grams of formula earlier that morning. She could not feed him smaller quantities at closer hours, for her pediatrician had told her that she must wait at least three hours after any feeding, no matter how small, because "that is how long it takes to digest the milk." Her mother makes sure that Clara obeys such rules. The day after the four-month-old baby's routine visit to the pediatrician's office, during which Clara was told to start giving him smashed apple and banana, her mother was out in front of the house feeding the baby the correct amount of apple puree.

Stress and Anxiety

A few women who have had frustrating or disappointing experiences with breast-feeding connect the loss of their milk to anxiety and stress, though it is rare for anyone to directly implicate the double weighings and feeding schedule. One woman blames the loss of her milk supply after a couple of weeks upon a stressful pregnancy due to separation from her husband. She does not attribute it to the distress she felt at forcing her baby to sleep in a separate room for the first year in spite of his constant crying. Another mother, who was kept from breast-feeding her first child in the late 1970s because he had meningitis and was sent to another hospital, had milk for only two weeks after her second child was born a decade later. She describes feeling stress at the hospital, given the staff's extreme attention to the quantity of milk mothers produced. Respecting the orario meant that she often had to wake her baby or "resist" and wait for hours when he cried. Although she now believes her mother was right to advise against these practices, she does not think she would have had the courage to resist the pressure—considering that when the ostetrica comes to visit she immediately wants to see the scale, while the pediatrician (and everyone else) continually asks about milk production.

As a mother named Cristina explains, the doppia pesata "gives a sense of despair . . . you are tied to this scale and besides, some days the baby is hungrier than others. . . . Yet the pediatrician gives you a range with a maximum and minimum for each poppata and says that the infant's feeding should stay within that range." The infant "becomes nervous" between meals because of hunger while the mother "becomes nervous" during meals because of having to prepare and heat up the supplement. When she stopped breast-feeding because the milk was all gone at two months, Cristina was relieved. She had given birth in a different hospital from the two most women in Santa Lucia use, where she was exposed to a shorter stay of only four days and new courses on massage, music, and physical contact for newborns. This may have contributed to making her more critical, but her controlled resistance generated mixed feelings. In spite of her awareness of its effects, she had been unable to completely give up the doppia pesata. She allowed her infant son to sleep in his carriage in her room at night, but describes this as a weakness in herself.

Mothers may be haunted by misgivings about their ability to breast-feed properly not only while they are doing so, but also many decades later. A woman from Florence named Serena had a daughter, Anna, in the early 1950s. A few years ago, Anna developed a painful and irritating skin condition, which was diagnosed as an allergic reaction. Her physician suggested that the cause may be the way in which she was breast-fed. For years, Serena has been anguished at this possibility, going over again and again how she was attentive during breast-feeding and did what she was told. She gave Anna toasted barley and sugar dissolved in boiled water before feeding her because her milk was "fatty." After six months, she had to stop because of a worm infection, for which she was treated with abundant dietary garlic and other medicines.

At the same time as the skin condition appeared, Serena's husband's health was deteriorating without any apparent reason, and he lost the use of his legs. In spite of this, Anna, who has lived in an extremely polluted and crowded city all her life, was encouraged to believe that her allergies were the result of an error in breast-feeding in the first months of life. This updated version of the ancient idea that all skin ailments in the nursling are due to defects in the mother's milk seems a cruel misuse of the knowledge that breast-feeding confers some protection against allergies. A mother who was told to breast-feed in a way contradictory to the prolonged, intensive, and exclusive breast-feeding that actually does protect against allergies was now blamed for having breast-fed in an improper manner. In the end, the cause may have been stress related to Anna's father's illness, for her condition improved dramatically several months after his death.

On average, women do not breast-feed for the amount of time they consider ideal or for as long as they would have liked. The elation they describe at reaching the target number of grams during a feeding turns to a feeling of unworthiness or betrayal by the body when the milk disappears. Yet, at the same time, mothers welcome the cessation of breast-feeding as the end of strict medical surveillance and the beginning of greater liberty in parenting. Ironically, there is little if any recognition of the role of regimented methods including the doppia pesata and orario in obstructing women from being able to produce milk.

Politicoeconomic Change, Family Life, and Generational Differences

Changes in the Postwar Economy

Now that we have sketched various infant feeding behaviors, we will try to explain how material and cultural changes have created the conditions that favor regimented methods.

For a decade or more after the war, health and living conditions were even worse than before, for many people's housing and livelihood had been destroyed. In Santa Lucia, six months of bombing demolished more than 200 buildings. Then, the postwar economic boom—stimulated by foreign aid, combined with government policies that promoted industry and industrialized agriculture—rapidly absorbed (or pushed) people out of the countryside. The balance in terms of inputs and revenues was tipped in favor of sharecroppers, sharecropping itself was outlawed (except in the case of families working the same land for generations), and landowners divided their holdings and left the business, even at unfavorable prices.[21] The common refrain of the day became *la terra ai contadini* (land to the farmers).

The construction industry grew enormously thanks to easier access to credit and the need for renovated or new domestic, government, and commercial buildings. Agriculture was and has been sustained by government support and protection, allowing for a relatively high proportion of the population to remain in farm work. Many government services and institutions introduced in the fascist period have grown, along with new ones.

In Santa Lucia, the roads were paved in the 1950s. The roads made it easier for children to attend upper-level schools in nearby towns and cities. They further opened the town to the outside, and commerce and tourism have brought people into it. Young people come and go, but much of the older generation rarely leaves town. This contributes to a palpable difference in beliefs and behaviors, including those related to reproduction and child rearing. The memory of hunger and deprivation has not been lost, contributing to a strong cultural tradition revolving around food which infuses ongoing concerns about infant feeding.

The immediate postwar reaction against fascism was violent and extreme. At the local level, communist administrations often ruled continuously until the middle 1980s or later. National government eventually took the form of the *pentapartito* (five-party) system, made up of coalitions of several parties with their own interests to defend and promote. The parties were unified in rejecting the moral philosophy of fascism, quickly eliminating or modifying many fascist provisions, such as certain demographic laws and regulations. Nevertheless, much fascist legislation and many fascist institutions have remained intact, their influence extended by decades.

One of the most pronounced legacies of fascism has been an enormous increase in state intervention in the private sphere and the domestic economy, even beyond the vision of the fascists themselves. The original meaning of fascist-born social welfare institutions and legislation has been dismissed as the institutions have adapted to new conditions. They are exploited for personal gain, but at the same time they impose their vision and capture the self-reliance and autonomy of individuals. Everybody has been absorbed into the state welfare system, whether they work for the government or not. This has led to expectations of public provision or protection of early pensions, health care, a "thirteenth" month of pay each year, and other services and benefits. The government or private employer is expected to provide for all needs.

While the economic boom has considerably narrowed the gulf between the rich and the poor, it has been a false, borrowed one and seems unsustainable. Critics point out that public assistance has not succeeded in proportion to its high costs and has failed to liberate the population of the fear of old age, ill health, and poverty.[22] Abuses are notorious; there are bus drivers who have been drawing benefits for blindness for years.

Over the past half-century, the state and its medical system have acquired unquestioned, implicit moral leadership in many areas, leaving the Church with little authority or practical influence compared to the past. This is due, at least in part, to widespread dissatisfaction with Church teachings about gender and morality. The traditionalistic model of separate male and female roles shared by fascist and Catholic ideology was carried into the postwar period. New social movements of the 1960s and 1970s demanded greater recognition of women's place in the public sphere and men's in the domestic sphere, and they cast off the overly rigid categories of the Church.

Today, most Italians describe themselves as Catholic, and there are still many active religious schools, parishes, and youth groups. Participation in religious processions, holidays, and rites such as marriage or baptism remains strong. However, church attendance is low, and priests, monks, and nuns are rapidly declining in number. The Church has been largely pushed out of health care, education, job training, and counseling, areas in which it used to have a monopoly.

The prosperity of the postwar period has had direct impacts on parents' ability and inclination to follow scientized norms for breast-feeding. The narrowing of the gap separating people in economic and educational opportunities has increased cultural uniformity and access to the national medical system, itself bolstered by the expansion of the state. The rise in disposable income means that most parents are able to afford the hospital-quality scale (rental fee of about $15 per month) and other paraphernalia for modern infant feeding. The transition from traditional and religious to state-medical moral authority is evident in the rise of standardized, medicalized approaches to reproduction and parenting.

Economic Change, Women's Work, and Family
Structures and Relationships

The socioeconomic changes of the postwar period have brought a more pronounced separation of women's and men's labor. Families have become small and uniformly simple or extended, in contrast to the wide variation in family sizes and structures of the past. Earlier this century, husbands and wives shared economic and domestic responsibilities, different as they may have been. Income and expenditures were pooled and organized on a yearly or longer basis. Women also often brought property and other capital to marriage. This applied not just to sharecropping families, but also artisans and landowners. By contrast, under the industrial economy, the income of family members is discrete and earned on an hourly or salaried basis unrelated to earthly cycles. Expenditures likewise tend to be individualized.

Husbands' labor, which earns more money for the same work, is valued more than wives' labor in terms of bolstering authority within the household. This has occurred in spite of (or perhaps because of) the subtraction of men from domestic responsibilities. Women's work is considered secondary to men's; even if spouses have the same jobs the partnership is not structured economically and socially the same way as in the past. This is also true for agricultural labor, since it usually means working at some distance from home as a laborer. The number of farm families working as an economic unit is very small.

The postwar economic boom allowed large numbers of women to renounce work and dedicate themselves entirely to home and family, for the first time in Italian history. Even in the 1950s, experts were concerned about emotional damage caused by the ever more common bourgeois family, in which the mother did not work and both parents projected "neuroses" on the children.[23] On the other hand, this is the context in which "productive," scientific mothering flourishes. The rapidity of the transition to middle-class homemaking in Italy contributed to wide acceptance of rising standards of bourgeois housekeeping. Husbands and children learned not responsibility or duty in family life, but rather entitlement to the labor and attentions of the wife/mother.

There is a strong, widely held, but erroneous belief in Italy that the fall in the birthrate is due to women's work outside the home and could have been prevented if day care had been expanded in the 1970s. In the past, when it was necessary for almost everyone to work, women were fully employed, if uncounted. Even official statistics show that after Unification there was a progressive decline in the proportion of women in the active population, with the lowest values reached in the 1950s—it fell from 32.4 in 1901 to 24.7 in 1961 (as birthrates plummeted, not the reverse), but rose again to 32.7 in 1981. Besides, the number of active women for every 100 women has generally been lower in Italy (20 to 30) than the former socialist countries (40 to 50) and the highly industrial and postindustrial countries (30 to 40), all of which have higher birthrates.[24]

Whether they have jobs outside the home or not, women spend a considerable amount of time working. One study found that homemakers worked the lowest number of hours per week, at around 52, while working women put in a total of 66 to 79 hours inside and outside the home, depending upon their profession. Meanwhile, compared to other European countries, Italy had the lowest or near-lowest rates of participation of men in domestic and parenting functions.[25] In a contradiction set up during the fascist period, women's primary responsibility for the household sustains the considerable time commitment required by scientific mothering, but may also contribute to women's preference for a small number of children.

Socioeconomic Change, Birth Control,
and Fertility Transition

Postwar changes in sexuality and the meaning of family and children have also impacted upon parenting beliefs and behaviors. There was opposition to the concept of family limitation and to particular methods before the fascist period, but it was then that it was encoded in law. Combined with certain health beliefs, fascist morality and legislation affect the kinds of methods in use to the present day, even if political and religious ideologies have never been able to stop people from controlling births.

Many of the cultural concerns of the fascist period for controlling sexuality and promoting the patriarchal family were carried directly into the postwar period.[26] Even among birth control advocates such as the physician Georg, divorce was equated with antibiological practices such as sexual promiscuity, abortion, and the "abuse" of marriage, meaning the "fraudulent" limitation of offspring. The latter was likened to a disease, said to threaten up to 95 percent of all marriages and to corrode the nation's vital forces. Georg maintained that it was not the wealthy class, which had never amounted to more than 2 to 5 percent of society, that was to blame for the delay of procreation and the fall in natality rates. Instead, declining birthrates were the result of the ever more complex division of labor, the disappearance of the family as an economic unit, the complete dependence of workers, especially office workers (*dipendenti*), on their insufficient earnings, and the economic necessity of women's work (1950:7, 54–57).

Together with conservatives and the Church, proponents of family planning argued for measures that would allow married women to renounce work so that they might have more children. Unlike the former, the latter promoted birth control, so long as this meant the method of periodic continence known to the present day as Ogino-Knaus. These two scientists had demonstrated that the fertile period falls in the middle of the cycle, rather than the days before and after the menstrual period, as had been widely believed (Georg 1950:69–70). Family planning advocates explained that this method allowed women to space births one to two years apart and continue to benefit from spermatic impregnation, which was impossible with mechanical methods or withdrawal. Unlike prolonged breast-feeding, the method was effective and harmless.[27] But, in spite of all this, it had been suppressed for 20 years and was still resisted by many physicians.

The Catholic Church granted papal approval of the Ogino-Knaus method in the early 1950s. While some fascist moral legislation is still in effect today—continuing to impede publication of information about birth control methods in the popular press—parliament began to abrogate some provisions at this time. These included the penal code article that had punished anyone who publicly advocated the limitation of births, making the public sale of birth control methods very difficult. In 1978, the laws against induced abortion were overturned, making it legal within 90 days of conception and permissible thereafter under certain conditions. Sterilization, on the other hand, has not been unambiguously legalized. A law in 1982 abrogated the 1931 law against it, but without eliminating two other laws. One makes it illegal to dispose of one's own body (as in suicide), and the other prohibits the causing of grave bodily lesions. This gives a maximum punishment for patient and physician (12 years) that is six times higher than under the fascist sterilization law. It is little wonder that the operations are usually done in secrecy, and many people believe that sterilization is still illegal.[28]

As recently as 1979, a survey found that withdrawal was the preferred method of half of all women, followed by the pill, condom, and periodic abstinence, with the diaphragm and IUD in distant last place. Sterilization was not common enough to warrant a category of its own.[29] In my 1991–92 questionnaires, many parents responded that they did not use birth control at all, just after answering that they planned to have no more children. I soon learned that withdrawal, periodic abstinence, and natural family planning are not considered birth control methods like mechanical or chemical ones. Sterilization is unheard of, except after repeat caesarean sections. For men, it is unthinkable—the equivalent of castration.

The ostetrica Carolina, who is dismayed at the cultural resistance to the condom in Italy, explains that people over 40 or 45 generally use coito interrotto, or to a much lesser extent the IUD, whereas women between their teens and thirties almost unfailingly use the pill. This trend toward more intrusive methods may have to do with changing ideas about the body and increasing openness to medical intervention. In the 1960s, the midwife Marina found that some of her patients had endured painful infections or tumors for years without discussing them with anyone, not even their husbands. Even today, taboos against talking about sex may contribute to the popularity of the pill as opposed to other methods.

Many people interpret the culture change toward fewer births in terms of a shift from their parents and grandparents having many children out of ignorance, to their own not having children out of egoism. Women's supposed unwillingness to make maternal sacrifices is denounced in the popular press and faulted for the decline of the Italian population in the face of immigration from Africa and Albania.[30] Many people believe that women's work is to blame, but it is also said, in the words of a young mother with one child, that irrespective of work or career women "want to be able to go out and do whatever they want." Young people consider having many children at random a thing of the past, which is tightly connected with ignorance and la miseria. To consciously plan to have few children and care for them in the most modern way has become a widely shared cultural value, in which birth control and medical intervention are implicitly accepted.

Demographic Change and the Presence of the Past

Compared to early this century, most parents are now alive when their children marry and have families of their own. Life has changed dramatically, and this can bring conflicts in the ways in which the generations approach child rearing. Over the past five or six decades, there has been a rapid rise in literacy, school attendance, and educational levels. Compared to children today, the older generations had little choice about residence or profession, which depended strongly upon parental approval. Women were often denied education or work opportunities because they were needed to take care of a widowed father or other relative, or his children.

On the other hand, there are many continuities with the past. Children live with their parents until they marry, usually by choice rather than the lack of housing. As long as their mother is alive, they return to her table for lunch on Sunday, if not every day—a tradition that runs throughout society to the most senior politicians in Rome. Farm and Church traditions are maintained through an annual cycle of celebrations and processions. Meal preparation is rather strictly dictated by geographical region, season, and holiday. Children are raised to an awareness of agriculture and history through their books, songs, and school activities, including making wine in nursery school. Most children, whether in small towns or larger cities, see their grandparents every day or at least every week.

Nevertheless, there is a wide gulf in mentality and worldview between the young and old. The difference is widely considered to be marked by the Second World War. I learned from a class of city teenagers that they believed that postwar Italy was like the image of 1950s America in the television serial *Happy Days*. In reality, their parents and grandparents were living in bombed-out hovels as they slowly rebuilt their houses; millions of children were forced to leave school to work or beg, and were constantly hungry and undernourished, especially in the Po Valley.[31] People in their forties or older are more aware of this and remember eating donated food from America after the war. In my questionnaires, almost everyone agreed that their lives were better than those of their parents because the latter had lived through miseria and war. They were divided about the future, however, expressing concern about moral crisis and environmental degradation that could make their own children's lives worse.

Young people reject the older generations' willingness to give in to resignation, hypocrisy, or unhappiness.[32] They are much less burdened by the weight of the dead or the eyes of the living that are so well-known to small communities in southern Europe, where nothing goes unobserved, even during the ghostly hours at lunchtime. This force can feel so great to older people that they literally never leave their apartments, for years on end.

Older people witnessed death much more immediately and frequently, especially during the war. They are likely to dress in mourning for a longer period than younger people, and to visit the cemetery much more often. Older people frequently talk about resignation and God's will with respect to illness and old age. They calmly discuss their own death and prepare their place in the family tomb. Every time I leave Santa Lucia, several people tell me that they will no longer be alive when I return.

Older people seem frustrated by young people's unwillingness to work hard and sacrifice. Economic prosperity has brought unrealistic expectations, and there are few jobs in general but even fewer jobs that seem desirable or acceptable to the young. Many young people continue going to college for ten years or more, while others wait for a permanent government position, with its many benefits. The dangerous, hard labor their older relatives did would be absolutely inconceivable to them.

Material conditions have changed dramatically. Women as young as their middle forties embroidered their own linens in preparation for marriage. They remember the tradition of planting a cherry tree when a child was born so that there would be wood for the bedroom furniture when the child married. It was not long ago that electricity, running water, and paved roads reached throughout the country, but young people take these conveniences for granted as they speed past their bicycle-riding elders in expensive motorcycles and cars.

The older generations were raised to accept inequalities as immutable, natural, or God-given, as Silone's second novel illustrates with a scene in which fascist guards shoot at socialist *braccianti* demanding expropriation of the land. The protagonist, disguised as a priest, hears a landowner say that, in spite of their poverty, the *braccianti* are better off than he. "Flesh used to suffering, does not feel pain" (1955 [1936]:118). The false priest asks a pious young woman if things could not change to eliminate poverty and misery. She responds that the Church's official teaching says otherwise: "The social inequalities themselves were also created by God and we must humbly respect them" (120).

When asked about social class differences in Santa Lucia today, two young college-educated sisters answered that they were minimal or nonexistent. Their parents remained silent. After a long pause, all four then named the families that used to form the aristocracy or produced illustrious personages, noting that one family still has titles. This episode reflects young people's blindness to or rejection of the fixed social categories and inequalities which older generations fatalistically accepted or upheld. Similarly, younger people consider life and death to be controlled by human agency rather than fate or divine will, a difference that affects their perceptions of parenthood.

As recently as the 1950s, Monsignor Prosperini wrote about the midwife's duty to give extreme unction to the woman dying in childbirth and to suggest to her sentiments of the *"perfect pain* of her sins"—that is, "resignation to the will of God and childlike abandonment to his mercy" (1954:184). This is quite a different attitude from that found today, when death in childbirth is extremely rare, priests are no longer found on the faculty of medical schools, and medical assistance is expected to overcome all possible complications. Parenthood has come to be seen as an active choice mediated by technological interventions. Any residual infant mortality including stillbirth is thought to be the result of deficiencies in medical treatment, except in the case of untreatable congenital disorders and diseases.[33] The care of children is considered effective and informed, though possibly excessive now that there are relatively few of them.

A teacher and mother of two school-age children describes the current approach to procreation and child rearing as *uno scontro* (a clash) between tradition and modernity, between holding on to past ways of life and reaching out for the latest trends. While women embrace medicalized childbirth, they still pray to saints for help. When it was proposed that the painting of the Madonna of Childbirth by Piero della Francesca be taken on tour, local women staged a sit-in. During breast-feeding, women uphold traditional beliefs about the harmful effects of certain foods on the milk, but at the same time they subscribe to modern notions about the timing and measurement of meals. A baby's ill-humor or inflamed skin may be blamed upon the mother's having eaten wild rabbit, which fits with the folk belief that attributes harelip in the infant to the mother's having eaten a hare during pregnancy. At the same time, the doppia pesata is esteemed because it is thought to be a postwar import from the United States.[34] The cultural memory is selective: America symbolizes technology and futurism, while the fascist period is better forgotten.

Now that it seems possible to avoid the disorders and diseases of the past, young parents seem to want to leave the world of their own parents and grandparents behind with respect to their own children. They associate the large families and high infant mortality rates of past times with la miseria and reject many of the child-rearing practices of the older generations. They invariably use single-use diapers: together with medical experts, they consider cloth diapers an anachronism, a symbol of backwardness, and "unhygienic" besides—even though some women made their own as recently as 25 years ago.

An article in a periodical distributed at pharmacies entitled "Grandmother is wrong when she says . . ." explains how two traditional treatments do nothing but comfort the patient, seconding the tendency to belittle older people's knowledge.[35] For their part, many older people speak disparagingly of young people's laxness toward their children, wishing they would use greater discipline. They often speak of fathers' distant relationship with their children with admiration, though this is sometimes tinged with regret given that they approve of young fathers' greater involvement. Older women who worked and kept the house and raised the children, saying, "*era una lotta*" (it was a struggle), seem both envious and disdainful of younger women's seemingly lesser burden. Some young parents would like to be more severe with their children but find that social pressure against it is too strong. Yet, discipline is still applied to children, if in opposite ways, for even if they are permissive with respect to behavior, parents today are strict about infant feeding.

To older people, today's parents have gained in some ways, but lost their ability to respond to their children spontaneously and with confidence. In other words, resignation and fatalism have been replaced by planning and a high level of parental engagement in reproduction and child rearing, but family authority and autonomy have given way to a need for expert advice and intervention.

Protecting Maternity and Infancy

Maternity and Work

Another area of historical continuity and change is the legislation "protecting" working women. The expansion and updating of the legislation in 1971 has left intact the principle that mandatory maternity leave is "a right but also an obligation."[36] Women's jobs are protected from the beginning of pregnancy until the child's first birthday. Mothers are prohibited from working for the last two months of pregnancy and the first three months after childbirth, for which they are compensated at 80 percent of their salary (paid through the government insurance system). This leave can be increased during pregnancy if the work presents health risks for mother or child. In theory, additional leave involves one or two periods of rest. In practice, women purposely obtain a medical certificate as early as the first month of pregnancy in order to stay home the entire time, even if their work is not hazardous and there is no real medical risk for the mother or fetus.

After the obligatory leave, the mother may take a "facultative abstention from work" at 30 percent of salary for a period which should not exceed six additional months within the first year, but quite often does—indeed, many people believe that the obligatory leave lasts six months. Leave may last up to three years if the child is ill. Upon returning to work, the mother is entitled to two fully paid half-hour daily rest periods if there is a day-care center or nursing room on site, or one-hour breaks if not. These can be combined to allow her to arrive two hours late, and as a result the nursing breaks have been transformed into a "reduced schedule."

Similar provisions to those in the past prohibit women from moving or lifting weights or doing dangerous, tiring, or health-threatening tasks from the beginning of pregnancy to the seventh month after childbirth. Instead, the woman must be transferred to other tasks without any loss of income (but with a gain if to a higher-paying job) or granted an extension of normal leave if all of the work is harmful, as in a paint factory. The categories of work forbidden to pregnant and nursing women are very similar to those outlined in previous legislation. They include jobs forbidden to children and adolescents, such as night work; jobs that expose workers to asbestos and silica, ionizing radiation, or causes of other occupational diseases; and those that require standing on stairs or scaffolding, making strong physical efforts, standing for more than half of the workday, or maintaining a tiring position.

In addition, the law prohibits pregnant women from using machines that shake or transmit intense vibrations, or are moved or operated by pedals if the movement is frequent or laborious. They are forbidden from agricultural labor involving the use of toxic or harmful substances in the care of crops or animals, and they may not work in the winnowing and transplantation of rice. They may not work with patients in wards for infectious or nervous and mental diseases, or aboard boats, airplanes, trains, trucks, and every other means of transportation.

The workers who benefit most from the legislation are those who work for state, parastate, and other public administrations, as well as businesses that are highly integrated with the state such as banks. By contrast, independent professionals, domestics, and autonomous workers, such as artisans, farmers, and shopkeepers, do not have the same rights (or obligations) and enjoy only some of the benefits or none at all.

The benefits to individuals have a social cost, in the widely recognized reluctance of firms and individual employers to hire women. Even though employers do not pay directly for leave, there are losses in time and money associated with the worker's absence during leave or a child's illness. Some people fear that abuses will lead to elimination of the provisions, to the harm of those who really need them.

When first introduced in the late nineteenth century and enlarged in the fascist period, legislation for women workers was sorely needed, for they worked in the most dangerous industries for long hours and insufficient pay. Infant mortality rates were high, and the fascist government resolved to reduce them by enabling mothers to breast-feed during a critical period in the child's early life. Today, few women breast-feed exclusively even for as long as they are required to stay at home, and many (particularly white-collar workers) work in jobs that could safely be continued throughout pregnancy. Most notably, the daily rest periods are not used for breast-feeding and are not known to have anything to do with it. Rather than responding to a real need to "protect" women, the legislation reinforces cultural concepts about the delicateness of maternity and acts as a disincentive to their employment.

ONMI in the Postwar Period

ONMI was one of many fascist institutions that survived the transition to the postwar republic. It continued to function for another three decades, under the same premise upon which it had been founded: the basis of civilized society is the moral and physical health of infants and mothers, and to safeguard its integrity is an essential objective of the state. Postwar writers continued to emphasize that the laws instituting ONMI and regulating women's work had the fundamental scope of "reorganizing the domestic hearth" and protecting the institution of the family, beyond meeting the essential necessities of life.[37] The emphasis of the organization remained the creation of healthy children for the good of the nation, not the improvement of conditions for women in their own right.[38]

However, there was a large gulf between these moral-spiritual goals and what ONMI could expect to accomplish in the immediate postwar period, given the population's great material needs and the organization's lack of resources. ONMI's budget in 1951 and 1952 was only 6 billion lire, less than half of what was needed.[39] Half of the money went in equal parts to Rome, Milan, and the central administration, leaving 3 billion lire for the rest of the country. Overall, the funds for institutions serving infants were stagnant or declining, which contemporaries attributed to a lack of political or social will and an insensitivity to the poor state of infancy.[40]

Meanwhile, employers calmly disobeyed the laws regarding maternity insurance and breast-feeding, in part because there were no provisions for noncompliance. The interenterprise asili did not exist even where the law required them, and employers made no attempt to respond to the needs of their employees. This was seen as damaging not because the laws failed to protect working women, but because they harmed the family in its role as the "natural social group in which the infant should find full assistance."[41]

A paradigm shift was taking place in the institutional care of infancy in the 1950s. The spotlight fell no longer upon breast-feeding, but immunization, prevention of contagion, reporting, and educational and psychological issues. The fall in infant mortality rates was now applauded as the outcome of a half-century of medical intervention in the fields of immunological therapy, chemotherapy, and antibiotic treatment.[42] References to

diet and life-style dwindled. In dozens of presentations at the First
National Conference for the Defense of Infancy in 1952, there was almost
no direct discussion of breast-feeding, except to say that passive immunity
protects infants against certain diseases for the first three or four months.[43]
ONMI clinics were criticized for functioning inadequately and limiting
themselves to the distribution of milk.[44]

New regulations for ONMI health professionals no longer highlighted maternal breast-feeding or the knowledge of infant feeding practices and puericultura once considered fundamental. Instead, training
focused upon clinical medicine and laboratory science, hygiene and infection, demographic and health statistics, pedagogy, and public assistance
and social and health legislation. Only the lower-level personnel were
expected to master notions of puericultura. The primary authority of specialist physicians over "auxiliary personnel" (midwife, nurse, social
worker, or assistente sanitaria visitatrice) was formally acknowledged.
This applied to ONMI clinics of all kinds (pediatric, obstetric-gynecologic,
prematrimonial and matrimonial, "social dermatology" [sexually transmitted disease], and "medical-psycho-pedagogic"), even though, in reality,
they often were staffed only by "auxiliary" personnel. ONMI's biomedical
emphasis was also reflected in norms specifying that women and children
must be seen in the clinics, rather than their homes.[45]

"Moral" intervention was abandoned or became less necessary
thanks to a broad culture change that left few infants or unwed mothers in
a state of extreme poverty and abandonment. As in the past, ONMI
defined the day-care centers and preschools that replaced the foundling
hospitals as locations for providing health services and recording data, as
well as educating parents in the hygienic-sanitary and civil-social fields.
Now, the children must be immunized, in addition to the old requirement
of being children of working mothers or families "gravely obstructed from
attending to their care." The schools would be visited periodically and
inspected every six months by the Provincial Health Director, who promoted "the adoption of always more modern methods of sanitary and
social assistance."[46] In practice, however, texts for day-care and preschool
teachers were often simply reprints of fascist-era writings. Even now, a lay
teacher says that her church-run preschool still uses course materials from
the 1920s.[47]

Until a generation ago, private organizations and the state ran most
day-care centers and preschools: in Santa Lucia, for example, the only
preschool was run by nuns until the communal school was opened in the
middle 1970s. Today, the communal and state schools are almost equal in
number, while the private (generally religious) schools are declining in
number and enrollments.[48] Emilia-Romagna and other central and northern regions are still favored with a disproportionate number of day-care

centers, preschools, and camps and summer programs. Emilia-Romagna has 104.3 places in preschool for every 100 children served, against a national average of 89.7. Emilia-Romagna and Lombardy together have more than one-third of the day-care centers and one-half of the camps and summer programs in the country.[49]

While the predominance of children's programs in Emilia-Romagna and nearby regions is now interpreted as the result of strong interest on the part of "local democratic administrations,"[50] we have seen that it is also an outgrowth of a century-old distribution of institutions for infancy that was accentuated during the fascist period. Such historical continuities have allowed ideas and attitudes rooted in the past to remain in full, if unacknowledged, force. For example, the maternity and work legislation in place today, together with the day-care system, continues to uphold the assumptions that women's work is the reason children need child care and that children must be protected through surveillance and control of their mothers' behavior. The progressive specialization and professionalization of medicine, and the development of the national health service, contribute to the diffusion of biomedical approaches in the care of maternity and infancy. Frequent, close contact between the population and the national biomedical culture reinforces conformity between medical and popular knowledge and practice.

As we will see, these historical processes, set within today's social and cultural context, have generated a crisis of confidence in the body and its management.

CHAPTER 9

A Crisis of Confidence
Modern Conflicts

Fascist-era norms of scientific mothering that initially could not take hold in the face of practical considerations related to women's work and the care of many children are now observed scrupulously. As their origins have been forgotten, parenting norms from the fascist period have become fixed in popular belief and practice.[1] There may be resistance to them, or variation in their application, but the norms have an enduring existence unaffected by individual interpretation. They have coercive power over people and are accepted implicitly and thought of uncritically.

The norms concern a biological function which, until very recently, belonged to a bounded private and family world. Breast-feeding has been brought into the public domain, where cultural concepts are enforced through social control. Mothers are monitored in their behavior by relatives, friends, acquaintances, and even strangers. This helps to maintain conformity with expert norms and beliefs, and it contributes to the maintenance of commonsense ideas about the nature of the world. Indeed, the need to time and meter feedings has become an unquestioned, natural, commonsense idea. However, unlike most commonsense knowledge, it is methodical and adherent to erudite knowledge, for the accessible has become the scientific and expert.[2]

While infant feeding itself is strictly confined to the home, its abstract manifestations—time schedules and milk rations—become the material of a public performance in which the mother demonstrates conformity with shared beliefs. Biopsychical processes are a powerful vehicle for mediating between the individual and society, shaping consciousness, and imparting cultural knowledge about time, gender, nature, and the authority of experts.[3] Further, the breast-feeding relationship is a liminal one—a pause between the social and biological identity of gestation and the independence of weaning—further lending itself to cultural elaboration. Through the ritual performance, the individual experiences a special consciousness that absorbs social and moral principles through biology and the emotions. The mother comes to find no conflict between herself and society, accepting scientific breast-feeding as an incontestable and suitable interpretation of the necessities of life.

Standardized, ritualized breast-feeding practices have emerged in the context of a generalized disenchantment with religious myths and rituals in favor of those of science and medicine. However, medical myths and rituals, and the experts who are their custodians, also draw their power from the mystery of life and death, and the mix of the corporeal and spiritual. Beneath the positivism and agency of current cultural and medical approaches to infancy, breast-feeding is still believed to profoundly influence infant survival, psychological development, and lifelong health.

Breast-feeding is a symbol, but unlike one with a fixed meaning, it has multiple and often conflicting meanings, giving it greater power to capture the imagination.[4] Mothers are both helpless, passive victims of internal and external forces and deliberate agents capable of harming their nurslings through improper or imprudent behaviors. The contradictory associations in Catholic tradition between maternity and chastity, sanctity and sexuality, converge upon the breast and breast-feeding. Fascist ideology presented the breast-feeding mother as a central symbol of the nation-state, but it confounded traditional loyalties to nature and family with a modern, unintentionally antiprocreative outlook.

These contradictions continue to affect attitudes about breast-feeding. The broader cultural opposition between reproduction and sexuality makes breast-feeding seem incompatible with sexual attractiveness and involvement—yet, at the same time, breast-feeding is eroticized. Meanwhile, the opposition between nature and culture, which all societies elaborate upon in some way or another, justifies an interventionistic approach to the body that interferes with the "nature" of breast-feeding and makes it difficult in biological terms. The body is alienated, as autonomy and self-sufficiency in its management are lost. Breast-feeding and parenting in general are highly intellectualized, and parents rely heavily upon experts and established ways of thinking and behaving. This creates a paradox. Since there is so much medical and social pressure to breast-feed, it is difficult to abandon it without regret or a sense of failure. Yet, by following medical norms mothers are forced to stop breast-feeding because their milk almost inevitably becomes scarce.

Sexuality, Procreation, and Parenthood

Sexuality and Sexism

As we have seen, today's social system is based on bounded simple families, in contrast to the wider families of traditional society. It tends to emphasize the conjugal sexual relationship, while minimizing the importance of offspring as workers, determinants of the parents' position in the larger family and community, and protectors of the couple's future well-being. Sexual images of women have proliferated in step with this change in social organization, especially since the Second World War. Nevertheless, although maternity is a much less frequent state for women, they continue to be defined by it.

This dual image leads to many contradictions. The popular book by Miraglia, Orlandini, and Micheletti tells readers that while in men the changes of puberty "are not remarkable," in women they are "much more important and striking." From the appearance of the breasts and menstrual periods through menopause, sexual and reproductive events constitute "so many crises imposed by nature which put into question the woman's body, her integrity, her identity" (1984:381). That is, maternal functions both define and subvert women's personhood.

The cultural preference for male offspring does little to validate a woman's identity during that phase, pregnancy, which is considered its very essence. Most advice books, under the pretense of preventing sex-linked diseases, provide instructions for "programming" the child's sex through dietary means, or by using a centrifuge to separate sperm. After birth, cultural biases affect the treatment of girls and boys. Some people say that girls should not learn to walk early because they will have more caesarean sections. Games, toys, and activities differ by sex, with the expected division between dolls and cars, or housework and sports.

As they grow up, girls are expected to clean up after their brothers and take on household tasks and errands that boys never deign to perform. A teenage girl said that her college-student brother does not even carry his laundry to the basket in the bathroom; he complains to his mother whenever his clothes are not cleaned and pressed. As several mothers of adolescent and young adult men have told me, grown children make for more work than little ones. One working mother spends an hour and a half each day ironing for her husband and three sons.

Girls are constrained to a much greater degree by discipline and punishment, and must quickly learn to compromise and be independent and mature. Boys' mischief and disrespectful or violent behavior are rewarded by implicit, if not overt, approval and admiration. Boys are encouraged to remain impulsive, self-centered, and dependent upon but prepotent with respect to their sisters, mothers, and wives for their entire lives. In short, females are assistants, males are actors. A television and print advertisement for mineral water accompanies the images of a pregnant woman with the word *protect,* a child with the word *grow,* and an older man with the word *live.*

Because they are destined to serve others, women are expected to fulfill their duty to improve themselves for the betterment or enjoyment of others. This problem becomes acute during pregnancy and breast-feeding, when, according to advice books, a conflict arises between the child and husband. Pregnant and puerperal women are told: "You will have to consecrate more time to your body, out of respect for your husband and for yourselves."[5] This means not only remaining thin, attractive, and available, but minimizing the offensiveness of increased sweating and genital secretions through extra devotion to personal cleanliness.

Women are advised to gain only 8 to 10 (or possibly 12) kilograms during pregnancy and keep their figures with a girdle for the abdomen and thighs, even if in theory it would be better not to. The weight should be gone within two months after childbirth, the physician consulted if it is not lost after the third month. Mothers are expected to bring a girdle to the hospital to wear after childbirth, to make themselves feel more secure, at ease, and agile. To make the most of their hospital stay they should think of themselves, which means "make yourselves pretty."[6] This is presented as an improvement on the past, when mothers had to resign themselves to a body ruined by maternity; now, they may calmly walk the beach in a bikini without embarrassing themselves when compared to young women.[7]

The scope of breast preparation during pregnancy and lactation is not just to make breast-feeding successful, but to avoid "antiaesthetical stretchmarks." This involves daily washing, massage, pinching and twisting of the nipple, and application of oils and creams. The message is that the breasts must be kept attractive, clean, and useful, while women must compete with one another as objects of sexual attention, even after they have become mothers.

During breast-feeding, the usefulness and attractiveness of the breasts come into conflict, and the child loses. Women must not forget their "duty of woman, of wife." Even a husband in love with his wife's body can become jealous of the "little intruder" attached to its breast. "The fact of breast-feeding for long weeks can upset conjugal relations, isolating the mother in her maternity."[8] The mother is told that she has no right to permit this, even if she mistakenly fears that she cannot have sex because the milk will go bad—just as she feared it would harm the unborn child during pregnancy. Instead, she should follow her physician's instructions regarding conjugal relations. This implies that the husband's right to sex is more valid than the wife's fear of it, and that the physician is best able to determine the length of time for which a woman should or may avoid it. Together with the idea that women remain overweight during breast-feeding, these attitudes contribute to the widespread renunciation of breast-feeding after a few days or "long weeks."

The primacy of the conjugal relationship is also reflected in the rising tendency to keep the child in its own crib and room. In the early 1950s, few people had any extra room, and 90 percent of families had their babies sleep in the parents' bed.[9] By the 1970s, couples who did not have the space would put their children in the kitchen or hallway. Today, no infant is permitted to sleep in the bed with its parents, although some are allowed to sleep in their strollers in the room for the first few weeks. Parents express fear of future problems getting the child to sleep in its own bed, but there is the underlying commonsense belief that the child should be left "alone and tranquil during the night, far from the affective and sexual life of the parents."[10] By the sixth week, the baby must be placed in another room, the door closed (or partitioned off from the parents if there is no other room).

On the other hand, the baby should not be isolated from the life of the couple and family during the day. "Look how the African children, whom the mother carries around on her back, are happy."[11] This is a very misleading comparison, since parents move their babies about and avoid putting them down anywhere else by keeping them in a stroller, not against their bodies. There, they are protected from sunlight, temperature, drafts, and physical or mental stimulation and pushed into a corner where they will be least disturbed. Their access to the breast is minimized by the feeding schedule and compensated with a pacifier. If infants are carried in a "marsupial," they are inserted face-forward even if too young to have head control, rather than on their stomachs close against the parent's body.

An early-1990s television advertisement for a device that claims to improve the shape of the breasts highlights the opposition between their maternal and sexual meanings. The *seno sano e bello* (healthy and beautiful breast) machine is said to be designed for breasts that have been damaged by breast-feeding or rapid weight loss. An electric current from a battery-operated power source athletically "trains" the pectoral muscles by making them contract and relax. This is accomplished—and demonstrated on a topless model—by placing a cup with a hole for the nipple on the breast five times a day. The price of 199,000 lire (then about $165) is said to be equivalent to one or two sittings at a beauty institute and to include a gift of a thin silicone-filled square for use in breast self-examination. Couples are then shown rejoicing in how much better the woman's breasts look and how happy the man is with them. The juxtaposition of a product for detecting breast cancer against one designed to improve the appearance drives home the message that the breasts must be cared for primarily in the interest of sexuality.

The virgin-whore fantasy pervading visual culture in the form of numberless semidressed young women shares the breasts as a central symbol with both cultural concepts of maternity and religious imagery regarding motherhood and virtue. The naked upper body with a baby attached to the breast is a frequent media image of maternity: as in pornography, it is often headless.[12] After Vatican II, the prayers of the rosary were changed to describe Jesus as the fruit of Mary's breast (*seno*) rather than abdomen or womb (*ventre*). Religious tradition compares the Church to a mother, the people to her neonate, with breast-feeding the metaphor for their mutual attraction.[13] We have already mentioned Saint Agata, whose breasts were severed under the orders of the angry official she rebuffed, and there are numerous stories of saints producing milk as virgins or having mystical experiences of breast-feeding the baby Jesus.

The message that woman exists for others and is not an agent in her own right is evidenced and reinforced in innumerable ways. Women's capabilities and aspirations are often unrecognized or ridiculed, while many highly visible women use sex as their main appeal, including actresses, singers, and politicians who have posed in lingerie for preelection publicity photographs. In an atmosphere that discourages women's ambition with respect to education, career, or athletics and disregards their achievements, it is difficult for women to feel that they have control over their lives or that they do anything worthwhile. This is especially true for homemakers, some of whom say that they just take their children to school and do "nothing." Thus, the things they do for others are also undervalued, even by women themselves.

Modern advice books warn women against becoming self-absorbed in maternity and turning into a "*mamma terribile*" who talks of nothing but herself and her children.[14] That is, they must accept their sacrifice and the effect it has upon their bodies, personalities, and activities, but not rejoice in it too much or they will annoy others and harm their children. As women have increasingly shouldered the domestic burden, but lost economic responsibility and authority within the family, scientific mothering has become a way to express industriousness, expertise, and productivity.

Parenthood and Responsibility

Fatherhood has changed along with motherhood over the past few generations. Until the middle of this century, fathers were present when their children were born in the home. Especially among farm families, they saw their children throughout the day and spent their evenings with them, sleeping in the same bed or room at night, although their relationships tended to be more formal. Today, parents and children spend much less time physically near each other, but may share greater emotional closeness.

As childbirth was hospitalized after the Second World War, fathers were excluded from the scene of birth. Over the past two decades, they have been invited back in response to a trend throughout Western societies. However, the practice has not been not fully accepted by men or women, and is motivated above all by an abstract recognition of the utility of having a trusted person in the delivery room. Consequently, if a father or partner is unprepared, he may be criticized by the mother, midwife, or physician for not helping, or even making childbirth harder. Childbirth has been so medicalized and decontextualized that it is seen as an individual performance aimed at best allowing the child to be brought to the light, rather than a family event at which the father may be present by his own right or interest.

Meanwhile, child rearing has been centralized in the person of the mother. Even women who work outside the home are responsible for housework and child care, almost to the complete exclusion of men. Many wives say they have trouble allowing their husbands to take a greater part in running the household, and social pressures tend to reinforce their reluctance to do so. Advice books and real-life situations tend to demarcate a limited domain for male participation in pregnancy, childbirth, and parenting, but blame this "error" on women. That men are pictured as amusingly incompetent in domestic matters is certainly no incentive to their assuming greater responsibility.

In the early months after a child is born, the new father is not expected to do anything at all, except perhaps to hold the occasional bottle. Mothers are told that the moment to involve the father is when it is time to take the baby out of the crib in the second month, for he is more an "important source of stimulation" than someone charged with less cerebral quotidian affairs.[15] Discussions of the father's role are often illustrated with an image of a man feeding a baby, contradicting the expert advice that mothers need not worry about the lost psychological benefits of breast-feeding as long as they always bottle-feed the infant themselves. While this enticement often justifies the decision to use bottle-feeding, many mothers find that their husbands do not end up feeding the baby after all.

One of the more pernicious assumptions about parenting stems from the fact that it is the mother who stays home from work for at least three months after childbirth (though in theory the father could do so in her place). During this time, she is expected to dedicate herself to the newborn and can scarcely expect assistance or relief. Once this pattern has been established, things change very little when she returns to work, and her work is what is thought to create the need for child care. It is she who must be available when the child is ill. This implies both that the mother's work outside the home is a choice that might as easily be renounced and that the father's work may not be interrupted for family obligations. Advice books address the "problem of the maternal substitute" by suggesting only female relatives or babysitters if parents prefer not to use a day-care center.

Moreover, the daily separation for work is presented as an event fraught with difficulty and suffering for both child and mother. There is no mention of paternal regret or guilt, and the cultural value of keeping the child home for a given ideal period of time (3 years in Santa Lucia, 12 to 18 months according to experts) plainly does not envision paternal care—though in practice grandfathers are often very active in taking care of small children. When the mother does not conform to this ideal, most parents and experts prefer to leave children with grandparents rather than a babysitter or day-care center. Very few people believe that children should be raised by several caretakers, as in the past when they grew up in "widened" families with many adults and older children, rather than a sole mother.[16]

The assumption that mothers, not fathers, are responsible for raising the young incorporates the belief that men must not be contaminated by association with the female role. In a rather extreme interpretation, Miraglia, Orlandini, and Micheletti explain that the secure, "active" father provides stability for the family through the exercise of his intellect and acts as guide and mediator between the primary mother-child unit and the sociocultural context. If this is lacking, the child will become fragile and insecure, and conjugal relations will be weakened. If the father identifies too closely with the "passive" female role in pregnancy, labor, and childbirth, they write, he creates a scene of "uncontrolled emotivity, regression, need for protection: all synonyms with femininity." He becomes nothing but an ugly mirror of the mother, to the detriment of his role in the upbringing of the child and the life of the couple (1984:335).

Ferrari and Bonelli proudly recall childbirth scenes from old films in which the physician comes out and asks the father, "do we save the mother or the child?" as (true) stories of another epoch, left behind thanks to modern medicine's ability to save both (1989:143). Images like these embody the conceit that women have their destinies and very lives decided through a consultation between men. While men are allowed to make high-level decisions, they are not permitted or expected to dirty their hands, as it were, in the low details of childbirth, child rearing, or housekeeping.

There are exceptions to the rule that women perform the domestic labor. For example, the presence of fathers in some aspects of child care, such as taking children to and from day care or school, is quite apparent. Couples vary among themselves and over time in their activities and relationships, and they are influenced in their perceptions of marriage and child rearing to different degrees by history and family. Nonetheless, it is difficult to escape the cultural contradictions that bind women to breast-feeding, but encourage them to abandon it.

Breast-Feeding and the Nature of the Body

Alienation of the Body

We have already discussed several ideas and practices illustrating the alienation of the body. For example, the knowledge that infant sucking stimulates milk production has been set aside to ensure that both mother and child behave in a controlled, regular manner. When milk production seems low, increasing the frequency of contact is not an option, and women instead hope for a pharmaceutical solution. Baby-led feeding is unthinkable because it would lead to feedings outside the home, away from the scale. This is a matter not of modesty—since women calmly expose their entire breasts to all present in their own homes—but of civilizing natural functions. Accordingly, nurslings, who are not yet civilized and, moreover, are being fed "naturally," are not allowed to sleep in bed with their parents, but older children are. They are not permitted to suckle at the breast whenever they wish, but may suck on a pacifier from the moment of birth until they are five or six years old.

Unregulated breast-feeding and nursing beyond the first few months evoke responses of disgust and disdain in many laypersons as well as medical professionals. To them, only vagabonds and gypsies breast-feed their infants for prolonged periods, and everyone knows that their behavior is not restrained by any cultural controls. On the other hand, a young pediatrician in Santa Lucia finds that these people have none of the problems in breast-feeding and child rearing that her patients report. The latter, "civilized" people, are separated from their children by many intermediaries and lack any intuition or instinct. They do not understand their children at all and do not know what their cries mean.

In fact, when I have described women's ability to influence and feel the let-down reflex to people in the town and cities nearby, they have found the idea incredible or even ludicrous. The only person to validate it was a woman considered to be gypsy-like who lived on a commune in the hills. Given their cerebral rather than naturalistic approach to child rearing, it is no wonder that the inducement that breast-fed infants develop a higher intellectual quotient appeals to parents, and biochemical explanations are favored over tactile or affective ones.[17]

It is considered more onerous to have too much milk than none at all, for excessive milk is said to be difficult to regulate and to cause the child to suffer. One woman remembers a hospital roommate who had too much milk, which was doubly bad because it was "heavy" and made the baby's face turn red. Whereas this woman ran out of milk and was happy to use formula because she could simply measure it out, her roommate had to find a way to feed her child less.

The culturally constructed schism in the mother-infant relationship contributes to the alienation of the body, for breast-feeding is seen as secretion of a product serving the child, which the mother can easily jeopardize. She must therefore act in specific ways, restricting physical activity and exposure to the elements; avoiding emotions, thinking, or sweating; sterilizing her nipples; obeying dietary restrictions and food prohibitions;

and using intrusive means of regulating the intestine. Of course, before all
of that, she must present herself for judgment of anatomical suitability by
a physician and submit to the latter's decisions about her ability to breast-
feed in case of illness or fever.

That young women almost uniformly use intrusive, internal birth control methods such as the pill and IUD when they are increasingly being
rejected by women in other Western societies is a reflection of a broad cultural acceptance of bodily manipulation.[18] A print advertisement for an
"intimate hygiene" product (Infasil Intimo) shows a young woman holding
an anatomy book and saying that she is studying to become a physician.[19]
The message is that intervening chemically in genital functions is a reflection
of one's education and medical expertise. Another print advertisement for a
home urine test called "Family-Test" claims to give consumers a "concrete"
means for periodically verifying the family's health.[20] It shows a young
father leading his daughter, son, and lastly, his wife, all of whom are dressed
to look unmistakably American. Like the other advertisement, this one
implies that surveillance over bodily functions signifies modernity and scientific progress, in this case through their cultural association with America.

While women are alienated from their bodies, they are also victims of
them. Childbirth is said to be the cause of a large number of immediate
and delayed medical problems, including hearing loss, and there is a saying in Romagna that it displaces all of the bones in the body except for the
chin. Marital sterility is known to be due equally to men and women, but
invariably blamed upon the latter. Beyond physical defects, women's psychological tensions are said to act negatively upon their extremely delicate
and complex hormonal mechanisms. Women also cause sterility by being
ashamed to ask for treatment for genital infections. Men's sterility, by
contrast, is thought to be caused by external factors for which they are not
to blame, whether environmental pollutants, stressful conditions that
affect brain chemicals, or genital infections.[21]

Breast-feeding is considered antithetical to thinness, attractiveness,
and sex. It is taken for granted that one must eat and grow fat to breast-
feed, and that the fat reserve created in pregnancy is not lost until weaning.
Breast-feeding is said to make the breasts sag and put the husband and
nursling into conflict. Women and medical experts observe that some
mothers continue to refuse to have sex with their husbands throughout
lactation. Many decide to renounce or limit breast-feeding in order to
begin a weight loss program or resume the birth control pill.

However, the strong pressure to breast-feed—exerted by older people
complaining about young women's lack of commitment to maternity and
experts propagating the latest knowledge about its benefits—does not
allow women to renounce it in tranquillity. This is why almost all women

begin by breast-feeding, even if they abandon it soon after. Women express relief at the loss of their milk, but also regret, disappointment, or guilt. Knowing that their mothers breast-fed them and their siblings for many months or years can sharpen these feelings.

When a woman who wishes to breast-feed fails to do so, she may feel let down by her body, or, more specifically, her "bad glands." Mothers either blame their bodies directly or point to bad water, harmful additives in food, unhealthy life-styles, or an unhappy and unfortunate world. These sentiments imply that the body is helpless to defend itself against external threats and internal defects, and they contribute to women's uncertainty about their ability to breast-feed successfully. Women surely are not heartened by cultural concepts that presume women's deficiency or insufficiency as mothers and producers of milk.

Early this century, when gracile women were considered to have a defective anatomy ill-favored for maternity, Rasponi described witnessing as an adolescent a couple's heart-wrenching search for a wet nurse as their two-week-old baby's pleas for food went unanswered. The mother was out of milk, but her husband was convinced of the mortal danger of bottle-feeding. She wept silently and kissed the baby, which only increased her suffering as he lifted his little head, fixed imploring eyes on her, and opened his mouth seeking a nipple (1914:13–14). Though death no longer threatens as it did then, women today can feel a similar sense of helplessness when their milk is missing or begins to disappear.

The current belief in nursing women's inadequacy, and the delicateness and fragility of maternity in general, is implicit in the rules for breast-feeding—which actually produce the conditions they presuppose. The "necessity" of regulating breast-feeding has been incorporated into culture so unconsciously that the physiological mechanisms blocking milk production and release remain unacknowledged. Women find, in spite of their willingness and availability to breast-feed, that their bodies are as insufficient and defective as the method presumes. Although bottle-feeding is thought to require even greater rigidity about schedules and quantities, it frees the mother from having to scrutinize, coax, struggle with, or lose faith in her body.

No one questions the validity of the doppia pesata and orario, given parents' need for a tangible measure of their success in caring for their infants properly at a time in which the individual's knowledge and behavior is so thoroughly challenged by and relegated to the authority of experts. This is reinforced by the public aspect of breast-feeding. The mother's performance is constantly judged, the number of grams she produces volleyed about among laypeople and health professionals as though it, rather than the milk itself, were the true product of lactation.

Cultural Constructs of Nature and Culture

The alienation of the body that invites recourse to mechanistic interventions in breast-feeding fits within the context of civilized rather than naturalistic maternity and infancy, and stems from a particular cultural interpretation of the boundary between nature and culture. Time, social relationships, the body, the domestic and outside world, and the landscape are all ordered by culture in contrast to a perceived state of nature, and this is reflected in beliefs and behaviors regarding infant feeding methods.

In Italy, there is a strict agricultural cycle that dictates the timing of the burning, sowing, fertilizing and "poisoning," and harvesting of fields to the day and sometimes hour. The day is divided into quarter-hour intervals by town clocks, and schools, shops, and other businesses keep the same hours so that meals are taken at the same time by everyone each day. Housework, shopping, and cooking are time-consuming, daily chores often done on a schedule. Food preparation is standardized according to season and mealtime, and modified in determinate ways if for a sick person, child, or pregnant or lactating woman.

If something can be quantified, it is. Italians' cultural obsession with fever is well-known. It is measured enthusiastically and frequently, as the true sign of illness, or illness itself. One father, whose daughter felt well in spite of having a slightly elevated temperature in the middle of summer, insisted on being concerned about it because it was "still a half-degree of fever." Another man says that if he has the slightest degree of fever he cannot move, but when asked how he knows whether he has a fever he says that he measures it with a thermometer. Similarly, if an infant shows signs of discomfort, parents explain that it ate too much at the last feeding. When asked how they know this, they say that they measured the feeding.

Foods are sold and recipes are written in weights, on the justified assumption that every kitchen has a scale. Indeed, all household products involve a high degree of quantification and precision. This is evident in their instructions or descriptions, such as "doses" of dishwashing liquid or laundry soap in grams for a given number of liters of water, depending on its temperature and hardness.

Cooking is thought to transform foods that are harmful when raw into benign and sometimes more healthful products. Milk is always served warm with something (sugar, cookies, bread, coffee, chocolate, toasted barley) dissolved in it. Cooked fruit is considered better for digestion, while raw fruit is thought to take away the strength. Likewise, vegetables are rarely eaten raw or unseasoned, indicating that ease of digestion is more important than nutritional content.

In contrast to the fascist-era approach to infancy, which extended regimentation and order to all aspects of children's lives, today's scientific mothering pampers infants in some ways while restricting them in others. Infants are closed into their strollers for many months, where they will be rocked back and forth rather than picked up if they fuss. A "good" infant is one that never needs to be picked up out of its carriage. Sometimes, infants are taught to walk early with a sash wrapped under the arms and held from behind by an adult.

Children are fed mushy, specially prepared foods well into the second year and are not expected to handle a spoon or fork until that time. They may drink a mixture of warm milk and grated cookie and chocolate from a bottle into their third year. Their meals are always seasoned (with either salt, oil, and parmesan cheese, or honey or sugar), and they are bombarded with candies, pastries, and ice cream. In addition to the usual prepared infant foods, there are special teas and olive oils. Parents, and especially grandparents, repeatedly change infants into spotless, pressed clothes throughout the day. Toilet training is often delayed until the age of three or four (one of six varieties of Lines brand diapers, the *gigante,* fits children weighing 18 to 30 kilograms [40 to 66 pounds]).[22]

These attentions make the concern that infants can be spoiled by on-demand feeding seem contradictory, but regimented breast-feeding is not as much a repressive practice as a form of excessive vigilance aimed at managing digestive and other functions. This kind of care has become possible on a wide scale due to the economic prosperity of the postwar period. It includes not only the regimentation of women's and children's time and behavior, but also prohibitions against or fears of harming pregnancy or lactation through women's thinking too much, sweating, exercising, or experiencing emotions.

At the same time that people repeat the fashionable phrase "pregnancy is not a disease," they treat it as a precarious condition that imposes enormous changes in behavior, outlook, and relationships. Maternity is said to irrevocably alter the mother's personality, subsuming her identity into its duties. When asked about his children's birth, the first thing a 50-year-old urban husband said, with evident pride, was that within five minutes of coming home from the hospital his wife started cleaning house.

To some men, women's eternal duty is based in religion and biology, for it is "natural" for mothers to have a closer relationship with their children: the mother is tied to the children and therefore also to the house, and the spouses live in two separate worlds. One Santa Lucia husband gave further proof of this "natural" separation in the fact that his wife is not a blood relative. In this view, a relationship of parity is seen as a competitive division of duties and a threat to the natural order. However, the separation of male and female roles in the household is a relatively new one. Only with the emergence of wage labor and a cash economy, and the appearance of many more public meeting places, did men abandon their domestic duties to spend leisure time away from home. Today, women's attempts to do the same thing are considered unnatural, unjustified, and frivolous.

Throughout the growth of the middle class since the 1940s and 1950s, bourgeois motherhood has been recognized by those who live it as not sufficient to fill the day. Enter the time-consuming duties of scientific mothering. Some women carry them out to an extreme of heroic house-work, exalting in having devoted an entire day to ironing clothes in mid-summer heat or worked so hard that the house feels like a sauna. Doing so with scientific rationality gives the impression of productive work and capability with numbers that defends them against the derision of men such as a 50-year-old who says that "the Italian woman just isn't intelli-gent yet."

By participating in scientific breast-feeding and motherhood in gen-eral, women incorporate cultural knowledge and connect themselves, however unconsciously, to their own nation's history as well as the transnational phenomenon of medicalization.

The Medicalization of Maternity

Fascism and the Cultural Construction of Motherhood

One of the things people often say about fascism, both inside and outside Italy, is that the trains ran on time. While this epithet reduces fascism to an obsession with punctuality, and is not entirely accurate, it does hold a grain of truth. The concern for order and time scheduling was real. Ironically, it has been silently incorporated into some areas, such as infant feeding, where it originally failed, but flamboyantly refuted in others, most notably transportation (!). Fascism was not a phenomenon imposed from without, but a movement sprung from within. This explains its concordance with broader sociocultural and demographic forces in shaping understandings of maternity and breast-feeding, as well as its unacknowledged influence upon the structural and cultural underpinnings of Italian life.

Basic concepts about time, space, and the body have been shaped by social and political forces.[23] Industrialization and agricultural intensifi-cation brought a representation of time that emphasized discrete intervals rather than seasonal rhythms or longer cycles, and this came to be applied to breast-feeding. Fascist-era infant feeding practices expressed attention to boundaries, quality, and overflow, mapping the spatial concerns of an expanding, militaristic nation-state onto medical understandings of the body and its products. While the government was concerned to protect and expand external boundaries, it sought to overcome internal ones among autonomous local and regional cultures. Not just demographic

patterns, but agricultural and industrial production were to be rationalized, regulated, and turned inward, controlling the flow of people and
goods across borders.

The standardization of method, the control of excess, and the rationalization of production and consumption in breast-feeding mirrored
these concerns. For example, individual liberty in infant feeding methods,
unguided by medical supervision, was perceived by physicians and political leaders as unacceptable. As geographical differences would give way to
a unified national culture, so variety and diversity in infant feeding methods would be replaced by a universal, uniform method ensuring controlled
infant milk consumption and growth. Milk production was metered and
timed like industrial production, for it was not undernutrition that caused
infant disease and death, but women's irrational and unregulated habit of
giving the breast too often, for too long, and with heedless disregard for
breast cleanliness and the danger of stagnant milk. These norms reflect a
striking match between health beliefs and political concerns about the
feared emergence of an old, decaying race if emigration, internal migration, and the fall in birthrates were not controlled.

The precepts of fascist political demography are no longer overtly
upheld, but have diffused and settled to a subconscious level. Many fascist
social welfare policies and institutions have been carried forward through
the years, though their original meaning may have been lost or forgotten.
For example, many laypeople and health professionals are not aware that
the "reduced schedule" women work for a year after childbirth derives
from the nursing breaks, but consider it and other provisions to be postwar innovations.

As during the fascist period, paid leave before and after childbirth is
now presented less as a right than a duty owed by mothers to the national
society. Until recently, however, the legislation was either ignored or
respected unevenly. Today, compliance is high, but the "progressive" measures serve as a disincentive to women's employment. Moreover, they
reflect and perpetuate divisive gender ideologies, together with the idea
that pregnancy and breast-feeding are disease conditions requiring close
medical surveillance and near exclusion from social life.

Although the pronatalist side of fascist demographic policy failed to
produce higher birthrates, the effort to rationalize child rearing succeeded.
Given the structural changes under way at the time, it would have taken
much more strident economic and social measures to significantly affect
vital rates (birth, death, marriage, migration). Paradoxically, the obsessive
maternalism of fascist domestic policy may even have contributed to the
fall in natality by adding extra responsibility and work to procreation and
child rearing.

The rising bourgeois ideal of maternal duty and sacrifice meant that well-off mothers were increasingly expected to breast-feed and care for their children themselves, rather than hiring servants for these tasks. More careful attention to infancy was also evident in the blossoming of medical and scientific interest and the proliferation of reformers' writings which earnestly sought to overcome the public's sense of resignation with respect to births and infant deaths. These changes in attitudes toward parenthood preceded but were fueled by the decline in infant mortality rates and the increase in the effectiveness of fertility control. They brought ever greater trust in the efficacy of medical intervention.

While fascist political and medical initiatives for regimented breast-feeding were successful among those women most in contact with the state medical system, they were not able to immediately stamp out individual or family self-reliance in infant feeding practices, especially in the rural districts. Over time, though, ONMI influence expanded even to the most remote regions, where clinics opened and health workers traveled with their schedules and scales in hand. Families were meanwhile progressively absorbed into the national culture. As women's domestic and economic authority eroded, scientific mothering became a way of demonstrating activity and productivity. Yet, there persists a naturalistic cultural representation of motherhood, which is all the more striking given Italy's record-low birthrates. Regimented breast-feeding continues to represent tradition together with an ideology of progress.

The social changes of the early twentieth century brought a sexualization of the breasts as part of a new ideal female body type that stressed youthful thinness and appeal to fashion, rather than the traditional "maternal" look. Fascist leaders opposed these trends as yet another frivolous aspect of the odious bourgeois worldview—and contrary to the sanctity of the family. They responded by making breast-feeding a central symbol of domestic politics.

Mother's milk was described as a biological and spiritual food, which in its giving was a testimony to the mother's devotion to her child and to maternity itself. However, there was a contradiction. The fascist regime exalted the virtues of mothers able and willing to devote themselves entirely to child care and housework, but in practice these were women of the wealthier classes in which birthrates were low and still falling, and breast-feeding was relatively rare or short-lived. Paradoxically, the rewards for prolific reproduction went to rural families, who were the ones most resistant to and isolated from the cultural values and health norms of professional medicine and among whom there was little room for bourgeois ideas about aesthetics or sexuality.

Today, maternity continues to be valued as the supreme self-sacrifice and evident expression of women's devotion to the husband and family, but at the same time women's attractiveness and appeal to men are strong cultural values. The social and economic context for large families has disappeared, but the ideology of maternity as the determinant of social standing and worth has not. While the breast continues to signify maternity, its erotic aspect is heavily exploited in the public arena. Even though infant mortality rates have fallen dramatically, medical surveillance of and attention to infants continues to grow. The cultural value of infancy contrasts against the reality of their low numbers, while the cultural value of maternity contrasts against the perception of women as sex objects. These contradictions contribute to the ambiguous meanings associated with breast-feeding and to its early renunciation.

Changes in Medical Authority and Organization

Over the past few generations, older women's knowledge of maternal events and functions has been eclipsed by that of biomedical experts. The multiple and extended family households of traditional Italian society were resistant to outside, expert authority, and mothers-in-law and other female relatives exercised their own authority over younger mothers. This was recognized by fascist leaders and physicians, who understood that the isolated, autonomous households impeded progress in building a uniform national culture. In the postwar period, nearly all families came to be organized on the simple family model and to look to the outside for guidance in reproduction and parenting, just as urban bourgeois and working-class families had begun to do a generation or more before.

Through the nineteenth century, the Church and local philanthropical societies had been the primary institutions caring for the sick, abandoned, and needy, including abandoned infants and unwed mothers. Over the second half of the nineteenth century, institutions for infants and mothers responded to economic and cultural changes by providing day care for children and medical and nutritional services for both. The state became more active in these areas through legislation, a limited degree of direct involvement, and regulation of the wet-nursing industry. In the fascist period, charitable institutions were brought under state control and direction, together with new day-care centers, maternal refectories, and pediatric and obstetrical clinics under the auspices of ONMI.

All of these institutions were supervised by medical professionals and became the podium for the transmission of their values and knowledge. Maternal breast-feeding was a requirement for public assistance, and regimented methods were written into new legislation, the organization and activities of ONMI, and the responsibilities and duties of health professionals. ONMI personnel made every effort to keep "illegitimate" mothers and children together so that all children would be breast-fed. Health professionals were forbidden to distribute information or implements for artificial feeding, unless the mother had a medical certificate.

As the need to care for illegitimate children and orphans of war diminished, ONMI focused upon preventive medical care. This went on for another three decades after the Second World War, during which the organization served as a powerful agent of culture change, fostering public acceptance of medical authority in family life.

Meanwhile, the presence of the state in public health has shifted from minimal intervention, limited largely to data collection, to a massive public health service. The network of local physicians and midwives has given way to the urban laboratory and hospital-based system of biomedicine, with its fondness for technological interventions. This process was concentrated in the interwar period, when the group of health experts serving women and children expanded into a complex field of specialized physicians, midwives, and other health and social service workers employed in specialized ONMI clinics throughout the country.

The community health workers of the nineteenth and early twentieth centuries lacked most of the diagnostic and therapeutic equipment available today. There was also a fundamentally different cultural conception of their role, which was primarily that of providing care rather than a cure. Medical knowledge varied geographically and was admittedly empirical, rooted in popular knowledge and practice. Physicians and midwives, like priests, were leading members of society whose influence was grounded in personal relationships cultivated over long periods through extended home visits.

It was against these conditions that advocates of professional medicine fought so ardently beginning in the latter half of the nineteenth century. They sought to distance medical from lay knowledge and practice and to unify it through a distinct national medical culture. They viciously criticized the ignorance of local physicians, midwives, and untrained healers, while crediting professional medicine with all improvements in morbidity and mortality rates. To standardize medical care, they brought patients out of their homes and created social distance between physicians and patients. Medical training began to involve extended laboratory and clinical experience with procedures, equipment, assistance, and supervision that bore little resemblance to real-world conditions.

The new medicine rejected the classical concept of physiological and anatomical homology between women and men, children and adults. Consequently, the care of maternity and infancy was divided both according to the individuals and in time, with childbirth representing a decisive point of separation. Formerly, midwives had cared for both mothers and infants through the first months after childbirth. Now, this care was to be divided with obstetricians and pediatricians. Textbooks on puericultura had referred to mothers and infants together from conception to weaning. Instead, the field was split and said to be devoted to conditions of health, in contrast to the more glamorous role of pediatrics and obstetrics in dealing with disease and dysfunction. Maternity came to be seen as a pathological condition necessarily requiring close medical surveillance.

Since then, technology-intensive methods and interventions in medicine have grown in favor, and childbirth has been completely hospitalized. There has been an overproduction of health professionals and an intensification of preventive and curative treatment. These forces have led to frequent contact between patients and the medical system, and played no small part in the dissemination and acceptance of medical beliefs regarding maternity and breast-feeding.

Health Beliefs and Cultural Concepts of Maternity and Breast-Feeding

The blending of the germ theory of disease into older understandings of the humors, constitutions, and permeability of the body to atmospheric influences has widened the range of control over health and disease. However, it has also multiplied the factors in illness and intemperance, and expanded the categories of behavior that can be blamed for causing disease or prescribed for curing it. That is, people are subject to external influences over which they have little control, but at the same time they have the ability to control health through antimicrobial therapy and the maintenance or restoration of balance and equilibrium. Sinister microorganisms are thought to enter the body when the balance is upset or imprudent behavior causes exposure to an environmental insult, but behavioral or atmospheric factors alone may also cause disease.

For example, sweating, even in summer, is said to lead to fever, especially if the person is also struck by a gust of wind. In a lactating woman, this will damage the milk and harm the child. Excessive milk production is considered a grave malady ruinous to the health of both mother and baby, while milk or colostrum itself becomes a source of infection if left upon the breast to spoil. The digestive system has come to be seen as the seat of health and well-being, so that regulation of the intestine assumes great importance for milk production and consumption.

The interwar period brought a fundamental reconceptualization of the relationship between mothers and infants. In the traditional view, the mother's blood linked the two from conception to weaning. The excess blood that was otherwise discharged through menstruation first fed the fetus and then was sent to the breast to be "cooked" and purified and made into milk. The milk transmitted the mother's moral and physical qualities, and it mechanically influenced the development of the child's organs. Breast-feeding therefore completed gestation in a concrete way. To abstain was to experience half a maternity and to subject oneself to severe discomforts and diseases.

In the 1920s, studies of infant digestion and maternal milk production were hailed as proof that the milk was made in the glands and was not simply transformed blood. The blood-milk bond was severed. No longer a continuous intermediary between mother and child, the milk was now a disembodied product—albeit a valued one for its nutritional and immunological properties. It did not directly transfer maternal virtues, for it was the *act* of breast-feeding that was the true spiritual food. Method became more important than the lactating woman's constitution or other qualities.

Identity between mother and nursling was replaced by complementarity, through the notion of the universal "natural periodicity" of organic functions. This linked their digestive and secretory functions through a shared need for alternation between activity and rest. Mother and infant were kept in physiological balance, but considered independent organisms. The feeding schedule and double weighings were necessary to avoid overburdening the infant's digestive system with too-frequent feedings and excessive quantities of milk. Chemical testing allowed for detection of "deficiencies" in milk quality.

Breast-feeding came to be seen above all in terms of benefits to the child, thanks to the splitting of the blood-milk unity together with political ideas about protecting infants for the future of the nation-state. Benefits to the mother, such as protection from breast cancer, were ignored. Sexual and reproductive functions were necessary not because of old humoral ideas about the regular exercise of all physiological functions, but because spermatic absorption and conception transmitted "paternal elements" needed for physiological and psychological balance and "completion" of the female organism. Meanwhile, the logical incompatibility between lactation and menstruation, based on their deriving from the same humor, was denied and replaced by a concept of weak hormonal incompatibility. Today, the perceived utility of maternity to women is limited to psychological benefits. The contraceptive effect of lactation is vehemently refuted by most laypeople and medical experts, although the Pope recently recognized it in his opposition to the use of formula in developing countries.

During the fascist period, infant mortality rates were interpreted no longer in terms of the *conditions* of infant feeding, especially those associated with mercenary and artificial feeding, but rather in terms of imperfect *method* in breast-feeding. This supported the program of universal maternal breast-feeding for the first year of life, provided it was performed according to a scientific method and under medical supervision. Medical regulation of maternal behavior was further justified by the extension of the logic linking pregnancy loss to exposure to destabilizing influences, using it to claim that infant disease and death were rooted in maternal misbehavior during breast-feeding.

The necessity of maintaining balance and moderation in order to avoid excesses or deficits of all kinds, in all people, had once served to protect the moral and physical health of mothers and infants together, as an end in itself. Medical texts had stressed the importance of life-style, constitution, and behavior to breast-feeding and considered the qualities of prospective wet nurses in great detail. Methodological issues received little if any attention. In fascist-era medicine, the correlation of imprudence with dire health consequences was directed toward preventing women from harming their infants through "irrational" breast-feeding. This fit well with the political conception of maternity as sacrifice, while the splitting of the blood-milk bond uncoupled maternal well-being from mother-infant interactions.

The implication that maternal behavior directly impacts infant health in negative and even deadly ways gave force to the behavioral norms imposed by experts. It continues, if less openly, to induce mothers to seek and follow medical advice regarding everyday activities and concerns. Many people still believe that infants used to die because mothers worked in the fields in summer, sweated, and then fed their infants their altered, toxic milk.

Given the diverging social and economic roles of women and men in the first decades of this century, it seems no coincidence that on the biological level they were now considered separate and unique. This also sheds light on the medical discouragement of parent-infant cosleeping and nocturnal breast-feeding, even if in reality most families had no choice but to live and sleep together in few rooms. In contrast to traditional beliefs, which focused upon the good, milk-rich mother, there was a rising emphasis on the good wife, who was to be available for her husband and separated from her infant during the night. This was said to be beneficial to the child as well.

Fascist medical and political leaders hailed women's universal capacity to breast-feed as the biological basis for their insistence that every woman follow her "moral and humane duty" to do so for one year. Their appeal to tradition and natural law was contrasted against celebration of futurism and industrial culture, a tension that ran throughout fascism. The message was that all women are able and obligated to breast-feed, but if they do not respect modern methods they will be responsible for continued high levels of infant mortality. Medical authority became the antidote to maternal ignorance.

The medical contraindications to breast-feeding were reduced to a bare minimum, while the legislation regulating public assistance and women's work aimed to ensure women's availability to breast-feed and propensity to do so with scientific rationality. These efforts were undermined by the authority of physicians to judge women's suitability to breast-feed or the advisability of continuing in case of illness, and the stipulation that employers, not workers, establish the feeding schedule. There was also the continued elaboration of contraindications and disincentives to breast-feeding, such as milk insufficiency, which women were told to overcome but whose reality was hardened in the process.

As a result of these contradictions, cultural beliefs continue to include derisive notions juxtaposed against laudatory ones. Earlier this century, robust, prolific, milk-rich country women were the antithesis of gracile urban bourgeois and working-class women. Yet, the former were considered backward and recalcitrant with regard to the modernization of child-rearing practices. The notion of universal capacity has arisen alongside that of widespread inadaptedness for breast-feeding, just as the intrinsic quality of autoregulation does not preclude the necessity of regimentation and rationing. Breast-feeding exalts women by benefiting children; if it is done unlovingly or improperly, it is harmful. In other words, breast-feeding is necessary and natural, but destined to failure unless controlled by medical intervention and supervision.

Cultural manipulation comes full circle in its interference with the nature of lactation, bringing about the disorder and maladaptiveness it expects while obscuring their social and historical roots. Women's bodies fail them, not because of inherent physical deficiencies but because of culturally imposed regulations on maternal behavior.

Medicalization and Modern Life

The changes in medical orientation and organization in the interwar period created a gap between medical and popular knowledge, which has since been closed. Popular, commonsense notions about health and disease have come to adhere tightly to those which are considered modern and scientific in what is now a highly literate culture with close and frequent contact with professional medicine. Medicalized norms for breast-feeding conflict neither with common sense nor current scientific knowledge, as they did when they were first introduced. The former diffidence of isolated farm families has given way to active acceptance of expert assistance and advice in reproduction and child rearing. Geographical, social class, and personal variation in infant feeding methods has been replaced by a uniform method of breast-feeding, bottle-feeding, and supplementation and weaning.

Over the postwar period, breast-feeding mothers have increasingly respected the feeding schedule and standardized dosing of milk, but their proportion in the population has changed in line with shifts in expert opinion about the advantages of bottle-feeding (itself conducted according to rigorous methods). From the 1960s through the early 1980s, medical opinion and hospital practices advocated bottle-feeding. There was a massive rejection of breast-feeding as women learned that formula made babies "more beautiful," while lactation disfigured their bodies, worsened all possible medical conditions, and caused a generalized degradation of the body.

Medical preference has since shifted back, and the trend has turned around to nearly universal breast-feeding, at least in the first days. As in the past, breast-feeding is said to be extremely important for individual and social health and well-being, and since there is such high compliance with medical opinion women find it difficult to reject it outright. Because they comply with the feeding schedule and double weighings, they are unable to breast-feed for long. Most couples have very few children compared to the past; and their economic well-being allows them to show their dedication by acquiring technological implements for child rearing.

Old ideas about women's culpability for infant disease or death through immoderate behavior give parents little scope for rejecting medical management, and since they do not trust more subjective means, they refer to external standards for reassurance that they are feeding their child properly. The idea that breastmilk must be metered to ensure regular infant growth has become so entrenched that it prevents virtually everyone from attempting baby-led feeding of the kind suggested by the traditional wisdom of not so long ago: "babies must eat little and often."

This transformation in belief and behavior shows that the interpretation and manipulation of biological functions is rooted both in specific cultural idioms and concerns and in more universal structural forces. Across Western societies, the drawing of infant feeding into the public sphere has taken place at the same time as dramatic changes in the nature of marriage, family, and social life. Breast-feeding has come to be perceived as something disquietingly intimate, "natural," and physical, which conflicts with the conjugal relationship.

It should not be assumed that a male-dominated political and medical system is to blame, for professional midwives and female physicians and other health professionals were just as eager as their male counterparts to scientize reproduction and infant care practices. Mothers enthusiastically accepted the new norms and continue to advance them by complying and expecting others to do so. Men are equally invested in the current system of knowledge and practice of infant feeding and uphold its commonsense notions with the same commitment as women.

The changes have brought both gains and losses. Physical proximity and emotional distance have given way to emotional closeness and physical distance between spouses and other family members. Women and men have made many gains in employment, but women have lost authority while men have lost involvement in the family. There have been vast improvements in material conditions and medical therapies. Yet, the expansion of the state, with its ever-growing medical system and its requirement of total submission to medical authority, has reached into the most intimate and private corners of individual and social life. This has rendered people extremely dependent upon it, far beyond the needs of health maintenance and treatment. Health professionals complain both of patients' complete lack of self-reliance and of their bothersome inquisitiveness and demands for information.

Clearly, breast-feeding is inconvenient to health professionals because they cannot control it to the same extent as bottle-feeding. Taken as part of a larger intrusion into reproduction and child rearing, expert intervention in breast-feeding reflects the conceit that it is the health professional who gives and maintains life. Intimate matters that were once confined to the family, such as contraception, childbirth, or infant care, are now accepted as the proper field of medical experts, who have nearly squeezed out priests, elders, and other traditional authorities. The self-assurance of individuals and families has diminished in the process, in spite of the public's ever-greater access to information, which would seem to predict the opposite.

To surrender individual competence and confidence to outside experts is a high and unnecessary price to pay for improved medical care, even if some medical experts may trivialize these outcomes. Offended by my assertion that fascist-era physicians had a role in medicalizing breast-feeding practices, an older Italian physician retorted that modern medicine was responsible for the historical decline in infant mortality rates. In his view, it was ungrateful of me to blame medical intervention for women's anguish and "failures" in breast-feeding, as if the medical community's manifest successes give physicians free rein to speak out in ever-expanding spheres of influence. Yet, the physician's claim about infant mortality is only partially sustainable, while the intervention in breast-feeding was far removed from the kinds of medical care that actually improved health and survival.

Indeed, the cultural beliefs we have examined have serious health costs for both mothers and babies, which we discussed in the opening chapter. By curtailing or precluding breast-feeding, they compromise a natural contraceptive and deprive women and their infants of health benefits as well as physical and emotional pleasure and intimacy. In non-Western countries, the decline in breast-feeding already yields severe health outcomes for infants. Coupled with new diet and exercise patterns, it could bring a massive increase in cancers that used to be rare in these populations. Finally, modern cultural beliefs do nothing to help women feel confident about their bodies and their ability to manage them, except through the mediation of medical experts.

Submission to medical authority has gone so far that people accept as common sense certain notions that completely violate all that is known about human biology, even with reference to processes such as breast-feeding that are explicitly thought of as natural. People can be convinced that sterilizing the breasts several times a day is an absolute obligation of breast-feeding, that many women simply have no milk, and that infant meals must be scheduled and metered according to external standards. Yet, none of us would be here if infectious disease were caused by sloppy breast-feeding, if a large proportion of mothers were unable to feed their infants, or if infants did not thrive unless separated physically from their mothers and fed according to a fixed regimen.

Medicalization has been a broad process that has affected us all. Industrialization has brought the regimentation of time and production, as well as a sharper separation of work by gender and paid or unpaid status. The growth of modern nation-states has brought medicalization and the demise of traditional authority. State-sponsored rationalization and scientific management of parenting has concentrated upon mothers, isolating them in the home (in theory at least), where they have been targets for new cultural and medical norms. These changes have had wide implications for the Western societies, affecting not just infant feeding practices but also debates about abortion rights, public assistance to parents and children, mandatory immunization of children, parents' rights in the workplace, and patients' rights to refuse treatment. All of these concern the competing claims of individuals, medical experts, commercial interests, and the state over our bodies.

The study of breast-feeding practices in Italy demonstrates that the balance among these interests is not in the nature of things, but rather the outcome of historical processes. With some reflection, we can understand with greater clarity the forces that impinge upon us and achieve a more fine-tuned utilization of our health-care options. The reward will be greater control over and confidence in our behavior and choices.

Infant Mortality Tables for the Community of Santa Lucia

TABLE A1. Infant Deaths as a Proportion of All Deaths, Santa Lucia, 1866–1991 (0–1-year-olds and 1–3-year-olds)

Year	Total Deaths	Age 0–1		Age 1–3	
		Deaths	%	Deaths	%
1866	105	31	30	8	8
1871	121	42	35	10	8
1872	113	27	24	19	17
1881	115	26	23	13	11
1891	113	35	31	19	17
1901	87	31	36	3	3
1911	106	43	41	6	6
1921	96	30	31	3	3
1923	88	32	36	9	10
1924	81	17	21	3	4
1925	71	11	15	2	3
1927	63	13	21	0	0
1929	82	16	20	3	4
1931	57	8	14	1	2
1941	69	18	26	1	1
1951	45	9	20	1	2
1961	38	6	16	0	0
1966	49	5	10	0	0
1971	34	0	0	0	0
1981	31	0	0	0	0
1991	34	0	0	0	0

TABLE A2. Infant Deaths as a Proportion of All Births, Santa Lucia, 1871–1981 (0–1 year-olds, 1–3 year-olds, stillbirths)

Year	Total Births	Age 0–1		Age 1–3		Stillbirths	
		Deaths	%	Deaths	%	n	%
1871	159	35	22	13	8	12	8
1887	183	22	14	11	6	9	5
1892	190	35	18	9	5	14	7
1901	174	35	20	2	1	14	8
1910	177	20	11	1	—[a]	7	4
1917	126	18	14	0	0	8	6
1924	221	14	6	7	3	12	5
1925	192	12	6	2	1	10	5
1938	152	8	5	0	0	3	2
1955	93	4	4	0	0	3	3
1970	44	3	7	0	0	0	0
1981	31	0	0	0	0	0	0

[a]less than one-half of 1 percent

TABLE A3. Sex Differences in Infant Deaths, Santa Lucia, 1871–1981

Year	0–2 mos.			2 mos.–1 yr.			1–3 yrs.			Total 0–3 yrs.			Ratio of Births (M:F)
	M	F	Total	M	F	Total	M	F	Total	M	F	Total	
1871	9	11	20	5	10	15	5	8	13	19	29	48	49:51
1887	10	4	14	6	5	11	5	6	11	21	15	36	49:51
1892	9	11	20	6	9	15	7	2	9	22	22	44	57:43
Subtotal	28	26	54	17	24	41	17	16	33	62	66	128	52:48
1901	13	7	20	12	3	15	1	1	2	26	11	37	48:53
1910	6	2	8	6	6	12	0	1	1	12	9	21	53:47
1917	4	5	9	5	4	9	0	0	0	9	9	18	50:50
Subtotal	23	14	37	23	13	36	1	2	3	47	29	76	50:50
1924	3	3	6	4	4	8	2	5	7	9	12	21	54:46
1925	5	3	8	2	2	4	1	1	2	8	6	14	52:48
1938	1	0	1	5	2	7	0	0	0	6	2	8	55:45
Subtotal	9	6	15	11	8	19	3	6	9	23	20	43	54:46
1955	2	2	4	0	0	0	0	0	0	2	2	4	53:47
1970	0	3	3	0	0	0	0	0	0	0	3	3	48:52
1981	2	5	7	0	0	0	0	0	0	2	5	7	45:55
Subtotal	2	5	7	0	0	0	0	0	0	2	5	7	50:50
Total	62	51	113	51	45	96	21	24	45	134	120	254	52:48

TABLE A4. Seasonal Distribution of Births and Infant Deaths, Santa Lucia, 1871–1981 (0–3 year-olds)

Year	Births Total	Winter Births n	Winter Deaths n	Winter %	Spring Births n	Spring Deaths n	Spring %	Summer Births n	Summer Deaths n	Summer %	Fall Births n	Fall Deaths n	Fall %
1871	159	48	19	40	48	14	31	30	5	17	33	9	27
1887	183	58	14	24	62	16	26	44	4	9	19	3	16
1892	190	52	16	31	55	13	24	40	8	20	43	7	16
1901	174	46	16	35	55	8	15	34	4	12	39	9	23
1910	177	51	7	14	51	6	12	29	2	7	46	6	13
1917	126	28	4	14	39	3	8	23	2	9	36	9	25
1924	221	67	2	3	56	6	11	46	9	20	52	4	8
1925	192	44	4	9	52	1	2	51	4	8	45	5	11
1938	152	50	3	6	41	2	5	28	2	7	33	1	3
1955	93	29	2	7	25	0	0	20	0	0	19	2	11
1970	44	8	2	25	12	1	8	13	0	0	11	0	0
1981	31	12	0	0	7	0	0	4	0	0	8	0	0
1871–92	532	158	49	31	165	44	27	114	17	15	95	19	20
1901–17	477	125	27	22	145	17	12	86	8	9	121	24	20
1924–38	565	161	9	6	149	9	6	125	15	12	130	10	8
1955–70	137	37	4	11	37	1	3	33	0	0	30	2	7

TABLE A5. Average Age in Months of Infant
Deaths per Season, Santa Lucia, 1866–1970 (0–3
year-olds)

Year	Winter	Spring	Summer	Fall
1866–92	7.1	6.3	13	7.2
1901–21	7.3	5	12	3.1
1923–41	12.4	8.2	9.1	5.9
1951–70	—[a]	0.7	0.3	2.1

[a]less than one-twentieth of one month

TABLE A6. **Distribution of Infant Deaths by Parents' Profession, Santa Lucia, 1871–1981** (Observed minus expected values for stillbirth (sb), birth to 2 months, 2 months to one year, one to three years)

	1871–92				1901–17				1924–38				1955–81	
	sb	0–2m	2m–1yr	1–3yrs.	sb	0–2m	2m–1yr	1–3yrs.	sb	0–2m	2m–1yr.	1–3yrs.	sb	0–2m
Farming/service	-1.2	-6.9	-3.7	-11.4	-3.2	-3.0	-14.4	-4.4	-2.0	1.8	-2.2	-4.6	1.1	1.0
Professions/ landowning	-2.4	-0.5	-3.6	2.2	-2.0	-1.8	-0.4	1.4	-0.8	-1.1	-1.4	*	-0.8	-1.8
Trades/ artisan crafts	3.6	-1.1	0.4	3.4	-0.3	-0.2	2.2	0.4	0	-1.3	0.4	1.9	-0.7	-0.5
Day labor	0.3	8.1	2.5	5.2	3.8	4.4	2.1	0.7	3.0	0.7	3.4	1.9	0.4	1.5
Other	1.0	0	5.0	1.0	1.7	0.6	10.5	1.9	-0.3	-0.2	-0.2	0.9	-0.1	-0.1

*less than 0.05

TABLE A7. Infant Deaths by Cause of Death (Females), Santa Lucia, 1900–1959 (birth to one year, one to three years)

Females	1900–1909		1910–19		1920–29		1930–39		1940–49		1950–59		Total
	0–1	1–3	0–1	1–3	0–1	1–3	0–1	1–3	0–1	1–3	0–1	1–3	
Respiratory infection	10	14	22	11	19	11	11	12	9	4	2	2	127
Gastrointestinal infection	8	5	15	7	11	6	1		2	2	1	1	59
Stillbirth/prematurity/ complications of birth	28		33		3		9		5		12		90
Insufficient development/ congenital weakness	4		30		27	1	15		21		9		107
Diphtheria						2		1	1				4
Rickets	3					2							5
Insufficient feeding	18		2										20
Oral fungus	4			1									5
Meningitis	1					1		1		2	1		6
Skin infection			1						1				2
Burn/accident/injury		2		4		1						1	8
Eclampsia/asphyxia	1	3	13	2	4						1		24
Helminth infection		2	1										3
N/A		1		2	1	1	1			1			8
Other	1	2	3	1	1	1	1			1	1	1	14
Total	78	30	120	28	66	26	38	14	40	10	27	5	482

TABLE A8. Infant Deaths by Cause of Death (Males), Santa Lucia, 1900–1959 (birth to one year, one to three years)

Males	1900–1909		1910–19		1920–29		1930–39		1940–49		1950–59		Total
	0–1	1–3	0–1	1–3	0–1	1–3	0–1	1–3	0–1	1–3	0–1	1–3	
Respiratory infection	10	11	30	7	27	9	16	6	13	1	4	1	135
Gastrointestinal infection	11	2	13	8	12	8	2	2	7	3	1		69
Stillbirth/prematurity/complications of birth	35		47		12		13		15		15		137
Insufficient development/congenital weakness	6		29		34	1	22		33		9		134
Diphtheria						1							1
Rickets	1	1		1									3
Insufficient feeding	11		7		1								19
Oral fungus	7		6		1	1							15
Meningitis		4		2	1	5		2					14
Burn/accident/injury			2	2		2	1	2	2	1		2	14
Eclampsia/asphyxia		6	19		9				4	4	2		44
Helminth infection	3	2	1										6
N/A	3	2	3	1	2	1	2	1	1		1		17
Other	1	2	2	1	3	1	2	2	1			1	16
Total	88	30	159	22	102	29	58	15	76	9	32	4	624

Notes

Chapter 1

1. Regarding the relationship between cultural interference in breastfeeding and social and family organization, see Maher 1992:10–11. For studies of breast-feeding in various cultural and historical contexts, see Millard 1990 and the essays in Stuart-Macadam and Dettwyler (eds.) 1995 and Maher (ed.) 1992 (including the chapter by Balsamo et al. on Italy).

2. See Dau Novelli 1994:59.

3. See Foucault 1973 [1965], 1973; Kunitz 1991; Scheper-Hughes and Lock 1987; Starr 1982. Regarding Italy in particular, see Cambi 1988.

4. Even today, although they are expected to advise breastfeeding mothers, physicians in the United States receive little or no training in the subjects of nutrition and lactation. They often give incorrect or inappropriate advice regarding common problems such as mastitis, infant teething, or low milk supply (Freed et al. 1995:474–75).

5. See Quine 1996:54.

6. See Dau Novelli 1994; DeGrazia 1992; Horn 1994; Ipsen 1996; Quine 1996.

7. See Dau Novelli 1994:254.

8. Regarding these and other examples of coevolution, see Durham 1991.

9. This section is based on Cohen 1989; Eaton, Konner, and Shostak 1988a, 1988b; Lee 1979.

10. See Cassidy 1980; Cohen 1989; but see also Wood, Milner, Harpending, and Weiss 1992.

11. Nesse and Williams 1994; Williams and Nesse 1991.

12. Micozzi 1995:356.

13. Cunningham 1995:257.

14. Micozzi 1995:357.

15. Dettwyler 1995b:53; Jolly 1985:309.

16. National Center for Health Statistics 1997:97 tab. 19.

17. For a cross-cultural view of milk kinship, see Khatib-Chahidi 1992. Regarding the history of cultural practices limiting infant access to colostrum, see Fildes 1986, 1995.

18. Regarding breastfeeding and infant care practices among the !Kung, see Konner 1972; Konner and Shostak 1987; Konner and Worthman 1980. Regarding breastfeeding among the Gainj, see Wood et al. 1985.

19. Stuart-Macadam 1995b. One author gives a range of 2.5 to 7 years, calling 6 to 7 years an "evolutionary imperative" (Dettwyler 1995b). However, the

evolutionary perspective itself suggests that there should be downward pressure on weaning age, both for the mother's reproductive advantage in decreasing inter-birth intervals provided there is no threat to the infant's survival, and, for the infant's advantage in providing for itself as early as possible. The latter reduces maternal debilitation and risk of death, which directly affect infant survival, and becomes especially important as the infant grows (see Jolly 1985:323).

20. See Millard 1990:215–17.

21. See Auerbach, Riordan, and Countryman 1993:235–36; Gussler and Briesemeister 1980.

22. Cohen 1989:71, 180.

23. Regarding mechanisms of milk production and release, see Cunningham 1995; Daly and Hartmann 1995a, 1995b; DeCarvalho et al. 1983; Konner and Worthman 1980; Maglietta 1985:300–308.

24. These are only a couple of the many hormones involved in lactation, including ACTH, TSH, thyroid hormone, and insulin.

25. Victoria 1993.

26. See Woolridge 1995.

27. Jolly 1985:234–35, 279–80; see also Dettwyler 1995b:53.

28. See Klapisch-Zuber 1985. While the aristocracy led the way in choosing mercenary breastfeeding, it was also the first to abandon it beginning in the nineteenth century (see Ulivieri 1988:210–13).

29. Ellison 1995:331.

30. Regarding the mechanisms of postpartum infertility, see Ellison 1995; Konner and Worthman 1980; Short 1976; Vitzum 1994; Wood 1990; Wood et al. 1985.

31. Regarding health benefits and defensive properties of breastfeeding and breast milk, see Aniansson et al. 1994; Cunningham 1995; Lawrence 1994; Mestecky, Blair, and Ogra 1991; Riordan and Auerbach 1993; Sheard and Walker 1988; Stuart-Macadam 1995a:12, 15–16.

32. Nevertheless, a recent study found no evidence for a connection between infant feeding method and adult longevity (Wingard et al. 1994).

33. See Stuart-Macadam 1995a:20–22. Always responding to iron deficiency with supplements may not be an appropriate strategy in general, given that iron is a necessary mineral to many pathogens. Likewise, fever affects metabolic processes in response to infection, and it also promotes the sequestration of iron. For an evolutionary perspective on these and other adaptive responses to infectious disease, see Ewald 1988, 1994.

34. Davis, Savitz, and Graubard 1988.

35. For the former, see Lanting et al. 1994; Lucas et al. 1992. For the latter, see Gale and Martyn 1996.

36. Quant 1995:129–30.

37. Regarding these effects on mood and behavior, see Dettwyler 1995a:171; Stuart-Macadam 1995a:10–11.

38. This section is based on Eaton et al. 1994; Micozzi 1995. See also Adami et al. 1994; Lambe et al. 1994; LaVecchia 1991, 1992.

39. This is not to imply that oral contraceptives protect against breast cancer. The opposite may in fact be the case (see LaVecchia 1991).

40. Regarding the average age at menarche and menopause in Italy over the past centuries, see Ballotta 1857:462; Bertaccini 1922:138; Bompiani 1939:19; CFLI 1940:312; DeNapoli 1934b:313; Lanfranchi 1955:xxiv; Miraglia, Orlandini, and Micheletti 1984:81; Mercurii 1601:74; Romanini 1975:18.

41. See the obstetrics text by Marzetti, Enea, and Pecorini 1991:184.

42. These factors carry risk differentials between 1.0 and 3.9. The factors that carry the highest relative risks (over 4.0) are North American or European ancestry; premenopausal status; older age; cancer in the other breast; and first-degree relative with premenopausal cancer in both breasts (Micozzi 1995:350).

43. Ing, Petrakis, and Ho 1977.

44. This section is based on McKenna 1986, 1996; McKenna and Mosko 1990. See also Konner and Super 1987.

45. It was only in 1992 that the American Academy of Pediatrics agreed that physicians should recommend the back-down position (McKenna and Bernshaw 1995:277).

46. Frederickson 1995:413.

Chapter 2

1. For historical accounts of popular ideas and practices related to reproduction and child rearing in Emilia-Romagna, see Baldini 1991; Camprini 1978; Olivi 1997.

2. Brefotrofio degli Esposti di Faenza 1865:119–20.

3. Ballotta 1857:276.

4. Mandini 1805:48.

5. See Ballotta 1857:266; Mandini 1805:7, 10, 29, 54, 163.

6. See Mercurii 1601:13.

7. Battelli 1909:145. See also Cecchi 1910.

8. For an explanation of coction and menstruation, see Mercurii 1601: 72–76.

9. Mercurii also referred to the *puerpera* as the "*Impagliata,*" a name that agrees with an expression in Romagnan dialect traditionally used by husbands after their wives had given birth: "*a i'ho la moj int la pàia*" ["*ho la moglie nella paglia*" or "my wife is in the hay"] (Camprini 1978:237).

10. This story is recounted in Ballotta 1857:243–44. Yet, even in past centuries there were people who questioned whether birthmarks and birth defects really arose in this way. Mercurii (1601:89) describes three "imprudent" women experimenting and saying, "*hora vedrete quato* [*sic*] *sono ciarloni questi nostri filosofi*" ["now you will see how much these philosophers of ours are windbags"]. One of the women's children was born with birthmarks, two without (which he attributes to their having an unfocused imagination, insufficiently persevering to excite the spirits that would have migrated to the touched part and formed the image of the desired thing).

11. Ballotta 1857:455.

12. Regarding Saint Agata, see Gordini 1961.

13. Balocchi 1847:641.

14. Mercurii 1601:256.

15. Mercurii 1601:253 and Ballotta 1857:459, respectively.

16. Balocchi 1847:634–35.

17. Ballotta 1857:279.

18. Ballotta 1857:281, 484. See also Mandini 1805:31–33.

19. See Mandini 1805:33–34; Rasponi 1914.

20. Regarding extremes of germ consciousness or lack thereof, see Rasponi 1914:21–22.

21. Regarding the higher fat content of colostrum and mother's milk compared to diluted cow's milk, see Rasponi 1914:29.

22. For an illustration, see Mercurii 1601:200.

23. See Brefotrofio degli Esposti di Faenza 1865.

24. DeLucca (1983:105) reports a physician-to-population ratio of 1:2,520 dispersed over a large area around Rimini in 1865.

Chapter 3

1. See Rasponi 1914, especially 12–15, 28, 40; Mercurii 1601:107–8.

2. For example, see Rasponi 1914:22.

3. See Camprini 1978:59.

4. Battelli 1909:77 and 115, respectively.

5. Battelli 1909:18.

6. Della Peruta reports that in the mid–nineteenth century almost one-half of the children born to poor families in Milan were entrusted to country wet nurses or foundling homes, and that at the beginning of this century 43 percent of all infants born in Milan were fed by mercenary wet nurses (1980:719).

7. Rasponi 1914:20.

8. See Rasponi 1914 and the novels by Ginzburg, especially the autobiographical *Lessico Famigliare* (1963).

9. See Ascoli's 1994 book on wet nursing.

10. See Ballotta 1857:255; Mandini 1805:26–28; Mercurii 1601:104.

11. See Carozzi 1914a:232.

12. See DeNapoli 1934b:418.

13. See Mandini 1805:30–31.

14. Ballotta 1857:256, 276.

15. Bertaccini 1922:144.

16. See Borrino 1937:514; Gelli 1931:814, 839, 840.

17. Regarding the history of pellagra, see DeBernardi 1984; Whitaker 1992.

18. Battelli 1909:47–48.

19. See ISTAT 1997:35–36. In 1927, of every 1,000 inhabitants, 250 lived in isolated houses or towns of fewer than 2,000 inhabitants, and 328 lived in communities of 2,000–5,000 (Caratozzolo 1933:165).

20. Regarding women's role in industrialization, see Biagi 1934:103–4; Carozzi 1914a:52–60; DeBernardi 1984:132–45; DeMichelis 1937:90; Garzanti Ravasi 1931a:35–38. Writers in the fascist period almost always undercounted

female labor, as in Pende's (1933a:130) estimate of one million paid female workers in 1927. Even official statistics from the turn of the century that counted five times as many paid female workers understated their number (see Marconcini 1935:263).

21. L'Asilo Infantile di Forlì 1912:6, 18–19.

22. DeMichelis 1937:84.

23. See Forgacs 1990:17–19; Garzanti Ravasi 1931a:55; ISTAT 1991:166, 1997:671.

24. There is an old proverb about this: "*Fra suocera, e nuora la guerra sempre vi si trova*" ["Between a mother-in-law and a Daughter-in-law there is alwayes jarring"] (old English translation) (P.P. 1660:19). Regarding family life and household size and organization, see Barbagli 1984; Kertzer 1984.

25. In Caratozzolo 1933:22.

26. Regarding the history of marriage rites, see Antoniotti 1982.

27. Ulivieri 1988:206.

28. See, for example, Carli 1933; Battara 1935.

29. See Battelli 1909; Cecchi 1910.

30. Battelli 1909:82–83, 172–73. See also Ulivieri 1988:210.

31. See P.P. 1660; Silone 1955 [1936]:120.

32. See Battelli 1909; Cecchi 1910; Labriola 1918; Marconcini 1935, 1937; Palmieri 1935.

33. Regarding legislation concerning women's work, maternity, and wet nursing, see Agnoli 1987; Bertaccini 1922:142–43; Cappuccio 1939:265–311; Carozzi 1914a:230–33; Gravelli and Campanile 1933:72–73; Grossi 1935:169–71; INPS 1980:23–27, 97–101; *Maternità e Infanzia* 1928, 3 (2): 111–14; ONMI 1962:231–35, 246.

34. See Babini 1856; Mariotti 1896. For historical accounts, see Comune di Forlì 1989; Dattilo 1991; Kertzer 1993.

35. See Comune di Forlì 1989:58; Garzanti Ravasi 1931b:13.

36. For case studies, see Livi Bacci 1983; Schneider and Schneider 1984.

37. Regarding these transitions, see Knodel 1977; McKeown 1979; Omran 1971; Schofield, Reher, and Bideau (eds.) 1991.

38. Consiglio 1933:82.

39. In Saraceno 1979/80:199. See also Boldrini 1933:93–94; Comune di Faenza 1882; Federici 1984:40–41, 156; Marconcini 1935:209; Michels 1933:89; ISTAT 1983:18–19, 1990:52.

40. Psalm 90:10 of the Old Testament also says that people live 70 years, though some reach 80.

41. Livi Bacci (1986) suggests that the retreat of pellagra from the northern and central regions may have directly contributed to the rise in fertility rates in the late nineteenth century.

42. Borrino 1937:650; Dambrosio 1976:31–32; Grossi 1935:144; ISTAT 1990:106, 1991:165; Sori 1984:577–78.

43. ISTAT 1991:162–63, 1997:74.

44. DeLucca (1983:102) reports that in the outskirts of Rimini, infant mortality remained at the level of 30 to 40 deaths in the first year per 100 live births for

the entire period between 1714 and 1915. Of every 100 deaths, 50 to 70 were children under the age of five.

45. CFLI 1940:111.

46. See Bellettini 1987:186–92; Breschi and Livi Bacci 1986; Gelli 1931:739; Mandini 1805:17–18; *Maternità e Infanzia* 1928, 3 (3): 240; Palmieri 1935:152; Rosetti 1894:365.

47. Rasponi 1914:20. Rasponi's own grandmother had 18 children. The ten fed by balie all died (17).

48. Borrino 1937:651.

49. See Livi Bacci 1990; Lunn 1991; Schofield and Reher 1991:15–16.

50. See, for example, Hastrup 1992; Morel 1991.

Chapter 4

1. For historical studies of fascism and the interwar period, see Clark 1984; DeFelice 1977 (as well as his 7-volume biography of Mussolini [Turin: Einaudi, 1965–89]); Lyttelton 1988; Mack Smith 1969; Preti 1987; and the sources in chap. 1, n. 6.

2. Much has been written on this subject, which is a common theme in the anthropological literature on Italy. See the much-derided Banfield 1958, as well as DuBoulay and Williams 1987; Silverman 1968.

3. See Dau Novelli 1994:123, 127, 173–74, 178, 225; Quine 1996:40–41.

4. Oswald Spengler's book, *Decadence of the West,* was followed by an influential book by the young Bavarian sociologist Riccardo (Richard) Korherr. The latter's *Decline of births: Death of peoples* was published in Italian in 1928, with prefaces by Spengler and Mussolini. I read the copy kept by Leandro Arpinati, once known as the "second Duce," whose daughter, Giancarla Arpinati Cantamessa, kindly allowed me access to his library.

5. Maraviglia 1929:243, 244.

6. Fabbri 1933b:140.

7. Maraviglia 1929:244.

8. Caratozzolo 1933:51.

9. Gravelli and Campanile 1933:76–77.

10. Coruzzi 1933:68.

11. Davanzati, in Gemelli 1933:128.

12. Party members and their families were among those exempted from deportation. See the film *Il Giardino dei Finzi-Contini.* For accounts of internal exile, see Ginzburg 1964 [1944]; Levi 1947.

13. See Ipsen 1996:119–35, 187–90.

14. See DeNapoli 1934b:298, 301.

15. Ardali 1943:35; Pende 1933a:98.

16. Grossi 1935:218.

17. DeNapoli 1934b:395.

18. Grossi 1935:223.

19. See Fabbri 1933b:141; Grossi 1935:115; Korherr 1928.

20. Marconcini 1935:433.
21. Biagi 1934:100.
22. Vaccaro 1937:142–43.
23. Grossi 1935:221; Gelli 1931:xiv.
24. Gelli 1931:1.
25. Grossi 1935:149.
26. See Fabbri 1933a:42–44; LoMonaco-Aprile 1934:5; Pende 1933a:125; Rabaglietti 1935:27.
27. Coruzzi 1933:67–68; Grossi 1935:78; Marconcini 1935:24–26.
28. Gini and others like him proposed biological mechanisms for Herbert Spencer's notion that both among and within species intellectual progress brought a weakening of reproductive activity or generative power. Arsenio (Arsène) Dumont had added that not only did the capacity to procreate decline, but so did the will as one moved up the social scale (see Marconcini 1935:185–86; Palmieri 1935:54).
29. Ardali 1943:10; Santi 1928:351–52.
30. Coruzzi 1933:68.
31. Coruzzi 1933:68; Marconcini 1937:61.
32. Marconcini 1937:31.
33. Bertaccini 1922:142; Bertarelli 1936:571.
34. Gelli 1931:8–9, 13, 33. Gelli credits the "majority of anthropologists" for these notions about the size, shape, and abilities of the female brain, explaining that the frontal lobes (seat of "cerebral power") denoted the grade of civilization. These and the occipital lobes were smaller in women. However, the brain of civilized women weighed more than the brain of men from "inferior" races.
35. See Caratozzolo 1933:34–35; Pende 1933a:117, 196–206.
36. See Pende 1939:3.
37. Haydée 1934:50.
38. Lorenzoni 1933:73; Marconcini 1935:387–88.
39. See Martin 1987. For international studies published in an Italian journal, see *Maternità e Infanzia* 1928, 3 (2): 65 and 3 (3): 219–24.
40. For an example, see Lorenzoni 1933:70–71, who also cited a study showing that 63 percent of husbands as opposed to 41 percent of wives in sterile couples owed their sterility to gonorrhea.
41. Regarding the pernicious effects of particular industries, see Biagi 1934:105–6; Borrino 1937:671–73; Coruzzi 1933:66–67; Grossi 1935:165–68; Lorenzoni 1933:70–73.
42. Borrino 1937:671.
43. Coruzzi 1933:67.
44. Garzanti Ravasi 1931a:54.
45. Cappuccio 1939:266–67.
46. See Carli 1933:59; Maraviglia 1929:242; Panunzio 1933:137–39.
47. For the criminal and civil codes, see Cappuccio 1939; Pandolfelli et al. 1939.
48. See chap. 3, n. 33.
49. Caratozzolo 1933:20.

Chapter 5

1. Gelli 1931:559; see DeNapoli 1934b:423.
2. Gelli 1931:672.
3. See Gelli 1931:664; Vicarelli 1926a:8.
4. CFLI 1940:314.
5. CFLI 1940:314.
6. DeNapoli 1934a:175, 1934b:416–17.
7. Bumm 1923a:282; see also 283–86 and Bumm 1923b:433; Borrino 1937: 116–17.
8. Borrino 1937:133–34; see DeNapoli 1934b:315.
9. Gelli 1931:794; see also 101, 106, 751.
10. Gelli 1931:101–2, 688; Gusso 1930:69–70.
11. Caratozzolo 1933:14.
12. *Maternità e Infanzia* 1928, 3 (3): 229.
13. CFLI 1940:305.
14. DeNapoli 1934b:328; Marconcini 1935:434; Pende 1933a:206–8, 1939:3; Sfameni 1936:xlix–l.
15. Bumm 1923a:40; Sfameni 1936:li.
16. Marconcini 1935:435; see Gelli 1931:6, 446–47, 489.
17. DeNapoli 1934b:297.
18. Haydée 1934:265–66.
19. Gelli 1931:106.
20. Weininger in DeNapoli 1934b:333; see Borrino 1937:105, 155; Bumm 1923a:131; Gelli 1931:740.
21. Bertaccini 1922:140.
22. Gelli 1931:469.
23. See Bumm 1923b:120–21; Resinelli 1926:93–96; Gelli 1931:447–65, 470–87.
24. Resinelli 1926:94.
25. Borrino 1937:5.
26. Gelli 1931:464.
27. CFLI 1940:314; Cova 1939:14.
28. Borrino 1937:293.
29. CFLI 1940:315. See also the novel by Ginzburg (1947:48).
30. Gelli 1931:707, 767.
31. CFLI 1940:323.
32. Borrino 1937:291.
33. ONMI 1962:247.
34. Grossi 1935:175.
35. CFLI 1940:315.
36. Gelli 1931:789.
37. In *La Preparazione Materna* 1939, 1 (1): i.
38. Borrino objected to medical and popular restrictions on diet, arguing that they could not be valid since they varied from region to region (1937:156).
39. See ONMI 1962:242.

40. Regarding the latter, see Bumm 1923a:284; Gelli 1931:96.

41. Borrino 1937:673.

42. In addition to the authors cited directly in this and the next section, see Bertaccini 1922:152–53, 158; Bertarelli 1936:599–601; CFLI 1940:315; Bumm 1923a:294.

43. Regno d'Italia 1921:23.

44. CFLI 1940:319.

45. Borrino 1937:655.

46. See Borrino 1937:176–85; Gelli 1931:779–82.

47. Gelli 1931:781.

Chapter 6

1. See Bumm 1923a:293; Fabbri 1933a:108.

2. Caviglia, in Sebastiano 1939:18.

3. ONMI 1962:250.

4. Borrino 1937:688.

5. Caratozzolo 1933:41.

6. Borrino 1937:89.

7. CFLI 1940:316, 318.

8. Marconcini 1935:439.

9. Caratozzolo 1933:41.

10. Articles 13 and 14, which concern breastfeeding, are discussed in Gelli 1931:558–59.

11. See Gelli 1931:527.

12. CFLI 1940:312.

13. Gabbi 1924:103.

14. See Bumm 1923; Vicarelli 1926b.

15. Mercurii (1601:189–90) provides illustrations of obstetrical instruments, such as single- or double-hooked tools for cutting the fetus "into pieces" and forceps for pushing and straightening the fetus or pulling it out by its mouth or eye cavities.

16. Cova 1939:15.

17. The cost of living fell from an index level of 100 in 1929 to 75.52 in 1934, but rose to 82.57 in 1936. Between 1929 and 1936, the average hourly wage fell from 2.02 to 1.74 lire for industrial workers and from 1.54 to 1.15 for male and 0.86 to 0.68 for female agricultural workers; indexed to 1929, the latter were 86.14, 74.68, and 79.07, respectively (DeMichelis 1937:90). Regarding peasant landownership and other economic matters, see Clark 1984:263–67; Quine 1996:37; regarding housing, see Grossi 1935:128.

18. Salvatori and Mira 1956:538–39.

19. Santandrea 1992:22; see Cova 1939:13; *Maternità e Infanzia* 1928, 3 (2): 153.

20. Vaccari 1984:244.

21. See Preti 1984:211.

22. Santandrea 1992:48. Regarding urban versus rural medical care, see Cenni 1965:38–40; Gelli 1931:525–26; Santandrea 1992:68–69.

23. See Borrino 1937:57–59, 167–69; Grossi 1931:173.

24. The inspection of 128 institutions for illegitimate infants took place in 1931. Only 53 were considered good, while 44 were rated as mediocre and 31 were found to be very bad. For a study of the conditions of infancy in a southern region, see Zanotti Bianco 1926.

25. Report on infant feeding and enteritis, Ufficio d'Igiene e sanità, 1936:3.

26. Borrino 1937:133; DeNapoli 1934b:416.

27. See *Maternità e Infanzia* 1933, 8 (3): 251. For an illustration showing various types of substitute milk or nutritional supplement, see Rasponi 1925.

28. Corsi 1937:39.

29. Fabbri 1933a:84.

30. Panunzio 1933:138.

31. Gaetano 1958:200.

32. Haydée 1934:257, 260.

33. ONMI 1962:84.

34. DeNapoli 1934b:415.

35. See ONMI 1962:88.

36. Cappuccio 1939; DeNapoli 1934a:168; Fabbri 1933a:105–17, 132–37; Vaccaro 1937:168.

37. Vaccaro 1937:167.

38. Gaetano 1958:181; see also ONMI 1962:107.

39. See Borrino 1937:686 for the notice she kept on her clinic door, offering prizes of children's clothing in recognition of good mothering.

40. See ONMI 1962:38.

41. Gaetano 1958:231.

42. ONMI 1962:42.

43. Zanelli 1939:26.

44. Health and social workers had to classify infants as gracile or robust on the forms they compiled (see, for example, Borrino 1937:829). Pende (1933a: 57–72) wrote at length about robustness as an indicator of health, and false versus true robustness in infants. Regarding the relationship between natural treatments and political demographic goals, see Gestri 1934; Saetti 1938.

45. *Maternità e Infanzia* 1928, 3 (2): 128.

46. Regarding the number of ONMI institutes and activities, employees, and mothers and infants served, see Biagi 1934:101–2; CFLI 1940:109–11, 318; Corsi 1937:46, 86–93; Garzanti Ravasi 1931b; Haydée 1934:305; LoMonaco-Aprile 1934:23–27, 30–31; ONMI 1962:187, 198, 216, 218–21, 226; Squadrilli 1929: 214–15.

47. Regarding ONMI's effectiveness (or lack thereof), see Cicotero 1967, 1970; Fabbri 1933a:84–88; Gravelli and Campanile 1933:87; LoMonaco-Aprile 1934:18–22; ONMI 1962:11–14; Vaccari 1984:244–45; Salvatorelli and Mira 1956:535–38.

48. LoMonaco-Aprile 1934:46.

49. Borrino 1937:310–11.

Chapter 7

1. Plasmon 1991:53.
2. Dana and Marion 1989:216.
3. Georg 1950:16–17, 62–64.
4. See Berneri and Zaccaria 1957:15; Dana and Marion 1989:221; Georg 1950:48–49; Lanfranchi 1955:xxxi; Marzetti, Enea, and Pecorini 1991:184.
5. Ferrari and Bonelli 1989:224.
6. I acquired a list of conditions treatable by thermal cures from the Ufficio Informazione e Accoglienza Turistica of the town of Castrocaro Terme (1991).
7. The product, "Euchessina," is advertised in *Educazione alla Salute* 1992:2.
8. Rocchi 1991.
9. Misura 1992.
10. Valli 1990:5.
11. Valli 1990:37.
12. In addition to the sources in note 1, see also Viganò 1992.
13. Prénatal 1992:315.
14. Romanini 1975:108.
15. Catteruccia 1962:92.
16. See, for example, Boschetti et al.1975:79.
17. Lentini 1953:252.
18. Lentini 1953:250.
19. Boschetti et al. 1975:75.
20. Ferrari and Bonelli 1989:49.
21. Boschetti et al. 1975:76.
22. See Boschetti et al. 1975:79; Generoso et al. 1994:69; Lentini 1953:253; Plasmon 1991:56–57.
23. Lentini 1953:251–52.
24. Boschetti et al. 1975:74.
25. Plasmon 1991:57.
26. Maglietta 1985:313.
27. See Lentini 1953:255–56; Maglietta 1985:313; Plasmon 1991:57; Romanini 1975:95.
28. *Avere un Bambino* 1992b:29.
29. Ferrari and Bonelli 1989:210.
30. Lentini 1953:271.
31. *Avere un Bambino* 1992d:54.
32. Boschetti et al. 1975:90, 92.
33. Plasmon 1991:63.
34. In Boschetti et al. 1975:86.

Chapter 8

1. Fornara 1952:14, 17.
2. Sorcinelli 1985:47.

3. Boschetti et al. 1975: cover page.
4. Dana and Marion 1989:49.
5. Ferrari and Bonelli 1989:193.
6. Miraglia, Orlandini, and Micheletti 1984:23.
7. See Dana and Marion 1989:180–83; Ferrari and Bonelli 1989:134–36, 140–41; Miraglia, Orlandini, and Micheletti 1984:18.
8. Dana and Marion 1989:11.
9. Plasmon 1991:54, 58.
10. See Lentini 1953:163.
11. Dana and Marion 1989:200; see Ferrari and Bonelli 1989:138–39; Luzi 1992:30–31.
12. Parazzini 1992:20, 22; Piccone 1994:23.
13. See Luzi 1992:31.
14. *Corriere Salute* 1992, Aug. 31, p. 32.
15. See Valli 1990:67–68.
16. Lentini 1953:260, 270–71; see also Olivi 1997:93.
17. Catteruccia 1962:90.
18. Lentini 1953:253.
19. Boschetti et al. 1975:82.
20. Miraglia, Orlandini, and Micheletti 1984:328.
21. For an impression of the rural environment and the persistence of share-cropping in Emilia-Romagna, see the stories by Guareschi (1948, 1963, among others).
22. See Martino 1990:223.
23. Origlia 1952:68.
24. See Federici 1984:75, 83–84. Molina, Monteverdi, and Del Boca (1990: 81) explain that women's employment is low in Italy at least in part because of a lack of part-time work and flexible work schedules.
25. See Federici 1984:102, 95–96. The discrepancy between women's and men's time spent working does not seem to have narrowed over the past two decades. Today, women work an average of 64 hours per week, combining paid and unpaid labor, whereas men work 55.8 hours. The countries in Europe with the lowest birthrates in the world, Spain and Italy, have the scarcest participation of men in household labor (Barbagli in Di Caro 1999).
26. See Scremin 1948.
27. See Berneri and Zaccaria 1957:13–27.
28. See Berneri and Zaccaria 1957:5; Modona 1978:324; Prénatal 1992: 34–35.
29. Federici 1984:67.
30. See Bocca 1990; Chianura 1990; Ronchey 1994.
31. See Paccagnella 1952:54.
32. I have borrowed this set of words from a story by Natalia Ginzburg (1977:89).
33. See Maglietta 1985:382.
34. In response to this common belief, Albani (1990:15) points out that Americans had abandoned rigid schedules and quantities of milk by the 1930s.

35. Pignedoli 1992:31.

36. Regarding this legislation, see Agnoli 1987; *Avere un Bambino* 1992a; Prénatal 1992:127–37.

37. Cicotero 1970:206.

38. A public health official showed me the file of a family under ONMI care in the 1950s. The mother had married at the age of 16, separated from her brutal and unstable husband, and become a prostitute. She now lived with a man who worked only occasionally and had a low IQ, as she did. She lived under a bridge over the Po, while all but two of her seven children were in institutions. ONMI's concern was not the mother, but the placement of her children.

39. Gatto 1952:88.

40. See Agostino 1952:124–25; Consiglio Nazionale Permanente per la Difesa dell'Infanzia 1952:6.

41. Buschi 1952:128; see Agostino 1952:124.

42. Ritossa 1962:127.

43. Consiglio Nazionale Permanente per la Difesa dell'Infanzia 1952; see also ONMI 1970b.

44. Carnevali 1952:118.

45. See ONMI 1967, 1970b; ONMI (ed.) 1962.

46. ONMI 1970b:13.

47. See Agazzi 1974 [1929–30].

48. See Lombardi 1989:32.

49. Dattilo 1990:149; ISTAT 1990:110.

50. Dattilo 1990:149.

Chapter 9

1. In this sense, they are social facts like Durkheim's moral regulations or legal codes (see Durkheim 1938:1–46).

2. Regarding common sense knowledge, see Geertz 1983:85–92.

3. See Turner 1967:19–47, as well as Martin 1987.

4. On symbols, see Obeyesekere 1981:13–21.

5. Dana and Marion 1989:111.

6. Ferrari and Bonelli 1989:187.

7. Ferrari and Bonelli 1989:82.

8. Dana and Marion 1989:215.

9. Lentini 1953:227.

10. Dana and Marion 1989:148.

11. Dana and Marion 1989:148.

12. See, for example, the cover of Prénatal 1992.

13. See Silone 1955 [1936]:101.

14. See Ferrari and Bonelli 1989:225.

15. *Avere un Bambino* 1992c:36.

16. See Albani 1990:60.

17. See Porciani 1992.

18. See Mendelsohn 1984:xv.

19. In *Avere un Bambino* 1992, 94:118.

20. In *Educazione alla Salute* 1992, 4:52 (back cover).

21. See D'Amico 1994; Diena 1994.

22. See the advertisement in *Avere un Bambino* 1992, 94:33.

23. For a general discussion of this phenomenon, see Scheper-Hughes and Lock 1987.

Glossary

aborto: loss of embryo or fetus either spontaneous or procured
agalattia: lack of milk
allattare/allattamento: to breastfeed/breast-feeding
allevatore: breeder
asilo: day-care center
assistente sanitaria: health worker

balia: wet nurse
bonifica: reclamation
bracciante: day laborer
brefotrofio: foundling home

capoparto: return of menstruation after childbirth
colonia: camp
colpo di aria/colpo di vento: draft/gust of wind
comare: folk midwife
comune: town and surrounding areas
cottione: coction, cooking

divezzamento/divezzare/divezzo: weaning/to wean/weaned child
doppia pesata: double weighing

febbre lattea: milk fever

governo: direction (of children)

integrale/integrare: whole or complete/to complete; i.e., to supplement in
    reference to breast-feeding
ipogalattia: insufficient milk production

latifondo: large agricultural concern employing day laborers
latte/lattante: milk/nursling
levatrice: midwife
libero professionista: liberal professional, e.g., surgeon

medico/medico condotto: physician/district physician
la miseria: connotes poverty, ignorance, ill health, disempowerment

nipiologia: the discipline dealing with the care of the nursling
nutrice: nursing mother or wet nurse

opoterapia: replacement therapy
orario/orari: schedule/standardized feeding times
ostetrica: midwife

padrone: landowner
parto/partoriente: childbirth/woman in childbirth
patria: fatherland
poppata/poppare/poppante: infant meal/to suck milk (breast or
    bottle)/infant who takes milk
puericultura: the discipline dealing with the care of mothers and infants

quarantena: the puerperium, lasting 40 days

razza: race
ruota: wheel, revolving church door (where babies were abandoned)

sindacato: union; labor/management organization under fascism
stirpe: stock, breeding population

visitatrice: health or social worker who makes home visits
volontà: self-will

References

Adami, Hans-Olov, et al.
1994 Parity, age at first childbirth, and risk of ovarian cancer. *Lancet* 344:1250–54.

Agazzi, Rosa
1974 [1929–30] *Guida per le educatrici dell'infanzia.* Brescia: La Scuola.

Agnoli, Mario, ed.
1987 *Codice della maternità. La legislazione demografica dello Stato in materia di matrimonio e maternità.* 2d ed. Rimini: Maggioli.

Agostino, Renata
1952 Untitled contribution. In Consiglio Nazionale Permanente per la Difesa dell'Infanzia 1952, 124–25.

Albani, Roberto
1990 *Capire tuo figlio.* Milan: Eurotrend.

Aniansson, G., et al.
1994 A prospective cohort study on breast-feeding and otitis media in Swedish infants. *Pediatric Infectious Disease Journal* 13:183–88.

Antoniotti, Ferdinando
1982 Matrimonio. In *Enciclopedia Medica Italiana,* vol. 9. 2d ed., 507–14. Florence: Edizioni Scientifiche.

Ardali, Paolo
1943 *La politica demografica di Mussolini.* Mantua: Franco Paladino.

Ascoli, Giulietta
1994 *Balie.* Palermo: Sellerio.

L'Asilo Infantile di Forlì
1912 *Resoconto degli esercizi 1909–1910.* Forlì: G.B. Croppi.

Auerbach, Kathleen, Jan Riordan, and Betty Ann Countryman
1993 The breastfeeding process. In Jan Riordan and Kathleen Auerbach, eds., 215–52.

Avere un Bambino
1992a Maternità e lavoro. Supplement to *Io e il mio Bambino* 94:119–28.
1992b Primo mese. Supplement to *Io e il mio Bambino* 94:29–32.
1992c Secondo mese. Supplement to *Io e il mio Bambino* 94:35–38.
1992d Quinto mese. Supplement to *Io e il mio Bambino* 94:53–56.

Babini, Paolo
1856 *Del brefotrofio degli esposti di Faenza e della Chiesa di Santa Maria anticamente detta Foris Portem.* Faenza: P. Conti.

Baldini, Eraldo
  1991   *Riti del nascere. Gravidanza, parto e battesimo nella cultura popolare romagnola.* Ravenna: Longo.
Ballotta, Francesco
  1857   *Igiene popolare.* Ravenna: Ven. Seminario Arcivio.
Balocchi, Vincenzo
  1847   *Manuale completo di ostetricia.* Florence: Giorgio Steininger.
Banfield, Edward C.
  1958   *The moral basis of a backward society.* Glencoe, IL: Free Press.
Barbagli, Marzio
  1984   *Sotto lo stesso tetto: mutamenti della famiglia in Italia dal XV al XX secolo.* Bologna: Il Mulino.
Battara, Pietro
  1935   *Fattori psicologici e morali di denatalità.* Florence: Le Monnier.
Battelli, Giuseppe
  1909   *La guerra tra il pane e l'amore colla critica e igiene dei sistemi antifecondativi e descrizione di un nuovo sistema.* Rome: Cooperativa Sociale.
Bellettini, Athos
  1987   *La popolazione italiana. Un profilo storico.* Turin: Einaudi.
Berneri, Giovanna, and Cesare Zaccaria
  1957   *Controllo delle nascite. Mezzi pratici per avere figli solo quando si vogliono.* Milan: ETOS.
Bertaccini, Colombano
  1922   *Nozioni elementari d'igiene ad uso delle scuole e delle famiglie.* Bologna: Cappelli.
Bertarelli, Ernesto
  1936   *Difendi te stesso. Guida alla conoscenza del corpo umano.* Milan: Fratelli Treves.
Biagi, Bruno
  1934   La madre ed il fanciullo nella concezione sociale del fascismo. *Civiltà Fascista* 1 (2): 97–110.
Bocca, Giorgio
  1990   Italiani, crescete e moltiplicatevi. *La Repubblica,* 6 June, 8.
Boldrini, Marcello
  1933   La fertilità delle classi povere. *L'Economia Italiana* 1:92–95.
Bompiani, R.
  1939   La sifilide ereditaria nella genesi dei disordini mestruali. *La Preparazione Materna* 1 (1): 17–21.
Borrino, Angiola
  1937   *Puericoltura ed assistenza sanitaria dell'infanzia.* Turin: UTET.
Boschetti, Enrico, Rita Dorigo, Valeriana Girolami, and Luisa Paschini
  1975   *Professione donna.* Vol. 3. Milan: Fratelli Fabbri.
Brefotrofio degli Esposti di Faenza
  1865   *Regolamento.* Faenza: Brefotrofio degli Esposti di Faenza.
Breschi, Marco, and Massimo Livi Bacci
  1986   Stagione di nascita e clima come determinanti della mortalità infantile. *Genus* 42 (1–2): 87–101.

Bumm, Ernesto
1923a *Trattato completo di ostetricia.* Vol. 1. Milan: Società Editrice Libraria.
1923b *Trattato completo di ostetricia.* Vol. 2. Milan: Società Editrice Libraria.
Buschi, Renato
1952 Untitled contribution. In Consiglio Nazionale Permanente per la Difesa dell'Infanzia, ed., 128.
Cambi, Franco
1988 I medici-igienisti e l'infanzia: controllo del corpo e ideologia borghese. In *Storia dell'infanzia nell'età liberale,* Franco Cambi and Simonetta Ulivieri, 53–80. Florence: La Nuova Italia.
Camprini, Italo
1978 *Canta la cicala taglia taglia: il grano al padrone al contadino la paglia.* Milan: Emme.
Cappuccio, Achille
1939 *La legislazione demografica.* Cuneo: Bertello.
Caratozzolo, Annunziato
1933 *Lo stato allevatore.* Naples: Alberto Morano.
Carli, Filippo
1933 Popolazione e richezza. *L'Economia Italiana* 1:57–60.
Carnevali, Piera
1952 Untitled contribution. In Consiglio Nazionale Permanente per la Difesa dell'Infanzia, ed., 117–19.
Carozzi, Luigi
1914a *Il lavoro nell'igiene—nella patologia—nell'assistenza sociale.* Vol. I. Florence: G. Barbera.
1914b *Il lavoro nell'igiene—nella patologia—nell'assistenza sociale.* Vol. II. Florence: G. Barbera.
Cassidy, Claire M.
1980 Nutrition and health in agriculturalists and hunter-gatherers. In *Nutritional Anthropology,* Norge Jerome, Randy Kandel, and Gretel H. Pelto, eds., 182–96. Pleasantville, NY: Redgrave.
Catteruccia, Crispino
1962 Igiene del lattante. In Opera Nazionale per la Protezione della Maternità e dell'Infanzia, ed., 88–93.
Cecchi, Ettorina
1910 *Come non aver figli. Teoria-pratica-consigli-metodi.* 6th ed. Florence: Il Pensiero.
Cenni, Gaspare
1965 *Diario di condotta.* Bologna: T.E.G.
Chianura, Carlo
1990 Martelli agli italiani "Dovete fare più figli" "E agli immigrati diamo il voto." *La Repubblica,* 5 June, 23.
Cicotero, Amilcare
1967 Maternità e infanzia (opera nazionale). *Nuovissimo Digesto Italiano* 10:325–28. Turin: UTET.

1970 Protezione della maternità e infanzia. *Grande Dizionario Enciclopedico* UTET, vol. 7, 206–7. Turin: UTET.

Clark, Martin
1984 *Modern Italy, 1871–1982.* New York: Longman.

Cohen, Mark Nathan
1989 *Health and the rise of civilization.* New Haven: Yale University Press.

Comune di Faenza
1882 *Censimento della popolazione,* vol. 8. Faenza: Comune di Faenza.

Comune di Forlì, ed.
1989 *Ad immagine e somiglianze. Riflessioni sull'infanzia in Romagna ed oltre.* Forlì: Comune di Forlì.

Confederazione Fascista dei Lavoratori dell'Industria (CFLI)
1940 *La cultura del lavoratore.* Florence: Lya L.

Consiglio Nazionale Permanente per la Difesa dell'Infanzia, ed.
1952 *La situazione dell'infanzia in Italia.* Rome: Tipografia dell'Orso.

Consiglio, Vincenzo
1933 La sterilità delle classi ricche. *L'Economia Italiana* 1:81–87.

Corsi, Pietro
1937 *La tutela della maternità e dell'infanzia in Italia.* Rome: Società Editrice di Novissima.

Coruzzi, Cesare
1933 Urbanesimo e sterilità. *L'Economia Italiana* 1:65–68.

Cova, Ercole
1939 La medicina ai servizi della politica demografica nello Stato Fascista. *La Preparazione Materna* 1 (1): 13–16.

Cunningham, Allan S.
1995 Breastfeeding: Adaptive behavior for child health and longevity. In P. Stuart-Macadam and K. Dettwyler, eds., 243–64.

Daly, S. E. J., and P. E. Hartmann
1995a Infant demand and milk supply. Part I: Infant demand and milk production in lactating women. *Journal of Human Lactation* 11 (1): 21–26.
1995b Infant demand and milk supply. Part II: The short-term control of milk synthesis in lactating women. *Journal of Human Lactation* 11 (1): 27–37.

Dambrosio, Francesco
1976 Maternità, contraccezione, aborto: problema di classe. In *Maternità cosciente,* F. Dambrosio, E. Badaracco, and M. Buscaglia, eds., 23–44. Milan: G. Mazzotti.

D'Amico, Arnaldo
1994 Il problema di una coppia su cinque. *La Repubblica,* 4 July, p. 23.

Dana, Jacqueline, and Silvia Marion
1989 *Avere un figlio. Nove mesi di vita della coppia.* Milan: Feltrinelli.

Dattilo, Cosetta
1990 Una mostra storico-pedagogica sull'infanzia fra otto e novecento. *Bollettino dell'Istituto Storico della Resistenza* 1:143–52.

Dau Novelli, Cecilia
 1994 *Famiglia e modernizzazione in Italia tra le due guerre.* Rome: Edizioni Studium.
Davis, Margarett K., David A. Savitz, and Barry I. Graubard
 1988 Infant feeding and childhood cancer. *Lancet* 2:365–68.
DeBernardi, Alberto
 1984 *Il mal della rosa. Denutrizione e pellagra nelle campagne italiane fra '800 e '900.* Milan: Angeli.
DeCarvalho, M., et al.
 1983 Effect of frequent breast-feeding on early milk production and infant weight gain. *Pediatrics* 72:307–11.
DeFelice, Renzo
 1977 *Interpretations of Fascism.* Cambridge, MA: Harvard University Press.
DeGrazia, Victoria
 1992 *How fascism ruled women.* Berkeley: University of California Press.
Della Peruta, Franco
 1980 Sanità pubblica e legislazione sanitaria dall'Unità a Crispi. *Studi Storici* 4:713–59.
DeLucca, Oreste
 1983 Mortalità infantile e condizioni sociali nella periferia riminese fra il 1714 e il 1915. *Romagna Arte e Storia* 3 (7): 99–114.
DeMichelis, Giuseppe
 1937 *Alimentazione e giustizia sociale.* Rome: Istituto Nazionale di Cultura Fascista.
DeNapoli, Ferdinando
 1934a *Da Malthus a Mussolini.* Vol. 1. Bologna: Cappelli.
 1934b *Da Malthus a Mussolini.* Vol. 2. Bologna: Cappelli.
Dettwyler, Katherine A.
 1995a Beauty and the breast: The cultural context of breastfeeding in the United States. In P. Stuart-Macadam and K. Dettwyler, eds., 167–216.
 1995b A time to wean: The hominid blueprint for the natural age of weaning in modern human populations. In P. Stuart-Macadam and K. Dettwyler, eds., 39–74.
Di Caro, Roberto
 1999 È uno sciopero di protesta (interview with Marzío Barbagli). *L'Espresso* 44 (11): 32–34.
Diena, Daniele
 1994 La sterilità non fa più paura. *La Repubblica,* 4 July, 23.
DuBoulay, Juliet, and R. Williams
 1987 Amoral familism and the image of the limited good: A critique from a Mediterranean perspective. *Anthropological Quarterly* 60:12–24.
Durham, William H.
 1991 *Coevolution: Genes, culture, and human diversity.* Stanford: Stanford University Press.

Durkheim, Emile
1938   *The rules of sociological method.* 8th ed. New York: Free Press.
Eaton, S. Boyd, et al.
1994   Women's reproductive cancers in evolutionary perspective. *Quarterly Review of Biology* 69 (3): 353–67.
Eaton, S. Boyd, Melvin Konner, and Marjorie Shostak
1988a   *The paleolithic prescription.* New York: Harper and Row.
1988b   Stone agers in the fast lane: Chronic degenerative diseases in evolutionary perspective. *American Journal of Medicine* 84:739–49.
Ellison, Peter T.
1995   Breastfeeding, fertility, and maternal condition. In P. Stuart-Macadam and K. Dettwyler, eds., 305–46.
Ewald, Paul W.
1988   Cultural vectors, virulence, and the emergence of evolutionary epidemiology. *Oxford Surveys in Evolutionary Biology* 5:215–45.
1994   *Evolution of infectious disease.* New York: Oxford University Press.
Fabbri, Sileno
1933a   *L'assistenza della maternità e dell'infanzia in Italia.* Milan: Chiurazzi e Figlio.
1933b   La difesa della famiglia e della stirpe. *L'Economia Italiana* 1:140–42.
1933c   *L'Opera Nazionale per la Protezione della Maternità e dell'Infanzia.* Milan: Mondadori.
Federici, Nora
1984   *Procreazione, famiglia, lavoro della donna.* Turin: Loescher.
Ferrari, Maria Pia, and Paolo Bonelli
1989   *La gravidanza. Nove mesi da vivere bene.* Milan: Mondadori.
Fildes, Valerie
1986   *Breasts, bottles, and babies: A history of infant feeding.* Edinburgh: Edinburgh University Press.
1995   The culture and biology of breastfeeding: An historical review of Western Europe. In P. Stuart- Macadam and K. Dettwyler, eds., 101–26.
Forgacs, David
1990   *Italian culture in the industrial era, 1880–1980: Cultural industries, politics, and the public.* Manchester: Manchester University Press.
Forleo, Romano, and Giulia Forleo
1989   *Figlio figlia. Guida a una gravidanza e a un parto felice.* Milan: Feltrinelli.
Fornara, Piero
1952   L'urgenza dei provvedimenti sanitari a favore dell'infanzia. In Consiglio Nazionale Permanente per la Difesa dell'Infanzia, ed., 14–20.
Foucault, Michel
1973   *The birth of the clinic: An archeology of medical perception.* New York: Pantheon.
1973   [1965] *Madness and civilization: A history of insanity in the age of reason.* New York: Vintage.

Frederickson, Doren
    1995   Commentary. Breastfeeding study design problems—health policy, epidemiologic and pediatric perspectives. In P. Stuart-Macadam and K. Dettwyler, eds., 405–18.

Freed, Gary L., Sarah J. Clark, James Sorenson, Jacob A. Lohr, Robert Cefalo, and Peter Curtis
    1995   National assessment of physicians' breast-feeding knowledge, attitudes, training, and experience. *Journal of the American Medical Association* 273 (6): 472–76.

Gabbi, Umberto
    1924   *Per il fascismo.* Milan: Istituto Editoriale Scientifico.

Gaetano, G. Paolo
    1958   *Codice della beneficenza ed assistenza pubblica.* Rome: Jandi Sapi.

Gale, Catharine R., and Christopher N. Martyn
    1996   Breastfeeding, dummy use, and adult intelligence. *Lancet* 347: 1072–75.

Garzanti Ravasi, Sofia
    1931a *Inchiesta sulle condizioni dell'infanzia. La Lombardia.* Vol. 1. Florence: Vallechi.
    1931b *Inchiesta sulle condizioni dell'infanzia. La Lombardia.* Vol. 2. Florence: Vallechi.

Gatto, Simone
    1952   Untitled contribution. In Consiglio Nazionale Permanente per la Difesa dell'Infanzia, ed., 86–89.

Geertz, Clifford
    1983. *Local knowledge.* New York: Basic Books.

Gelli, Gino
    1931   *La guida medica. Ad uso delle donne spose e madri.* Florence: Bemporad.

Gemelli, Agostino
    1933   La "sterilizzazione coattiva e preventiva" nell'insegnamento degli studiosi italiani. *L'Economia Italiana* 1:117–28.

Generoso, Massimo, Paolo Becherucci, Silvia Pettini, and Vincenza Gancitano
    1994   *Puericultura neonatologia pediatria con assistenza.* Florence: S.E.E.

Georg, J. E.
    1950   *Agenesi e fecondità nel matrimonio. Il controllo delle nascite mediante la continenza periodica secondo il metodo Ogino-Knaus.* Turin: Marietti.

Gestri, Romano
    1934   Le cure idro-climato-talassologiche nella battaglia per l'incremento demografico. *Rivista di Idroclimatologia, Tassologia, e Terapia Fisica II.*

Gini, Corrado
    1930   *Nascita, evoluzione e morte delle nazioni. La teoria ciclica della popolazione e i vari sistemi di politica demografica. Quaderni dell'Istituto Nazionale Fascista di Cultura.* Rome: Libreria del Littorio.

Ginzburg, Natalia
    1947   *È stato così.* Turin: Einaudi.
    1963   *Lessico famigliare.* Turin: Einaudi.
    1964   [1944] Inverno in Abruzzo. In *Le piccole virtù,* Natalia Ginzburg. Turin: Einaudi.
    1977   *Famiglia.* Turin: Einaudi.
Gordini, Gian Domenico
    1961   Agata, santa, martire. *Bibliotheca Sanctorum,* 320–27. Rome: Istituto Giovanni XXIII nella Pontificia Università Lateranense.
Gravelli, Asvero, and A. Campanile
    1933   *Primi elementi di cultura fascista.* Florence: Vallecchi.
Grossi, Giuseppe
    1935   *Legge e potenza del numero.* Bologna: Zanichelli.
Guareschi, Giovannino
    1948   *Don Camillo.* Milan: Rizzoli.
    1963   *Il compagno Don Camillo.* Milan: Rizzoli.
Gussler, J., and L. Briesemeister
    1980   The insufficient milk syndrome: A biocultural explanation. *Medical Anthropology* 4 (2): 145–74.
Gusso, Aldo
    1930   *Sulla natura e sul trattamento delle amenorrea, con particolare riguardo alla idroterapia salsoiodica.* Ancona: Ospedale Civile Umberto I.
Hastrup, Kirsten
    1992   A question of reason: Breast-feeding patterns in seventeenth- and eighteenth-century Iceland. In V. Maher, ed., 91–108.
Haydée
    1933   *Il libro della mamma e del bambino.* Trieste: Casa Editrice Triestina.
Horn, David G.
    1994   *Social bodies: Science, reproduction, and Italian modernity.* Princeton: Princeton University Press.
Ing, Roy, Nicholas L. Petrakis, and J. H. C. Ho
    1977   Unilateral breast feeding and breast cancer. *Lancet* 2 (8029): 124–27.
Ipsen, Carl
    1996   *Dictating Demography: The problem of population in Fascist Italy.* New York: Cambridge University Press.
Istituto Nazionale Previdenza Sociale (INPS)
    1980   *Mezzo secolo di attività assicurativa e assistenziale (1898–1948).* Rome: INPS.
Istituto Centrale di Statistica (ISTAT)
    1962   *Annuario di statistiche demografiche.* Vol. IX. Rome: A.B.E.T.E.
    1983   *12ismo censimento generale della popolazione 25 ottobre 1981.* Vol. 2. *Dati sulle caratteristiche strutturali della popolazione e delle abitazioni.* Rome: ISTAT.
    1990   *Annuario statistico italiano.* Rome: ISTAT.
    1991   *Le regioni in cifre.* Rome: Rubbettino.
    1992   *Statistiche demografiche.* Vol. 35/36, tome 2, part 1. Rome: Rubinetto.

1996 *Conoscere l'Italia.* Rome: ISTAT.

1997 *Annuario statistico italiano 1997.* Rome: ISTAT.

Jolly, Alison

1985 *The evolution of primate behavior.* 2d ed. New York: MacMillan.

Kertzer, David I.

1984 *Family life in Central Italy, 1880–1910: Sharecropping, wage labor, and coresidence.* New Brunswick, NJ: Rutgers University Press.

1993 *Sacrificed for honor: Italian infant abandonment and the politics of reproductive control.* Boston: Beacon Press.

Khatib-Chahidi, Jane

1992 *Milk kinship in Shi'ite Islamic Iran.* In V. Maher, ed., 109–32.

Klapisch-Zuber, Christine

1985 *Women, family, and ritual in Renaissance Florence.* Chicago: University of Chicago Press.

Knodel, John

1977 Family limitation and fertility transition: Evidence from the age patterns of fertility in Europe and Asia. *Population Studies* 31:219–49.

Konner, Melvin

1972 Aspects of the developmental etiology of a foraging people. In *Ethnological studies of child behavior,* N. Blurton Jones, ed., 285–304. Cambridge: Cambridge University Press.

Konner, Melvin, and Marjorie Shostak

1987 Timing and management of birth among the !Kung: Biocultural interaction in reproductive adaptation. *Cultural Anthropology* 2 (1): 11–28.

Konner, Melvin, and C. Super

1987 Sudden Infant Death Syndrome: An anthropological hypothesis. Reprint, Academic Press, Inc., 95–108.

Konner, Melvin, and Carol Worthman

1980 Nursing frequency, gonadal function, and birth spacing among !Kung hunter-gatherers. *Science* 207:788–91.

Kunitz, Stephen J.

1991 The personal physician and the decline of mortality. In R. Schofield, D. Reher, and A. Bideau, eds., 248–61.

Labriola, Teresa

1918 *I problemi sociali della donna.* Bologna: Tanichelli.

Lambe, M., C. C. Hsieh, D. Trichopoulos, A. Ekbom, M. Pavia, and H. O. Adami

1994 Transient increase in breast cancer following birth. *New England Journal of Medicine* 331:5–9.

Lanfranchi, Luciana

1955 Guida alla vita coniugale. Insert to no. 18 of *Bella,* no. 4.

Lanting, C. I., V. Filder, M. Huisman, B. C. L. Touwen, and E. R. Boersma

1994 Neurological differences between 9-year-old children fed breast-milk or formula-milk as babies. *Lancet* 344:1319–22.

LaVecchia, Carlo

1991 Il carcinoma della mammella. *Dizionario della Salute* 11:253–55.

1992 Oral contraceptives and breast cancer. *Breast* 1:76–81.

Lawrence, Ruth A.
  1994   *Breastfeeding: A guide for the medical profession.* 4th ed. St. Louis:
         C. V. Mosby.
Lee, Richard Borshay
  1979   The !Kung San: Men, women, and work in a foraging society. New
         York: Cambridge University Press.
Lentini, Diego
  1953   *Matrimonio e maternità.* Bologna: Cappelli.
Levi, Carlo
  1947   *Christ stopped at Eboli.* New York: Time.
Livi Bacci, Massimo
  1983   Ebrei, aristocratici e cittadini: precursori del declino della fecondità.
         Quaderni Storici 54/a.18 (3): 913–39.
  1986   Fertility, nutrition and pellagra: Italy during the vital revolution. *Jour-
         nal of Interdisciplinary History* 16 (3).
  1990   *Population and nutrition: An essay on European demographic history.*
         Cambridge: Cambridge University Press.
Lombardi, Bruno
  1989   Scuola dell'infanzia dall'assistenza al progetto pedagogico. In Comune
         di Forlì, ed., 20–33.
LoMonaco-Aprile, Attilio
  1934   *La protezione della maternità e dell'infanzia.* Rome: Istituto Nazionale
         Fascista di Cultura.
Lorenzoni, Andrea
  1933   L'impiego delle donne nell'industria e sue conseguenze sulla natalità.
         L'Economia Italiana 1:29–73.
Lucas, A., R. Morley, T. J. Cole, G. Lister, and C. Leeson-Payne
  1992   Breast milk and subsequent intelligence quotient in children born pre-
         term. *Lancet* 339:261–64.
Lunn, Peter G.
  1991   Nutrition, immunity and infection. In R. Schofield, D. Reher, and
         A. Bideau, eds., 131–45.
Luzi, Ernesto
  1992   Nascere in famiglia. *L'Educatore Sanitario* 1:30–31.
Lyttelton, Adrian
  1988   *The seizure of power: Fascism in Italy, 1919–1929.* 2d ed. Princeton:
         Princeton University Press.
Mack Smith, Denis
  1969   *Italy: A modern history.* Ann Arbor: University of Michigan Press.
Maglietta, Vittorio
  1985   *Puericultura. Pediatria preventiva e sociale.* 2d ed. Milan: Ambrosiana.
  1989   *Terapia pediatrica pratica.* 2d ed. Milan: Ambrosiana.
Maher, Vanessa
  1992   Breast-feeding in cross-cultural perspective: Paradoxes and proposals.
         In V. Maher, ed., 1–36.

Maher, Vanessa, ed.
 1992 *The anthropology of breastfeeding.* Oxford: Berg.

Mandini, Antonio
 1805 *L'infanzia.* Rimini: Marsoner.

Maraviglia, Maurizio
 1929 *Momenti di vita italiana.* Rome: Linciana.

Marconcini, Federico
 1935 *Culle vuote.* Como: Cavalleri.
 1937 *Perché la patria viva.* Turin: Benuti.

Mariotti, Gaspare
 1896 *Istituto materno infantile. Progetto di un nuovo ordinamento degli istituti infantili in Italia.* Girgenti: Cav. Carini e Sorella.

Martin, Emily
 1987 *The woman in the body: A cultural analysis of reproduction.* Boston: Beacon Press.

Martino, Antonio
 1990 Il "Welfare State": a vantaggio di chi? In *Le paure del mondo industriale,* S. Ricossa, ed., 199–226. Bari: Laterza.

Marzetti, Luigi, Domenico Enea, and Francesco Pecorini
 1991 *Manuale di ginecologia e ostetricia.* 2d ed. Rome: Edizioni Universitarie Romane.

McKenna, James J.
 1996 Sudden Infant Death Syndrome: Making sense of current research. *Mothering,* no. 81 (winter): 73–80.
 1986 An anthropological perspective on the Suddent Infant Death Syndrome (SIDS): The role of parental breathing cues and speech breathing adaptations. *Medical Anthropology* 10 (1): 9–53.

McKenna, James J., and Nicole J. Bernshaw
 1995 Breastfeeding and infant-parent co-sleeping as adaptive strategies: Are they protective against SIDS? In P. Stuart-Macadam and K. Dettwyler, eds., 265–304.

McKenna, J., and S. Mosko
 1990 Evolution and the Sudden Infant Death Syndrome (SIDS). Part 3: Infant arousal and parent-infant co-sleeping. *Human Nature* 1 (3): 291–330.

McKeown, Thomas
 1979 *The role of medicine: Dream, mirage, or nemesis?* Princeton: Princeton University Press.

Mendelsohn, Robert S.
 1984 *How to raise a healthy child . . . in spite of your doctor.* New York: Ballantine Books.

Mercurii, S. Scipion
 1601 *La commare o riccoglitrice.* Venice: Giovanni Battista Giotti.

Mestecky, Jiri, Claudia Blair, and Pearay L. Ogra, eds.
 1991 *Immunology of milk and the neonate.* New York: Plenum Press.

Michels, Roberto
1933   Le classi medie e la natalità. *L'Economia Italiana* 1:88–91.
Micozzi, Marc S.
1995   Breast cancer, reproductive biology, and breastfeeding. In P. Stuart-Macadam and K. Dettwyler, eds., 347–84.
Millard, Ann V.
1990   The place of the clock in pediatric advice: Rationales, cultural themes, and impediments to breastfeeding. *Social Science and Medicine* 31 (2): 211–21.
Miraglia, Ferruccio, Ezio Orlandini, and Giuseppe Micheletti
1984   *Sarò madre. La donna dall'adolescenza alla maternità.* Milan: Rizzoli.
Misura
1992   Informazioni nutrizionali. Il benessere vien mangiando. *Corriere Salute* 4 (31): 9.
Modona, Guido Neppi
1978   Tutela penale della maternità. *Enciclopedia Europea,* vol. 7, 324. Milan: Garzanti.
Molina, S., S. Monteverdi, and D. Del Boca
1990   Il lavoro. In *Il futuro degli italiani. Demografia, economia e società verso il nuovo secolo,* Fondazione Giovanni Agnelli, ed., 51–94. Turin: Fondazione Giovanni Agnelli.
Morel, Marie-France
1991   The care of children: The influence of medical innovation and medical institutions on infant mortality, 1750–1914. In R. Schofield, D. Reher, and A. Bideau, eds., 196–219.
Mortara, Giorgio
1933   La fecondità dei matrimoni in Italia nel 1930 e nel 1905. *L'Economia Italiana* 1:36–37.
Mussolini, Benito
1928   Prefazione. In *Regresso delle nascite: morte dei popoli,* Riccardo Korherr, 7–30. Rome: Libreria del Littorio.
1933   Urbanesimo e denatalità. *L'Economia Italiana* 1:56.
National Center for Health Statistics
1997   Health, United States 1996–97 and Injury Chartbook. Hyattsville, MD: National Center for Health Statistics.
Nesse, Randolph M., and George C. Williams
1994   *Why we get sick: The new science of Darwinian medicine.* New York: Random House.
Obeyesekere, Gananath
1981   *Medusa's hair: An essay on personal symbols and religious experience.* Chicago: University of Chicago Press.
Olivi, Alessandra
1997   Mangiare "per due" o mangiare "quel che c'è". Regimi alimentari della madre in Italia (1930–1950). In *Donne e microcosmi culturali,* Adriana Destro, ed., 77–106. Bologna: Pàtron.
Omran, Abdel
1971   The epidemiologic transition. A theory of the epidemiology of population change. *Milbank Memorial Fund Quarterly* 49 (4): 509–38.

Opera Nazionale per la Protezione della Maternità e dell'Infanzia (ONMI)

1962   *L'Opera Nazionale per la Protezione della Maternità e dell'Infanzia dalla sua fondazione.* Rome: ONMI.

1967   *Regolamento organico del personale impiegatizio.* Rome: Vichi e Pinzi.

1970a *Libretto sanitario infantile.* Rome: ONMI.

1970b *Norme sul funzionamento delle istituzioni Onmi.* Rome: Ugo Quintily.

Opera Nazionale per la Protezione della Maternità e dell'Infanzia (ONMI), ed.

1962   *Primo seminario di studio e di informazione per le assistenti sociali dell'O.N.M.I.* Rome: Carlo Colombo.

Origlia, Dino

1952   La difesa del fanciullo nella famiglia. In Consiglio Nazionale Permanente per la Difesa all'Infanzia, ed., 67–76.

Paccagnella, Elsa Bergamaschi.

1952   Il dovere sociale dell'assistenza all'infanzia. In Consiglio Nazionale Permanente per la Difesa all'Infanzia, ed., 52–58.

P.P.

1660   *Choice proverbs and dialogues in Italian and English. Also, delightfull stories and apophthegms, taken out of famous Gucciardine.* London: E.C.

Palmieri, Vincenzo

1935   *Denatalità—La grande insidia sociale vista da un medico.* Milan: Società Palermitana Editrice Medica.

Pandolfelli, G., G. Scarpello, M. Stella Richter, and G. Dallari

1939   *Codice civile,* vol. 1. Milan: A. Giuffre.

Panunzio, Sergio

1933   L'azione morale e legislativa. *L'Economia Italiana* 1:135–39.

Parazzini, Fabio

1992   Abuso di cesareo? *Educazione alla Salute* 4:20–22.

Pende, Nicola

1933a *Bonifica umana razionale e biologia politica.* Bologna: Cappelli.

1933b Eugenica e politica demografica. *L'Economia Italiana* 1:113–16.

1939   La donna totale. Maternità fisiologica e maternità spirituale. *La Preparazione Materna* 1 (1): 2–4.

Piccone, Marina

1994   Mi sono accovacciata e Paolo è sguasciato fuori. *La Repubblica,* 4 July, 22–23.

Pignedoli, Tito

1992   La nonna ha torto quando. . . . *Educazione alla Salute* 4:31.

Pini, Giorgio

1923   *Famiglia e matrimonio.* Milan: Imperia.

Plasmon

1991   *È nato. Manuale di puericultura per i primi anni di vita del bambino.* 8th ed. Milan: Scotti Bassani.

Porciani, Franca

1992   Tutti i geni col latte di mamma. *Corriere Salute* 4 (8): 2–3.

Prénatal

1992   *La guida Prénatal alla nascita. Le cose da sapere da fare da decidere quando si fa un bambino.* Milan: Arcadia.

Preti, Domenico
1984   Le condizioni di vita: la tutela della salute (durante il ventennio fascista). In Roberto Finzi, ed., 203–13.
1987   *La modernizzazione corporativa (1922–1940)*. Milan: Franco Angeli.
Prosperini, Ferdinando
1954   *L'ostetrica e la sua missione*. Rome: Studium.
Quant, Sara A.
1995   Sociocultural aspects of the lactation process. In P. Stuart-Macadam and K. Dettwyler, eds., 127–44.
Quine, Maria Sophia
1996   *Population politics in twentieth-century Europe: Fascist dictatorships and liberal democracies*. London: Routledge.
Rabaglietti, Giuseppe
1935   *Le istituti del regime*. Bologna: Nerozzi.
Rasponi, Contessa Augusta
1914   *La mia statistica. Piccolo studio sull'allevamento dei bambini*. Bologna: Stabil. Poligrafico Emiliano.
1925 (ca.) *Rosee pagine di Gugù, ai cari bambini appena nati*. Published by author.
Regno d'Italia
1921   Libretto di Famiglia. Forlì: Stab. Tip. Romagnolo della Rivista "Lo Stato Civile Italiano."
Resinelli, Giuseppe
1926   Alterazioni funzionali dell'utero nella gravidanza e nel parto. In *Trattato di ostetricia*, vol. II, Innocente Clivio, ed., 91–122. Milan: Casa Editrice Dottor Francesco Vallardi.
Riordan, Jan, and Kathleen Auerbach, eds.
1993   *Breastfeeding and human lactation*. Boston: Jones and Bartlett.
Ritossa, Pio
1962   La profilassi delle malattie infettive quale strumento di prevenzione sociale. In Opera Nazionale per la Protezione della Maternità e dell'Infanzia, ed., 126–35.
Rocchi, Francesca
1991   Per scordare il pancione. *Corriere Salute*, 9 December, 10.
Romanini, Carlo
1975   *Professione donna*. Vol. 12. Milan: Fratelli Fabbri.
Ronchey, Alberto
1994   Il mondo a conclave sulla bomba demografica. *La Repubblica* 19 (197): 1, 4.
Rosetti, Emilio
1894   *La Romagna. Geografia e storia*. Milan: Hoepli.
Saetti, Andrea
1938   *Igiene e natura o igiene naturale*. Milan: Fratelli Bocca.
Salvatorelli, Luigi, and Giovanni Mira
1956   *Storia d'Italia nel periodo fascista*. Turin: Einaudi.
Santandrea, Assuntina
1992   *Ricordi di una levatrice*. Faenza: Faenza Editrice.

Santi, Emilio
1928   Natalità a Trieste. *Maternità e Infanzia* 3 (4): 351–52.
Saraceno, Chiara
1979/80   *La famiglia operaia sotto il fascismo.* Annals of the Fondazione
Giangiacomo Feltrinelli, 20th year. Milan: Feltrinelli.
Scheper-Hughes, Nancy, and Margaret Lock
1987   The mindful body: A prolegomenon to future work in medical anthro-
pology. *Medical Anthropology Quarterly* 1 (1): 6–41.
Schneider, Jane, and Peter Schneider
1984   Demographic transitions in a Sicilian rural town. *Journal of Family
History* 9 (3): 245–72.
Schofield, Roger, and David Reher
1991   The decline of mortality in Europe. In R. Schofield, D. Reher, and
A. Bideau, eds., 1–17.
Schofield, Roger, David Reher, and Alain Bideau, eds.
1991   *The decline of mortality in Europe.* Oxford: Clarendon Press.
Scremin, Luigi
1948   *Matrimonio divorzio e biologia umana.* Milan: Istituto di Propoganda
Libraria.
Sebastiano, Baravalle
1939   *Maternità ed infanzia e previdenza sociale.* Vercelli: S.A.V.I.T.
Sfameni, Pasquale
1936   Prefazione. In *La dottrina umorale-ormonica di Sfameni in ostetricia,*
E. Barbanti-Silva, v–li.
Sheard, N. F., and W. A. Walker
1988   The role of breast milk in the development of the gastrointestinal tract.
Nutrition Reviews 46 (1): 1–8.
Short, R. V.
1976   The evolution of human reproduction. *Proceedings of the Royal Soci-
ety of London* 195:3–24.
Silone, Ignazio
1949   [1930] *Fontamara.* Verona: Mondadori.
1955   [1936] *Vino e pane.* Verona: Mondadori.
Silverman, Sydel
1968   Agricultural organization, social structure, and values in Italy: Amoral
familism reconsidered. *American Anthropologist* 70:1–20.
Sorcinelli, Paolo
1985   Il problema alimentare in Italia alla fine dell'Ottocento. In Roberto
Finzi, ed., 31–50.
Sori, Ercole
1984   Malattia e demografia. In *Storia d'Italia. Annali 7, Malattia e medicina,*
Franco della Peruta, ed., 541–89. Turin: Einaudi.
Squadrilli, Gaspare
1929   *L'Italia di Mussolini e gli Italiani nuovi.* Rome: Pinciana.
Starr, Paul
1982   *The social transformation of American medicine.* New York: Basic
Books.

Stuart-Macadam, Patricia
  1995a Biocultural perspectives on breastfeeding. In P. Stuart-Macadam and
        K. Dettwyler, eds., 1–38.
  1995b Breastfeeding in prehistory. In P. Stuart-Macadam and K. Dettwyler,
        eds., 75–100.
Stuart-Macadam, Patricia, and Katherine A. Dettwyler, eds.
  1995 *Breastfeeding. Biocultural perspectives.* New York: Aldine de Gruyter.
Turner, Victor
  1967 *The forest of symbols: Aspects of Ndembu ritual.* Ithaca: Cornell Uni-
        versity Press.
Ufficio d'Igiene e Sanità
  1936 *Indagini sulla mortalità infantile per enterite e sul modo di allattamento.*
        Archivio di Stato di Faenza, category IV, folder 12.
Ulivieri, Simonetta
  1988 La donna e l'infanzia: l'ambiguità dei sentimenti e delle pratiche. In
        Storia dell'infanzia nell'età liberale, Franco Cambi and Simonetta
        Ulivieri, 185–230. Florence: La Nuova Italia.
Vaccari, Ilva
  1984 L'Opera Nazionale Maternità e Infanzia. *Enciclopedia dell'Antifas-
        cismo e della Resistenza,* vol. 4, 243–45.
Vaccaro, Giovanni
  1937 *La madre. Il nome più santo, più immortale.* Milan: La Propaganda.
Valli, Fabio
  1990 *Guida all'alimentazione in gravidanza.* Milan: Giovanni de Vecchi.
Vicarelli, Giuseppe
  1926a Operazioni ostetriche. In *Trattato di ostetricia,* vol. III, Innocente
        Clivio, ed., 1–270. Milan: Casa Editrice Dottor Francesco Vallardi.
  1926b Malattie del sistema osseo e difetti di conformazione dello sceletro in
        rapporto con la gravidanza e col parto. Viziature pelviche. In *Trattato
        di ostetricia,* vol. II, Innocente Clivio, ed., 123–214. Milan: Casa
        Editrice Dottor Francesco Vallardi.
Victoria, Cesar G., Elaine Tomasi, Maria Teresa A. Olinto, and
  Fernando C. Barros
  1993 Use of pacifiers and breastfeeding duration. *Lancet* 341:404–6.
Viganò, Paolo Nannei
  1992 Così si rieduca l'intestino del bambino. *Corriere Salute,* 3 Feb., 4 (5):
        17.
Vitzthum, V. J.
  1994 Comparative study of breastfeeding structure and its relation to
        human reproductive ecology. *Yearbook of Physical Anthropology*
        37:307–49.
Whitaker, Elizabeth
  1992 Bread and work: Pellagra and economic transformation in turn-of-the-
        century Italy. *Anthropological Quarterly* 65 (2): 80–90.
Williams, George C., and Randolph M. Nesse
  1991 The dawn of Darwinian medicine. *Quarterly Review of Biology* 66 (1):
        1–22.

Wingard, D., et al.
    1994   Is breast-feeding in infancy associated with adult longevity? *American Journal of Public Health* 84:1458–62.
Wood, James W.
    1990   Fertility in anthropological populations. *Annual Review of Anthropology* 19:211–42.
Wood, James W., et al.
    1985   Lactation and birth spacing in Highland New Guinea. *Journal of Biosocial Science,* Suppl. 9:159–73.
Wood, J. W., G. R. Milner, H. C. Harpending, and K. M. Weiss
    1992   The osteological paradox: Problems of inferring prehistoric health from skeletal samples. *Current Anthropology* 33:343–70.
Woolridge, Michael W.
    1995   Baby-controlled breastfeeding: Biocultural implications. In P. Stuart-Macadam and K. Dettwyler, eds., 217–42.
Zanelli, C.F.
    1939   Preparazione materna e previdenza sociale. *La Preparazione Materna* 1 (1): 22–30.
Zanotti-Bianco, Umberto
    1926   *Inchiesta sulle condizioni dell'infanzia in Italia: La Basilicata.* Rome: Meridionale Editrice.

Index

and infant survival, 14, 19, 20, 30, 63, 81, 92–94, 101, 134, 157, 168, 276, 309n. 19; as natural and sacred duty/index of morality, 32, 133, 141–42, 158, 168, 223, 295; in non-human primates and other mammals, 13–14, 18, 30; and nutrition and digestion, 16, 22, 46–47, 53, 132, 134, 145–46, 151–53, 165, 196, 204, 213, 214–16, 221, 224, 228, 257, 283, 293; and performance on intelligence tests, 21, 283; physiology, 2, 16, 17–18, 45, 47, 146, 151, 153, 285; psychological dimensions of, 22, 204–5, 208, 223, 227–28, 237, 251, 276, 281; recent (Western) pattern of, 14, 23, 24; standards for scheduling and rationing of meals in, 159–60, 161–62, 229, 231; symbolism/ritual aspects of, 1, 2, 3, 7, 56, 95, 117, 131, 193, 275–76, 279–80, 290, 291; and transfer of moral or spiritual qualities, 32, 44, 133–34, 135, 151, 275, 290, 293–94. *See also* Allergies and breast- feeding; Breast cancer; Breastmilk; Emotions; Exercise, physical/physical exertions; Exhaustion/depletion/degradation of the body, and breast-feeding; Eyesight, and breast-feeding; Sexual intercourse, during pregnancy and/or lactation; Sleep; Supplementation; Weaning; Work
Breast fluid, 25–26
Breastmilk: age of, 52–53, 165; composition (nutritional and immunological), 14, 16, 18, 20–21, 26, 28, 45, 134, 144, 151–52, 161, 223–24, 232; effect of constitution on, 35, 44, 45, 46, 47, 49, 52, 151, 255; effect of emotions and exertions on, 17, 46, 47, 48, 51, 53, 56, 151, 157, 165, 220–21, 225, 283, 287; effect of infant suckling behavior on composition of, 18; effect of menstruation or menstrual cycle on, 33, 34, 47,

134, 136–37, 163, 165, 166, 208–9, 247; effect of pregnancy on, 33, 34, 137, 163, 181, 209; effect of sexual relations on, 136–37, 151, 166, 278; lack, disappearance, deviation of, 2, 3, 46, 47, 64, 68, 134, 136, 152, 156, 216, 234, 251, 252–53, 255, 257, 259, 261, 276, 285, 299; as medicine, 32; passage of noxious substances and flavors in, 2, 46, 53, 153, 181, 221, 224, 247, 269, 283; protection of, 42–43, 56, 74; in relation to other secretions, 32, 33, 34, 35, 36, 37, 39, 44, 53; secretion in virgins, old ladies, men, and saints, 45, 280; substances thought to increase production or improve quality of, 47, 152, 215, 225; susceptibility to alteration of, 55–56, 151–54, 165–66, 205, 223–24, 283; testing of, 45, 46, 152, 165, 186, 224, 232, 250, 251, 294; underproduction and overproduction of, 16, 35, 44–48, 66, 151, 155, 156, 159, 183, 186–87, 217, 228, 230, 236, 237, 245, 240, 283, 293, 296, 309n. 4. *See also* Fever; Work
Bumm, Ernesto, 134, 151, 173, 177–78

Caesarean section, 57, 61, 121, 176, 243–45, 246, 250, 266, 277
Calabria, 73
Calories, 13, 18, 23, 25, 161
Campania, 89
Camps, for children's health, 123, 191, 198–99, 273–74
Cancer, 13, 20, 21, 22, 25, 48, 87, 299
Capitalism, 69, 102,103, 108, 239
Capoparto, 33, 136, 209
Casa della Madre e del Bambino, 196, 197, 200
Casein, 134–35
Catholic Church/Catholicism: and fascism, 7, 96, 98, 105, 124, 263; and health care, charity work, education, and moral authority 63, 83, 98, 103, 176, 192, 263, 267, 268, 273, 291;

Coruzzi, Cesare, 120
Cosleeping, parent-infant, 14, 26–28,
 43, 50, 149, 252, 295. *See also* Sleep
Cost of living, 179, 317n. 17
Countryside. *See* Rural areas, hygienic
 and medical conditions of
Cow's milk, 13, 15, 20, 21, 54, 65, 151,
 152, 157, 163, 166, 187, 233, 235,
 236, 248–51, 253. *See also* Animal
 milk
Cradle cap, 36
Cribs, 4, 26–28, 43, 149, 226, 258, 278,
 281
Crying, infant, 15, 28, 43, 50, 75,
 149–50, 158, 159, 184–85, 186, 205,
 211, 226, 230, 232, 250, 254, 258,
 260, 283
Culle vuote, 106
Cultural unification/uniformity, 4, 9,
 30, 71, 73, 238–39, 247, 248, 263,
 289, 290, 291, 292

Darwin, Charles, 105, 169
Day care/day-care centers, 63, 76 , 83,
 84, 119, 123, 128, 189, 190, 191, 192,
 195, 196, 198–200, 202, 212, 264,
 271–74, 281–82, 291. *See also*
 Preschools
Day laborers, 57, 67, 69–72, 73, 86, 91,
 102, 264, 268, 306
Day of the Mother and Child, 125
Death rates, 5, 15, 16, 32, 68, 86,
 301–8. *See also* Mortality rates
Defeminization, 116–18
D'Efeso, Sorano, 49, 176
Demographic policies: in ancient
 Rome, 99; outside Italy, 6, 7, 9. *See
 also* Fascism
Demographic transition, 4, 10, 69,
 84–86, 239
DeNapoli, Ferdinando, 141, 142, 170
Dentition, 36, 53, 163, 195 , 234. *See
 also* Teeth/teething
De Stefani law, 125
Diarrhea, 33, 36, 46, 50, 51, 53, 137,
 146, 150, 151, 164, 167, 212, 220, 230

Dick-Read, Grantley, 241
dipendente, 70, 265
diphtheria, 92, 307, 308
Disease-causes, 29, 35, 39
Disinfection/sterilization, 55, 160, 175,
 180, 211, 213, 244, 246, 253. *See also*
 Cleanliness
Divorce, 107, 108, 265
Drafts, 35, 42, 138, 209–11, 279
Dry nurses, 67, 249
Dumont, Arsène, 315n. 28

Economic boom, postwar, 88, 251,
 261–62, 264
Elite families/women, 8, 22–23, 29, 44,
 48, 54, 65, 70, 76, 77, 80, 85, 91, 93,
 107, 123, 154, 157–58, 164, 178, 180,
 183, 184, 185, 187, 250, 265, 290
Emigration, 7, 88, 96, 100, 126, 179,
 289
Emilia-Romagna, 9, 10, 62, 69, 71, 73,
 76, 85, 86, 88, 89, 90, 91, 176, 202,
 273–74
Emotions, 35, 36, 38, 40, 41, 45, 46, 47,
 53, 120 , 143–44, 147, 148, 157, 217,
 275. *See also* Breastmilk; Pregnancy
Employment offices/assistance, 126,
 128, 197
Endometrial cancer, 24, 25, 37
Enemas, 38, 146, 150, 153, 174, 186,
 214, 216, 244, 245, 246
England, 7, 88, 99, 114, 185, 251. *See
 also* United Kingdom
Epidemic disease, 16, 41, 163
Epidemiologic transition, 4, 69, 87–88,
 202, 239
Estrogens, 17, 24, 25
Eugenics, 6, 7, 60, 104–5
Europe, 4, 7, 15, 16, 18, 26, 27, 49, 69,
 74, 77, 81, 82, 85, 94, 98, 99, 104,
 106, 107, 114, 154, 174, 241, 245,
 264, 268
Evil eye, 34
Evolution, biological, 4, 6, 11, 13, 14,
 15, 19, 23, 28, 30, 85, 94, 113, 139,
 309n. 19, 310n. 33